COPING WITH PHYSICAL ILLNESS

2: New Perspectives

COPING WITH PHYSICAL ILLNESS

2: New Perspectives

Edited by
Rudolf H. Moos
Stanford University and
Veterans Administration Medical Center
Palo Alto, California

In collaboration with
Jeanne A. Schaefer

PLENUM MEDICAL BOOK COMPANY
New York and London

Library of Congress Cataloging in Publication Data

(Revised for Vol. 2)

Main entry under title:

Coping with physical illness.

    Vol. 2 edited in collaboration with Jeanne A. Schaefer.

    Vol. 2 has additional title: New perspectives.

    Includes bibliographies and indexes.

    1. Sick — Psychology. 2. Adjustment (Psychology) I. Moos, Rudolf H., 1934–
II. Tsu, Vivien Davis. III. Schaefer, Jeanne A. [DNLM: 1. Adaptation, Psychological. 2. Attitude to health. 3. Stress, Psychological. BF335 C783]

R726.5.C68   616.08   76-26175

This edition is an unabridged reprint of the
hardcover edition, published by Plenum in 1984.

First paperback printing — 1989

ISBN 0-306-43350-8

© 1984 Plenum Publishing Corporation
233 Spring Street, New York, N.Y. 10013

Plenum Medical Book Company is an imprint of Plenum Publishing Corporation

Printed in the United States of America

Contributors

Sharon Price Aadalen, R.N., Ph.D., Continuing Education Consultant, Educator, and Researcher, Edina, Minnesota

Harry S. Abram, M.D., deceased, Former Professor, Department of Psychiatry, Vanderbilt University Medical School, Nashville, Tennessee

Ande Anderten, M.S.W., Department of Social Services, Massachusetts General Hospital, Boston, Massachusetts

William R. Beardslee, M.D., Harvard Medical School and Children's Hospital Medical Center, Boston, Massachusetts

Herbert N. Brown, M.D., Director, Adult Psychiatric Resident Training Program, Cambridge Hospital, Cambridge, Massachusetts

Donald Brunnquell, Ph.D., Staff Member, the Children's Health Center, Minneapolis, Minnesota

Denton C. Buchanan, Ph.D., Director of Psychology, Royal Ottawa Regional Rehabilitation Center, Ottawa, Ontario, Canada

Ned H. Cassem, M.D., Department of Psychiatry, Massachusetts General Hospital, Boston, Massachusetts

Lino Canzona, D.S.W., Department of Social Work, King's College, London, Ontario, Canada

Grace Hyslop Christ, C.W.S., Assistant Director, Department of Social Work, Memorial Sloan-Kettering Cancer Center, New York, New York

Martha Cleveland, Ph.D., Licensed Consulting Psychologist, 6185 Apple Road, Excelsior, Minnesota

David Ray DeMaso, M.D., Harvard Medical School and Children's Hospital Medical Center, Boston, Massachusetts

Stanley J. Dudrick, M.D., St. Luke's Episcopal Hospital, Houston, Texas

DeAnn M. Englert, M.S.N., R.N., Nutritional Support Nurse Consultant, Denver, Colorado

Dianne Fochtman, R.N., M.S.N., Clinical Specialist in Pediatric Oncology, the Children's Memorial Hospital, Chicago, Illinois

Earl R. Gardner, Ph.D., deceased, formerly of Department of Psychiatry, the University of Texas Medical School, Houston, Texas

Edward Goldson, M.D., Director, Family Care Center, the Children's Hospital and Department of Pediatrics, University of Colorado Medical Center, Denver, Colorado

Marian D. Hall, Ph.D., Staff Member, the Children's Health Center, Minneapolis, Minnesota

Richard C. W. Hall, M.D., Chief of Staff, Veterans Administration Medical Center, Memphis, Tennessee

Carl G. Kardinal, M.D., Department of Internal Medicine, Ellis Fischel State Cancer Hospital, Columbia, Missouri

Martin J. Kelly, M.D., Associate Director, Psychiatry Division, Peter Bent Bringham Hospital, Boston, Massachusetts

Lorrin M. Koran, M.D., Department of Psychiatry and Behavioral Sciences, Stanford University and Veterans Administration Medical Center, Palo Alto, California

Margarita Kutsanellou-Meyer, C.S.W., Staff Social Worker, Memorial Sloan-Kettering Cancer Center, New York, New York

Carolyn J. LaBarbera, Ph.D., Department of Psychiatry, Vanderbilt University School of Medicine, Nashville, Tennessee

Eleanor L. Levine, M.S.W., Social Service Department, Toronto General Hospital, Toronto, Ontario, Canada

Emanuel Lewis, M.D., Consultant Psychotherapist, the Tavistock Clinic and Consultant Psychiatrist, Department of Child and Family Psychiatry, Charing Cross Hospital, London, England

Courtney Rogers Malone, M.Ed., Learning Disabilities Specialist, Public School System, Falmouth, Massachusetts

Frederick Mandell, M.D., Children's Hospital Medical Center and the Massachusetts Sudden Infant Death Syndrome Center, Boston, Massachusetts

Bonnie Maslin, Ph.D., Consultant in Occupational Mental Health, New York, New York

Elizabeth McAnulty, R.N., M.P.H., Children's Hospital Medical Center and the Massachusetts Sudden Infant Death Syndrome Center, Boston, Massachusetts

Bernice Moos, B.S., Department of Psychiatry and Behavioral Sciences, Stanford University and Veterans Administration Medical Center, Palo Alto, California

Rudolf H. Moos, Ph.D., Department of Psychiatry and Behavioral Sciences, Stanford University and Veterans Administration Medical Center, Palo Alto, California

Elaine M. Musial, R.N., M.S.N., Nephrology Nurse Clinician, Duke University Medical Center, Durham, North Carolina

Yehuda Nir, M.D., Director of Pediatric Psychiatry, Memorial Sloan-Kettering Cancer Center and Associate Clinical Professor of Psychiatry, Cornell Medical Center, New York, New York

William Olson, M.D., Department of Neurology, University of North Dakota, School of Medicine, Fargo, North Dakota

Sally E. Palmer, M.S.W., Lecturer in Social Work, Faculty of Continuing Studies, University of Western Ontario, London, Ontario, Canada

Mark Perl, M.B.B.S., Department of Psychiatry, University of California Service, San Francisco General Hospital, San Francisco, California

Sylvia Poss, M.A., Chief Social Worker, Johannesburg Hospital, Johannesburg, South Africa

Beth S. Price, M.S.W., Social Service Department, Toronto General Hospital, Toronto, Ontario, Canada

Robert M. Reece, M.D., Children's Hospital Medical Center and the Massachusetts Sudden Infant Death Syndrome Center, Boston, Massachusetts

Judith A. Ritchie, R.N., Ph.D., Associate Professor, Graduate Program of the Dalhousie University School of Nursing, Halifax, Nova Scotia, Canada

Robert Roelofs, M.D., Department of Neurology, University of Minnesota School of Medicine, Minneapolis, Minnesota

Peter Rothstein, M.D., Department of Anesthesiology and Pediatrics, Yale University School of Medicine and Director, Pediatric Intensive Care Unit, Yale New Haven Hospital, New Haven, Connecticut

Judith B. Sanders, M.S.N., R.N., Director of Nursing, Fulton State Mental Hospital, Fulton, Missouri

Jeanne A. Schaefer, R.N., Ph.D., Department of Psychiatry and Behavioral Sciences, Stanford University and Veterans Administration Medical Center, Palo Alto, California

David Spiegel, M.D., Department of Psychiatry and Behavioral Sciences, Stanford University School of Medicine, Stanford, California

Sondra K. Stickney, R.N., Hermann Hospital, Houston, Texas

Florence Stroebel-Kahn, R.N., B.S.N., Independent Consultant, Speaker, and Educator, Minneapolis, Minnesota

I. David Todres, M.D., Joseph S. Barr Pediatric Intensive Care Unit, Children's Service, Massachusetts General Hospital, Boston, Massachusetts

Alice Stewart Trillin, Educational Consultant, New York City

Lokky Wai, M.A., Department of Social Work, University of Western Ontario, London, Ontario, Canada

David A. Waller, M.D., Director, Child and Adolescent Psychiatry, Department of Psychiatry, University of Texas Health Science Center, Dallas, Texas

Avery D. Weisman, M.D., Project Omega and Department of Psychiatry, Massachusetts General Hospital and Harvard Medical School, Boston, Massachusetts

Irvin D. Yalom, M.D., Department of Psychiatry and Behavioral Sciences, Stanford University School of Medicine, Stanford, California

Milford Zasslow, M.D., Department of Psychiatry and Behavioral Sciences, Stanford University and Veterans Administration Medical Center, Palo Alto, California

Preface

This book provides new ideas about how patients and their families cope with serious health crises. Biomedical knowledge has expanded abruptly in the past decade during which time diagnostic and treatment procedures have become unusually specific and effective. Similarly, important advances have taken place in our understanding of the central role of psychosocial factors in health and illness. Recent trends have sparked the formulation of useful concepts of *coping skills* and *social resources* and have emphasized the value of an active assertive role for patients in the process of obtaining health care. The emergence of subspecialties such as behavioral medicine and health psychology has stimulated renewed interest in these areas. Moreover, the growth of holistic medicine and a biopsychosocial orientation highlights the contribution of a psychosocial perspective in an integrated framework for providing health care.

To cover these diverse trends, I offer a unified conceptual approach for understanding the process of coping with the crisis of physical illness and identifying the underlying adaptive tasks and domains of coping skills involved in this process. The first half of the book covers coping with selected health crises, such as birth defects and perinatal death, childhood and adult cancer, and chronic physical disabilities. The second half of the book covers "the crisis of treatment" and emphasizes the coping tasks evoked by the hospital environment and radical new medical treatments as well as the stresses faced by health care staff and issues that are elicited by death and the fear of dying. As in my earlier book on this topic, the material highlights the fact that most individuals cope effectively with life crises, even though disturbing symptoms and disorganization sometimes occur. I emphasize the idea that a life crisis is a critical juncture—a key turning point—during which patients and their families are uniquely open to the influence of professional caregivers. Because such influence can be for better or for worse, health care staff assume a potent responsibility for promoting effective coping.

Coping with Physical Illness: New Perspectives is conceived broadly to meet the needs of a diverse audience. There is a wealth of existing knowledge about how human beings cope with physical illness and disability, but the information is scattered widely throughout the literature. The selections contained in this book were identified after a search of well over 100 journals and periodicals. The resulting material is relevant to selected courses in schools of nursing, medicine, and public health—particularly in departments of psychiatry, behavioral sciences, epidemiology, and family and community health—and in health education programs. It is also useful for selected courses in departments of psychology, sociology, and social work.

The concepts and practical ideas are of special value to nurses and nursing students, social workers, medical students, physical therapists, occupational therapists, and pastoral and other counselors who work in health care settings. They should also be useful in nurse practitioner, physician's assistant, and other paramedical training programs. Each of these groups is centrally concerned with the way in which patients and their families cope with the personal crises of illness, hospitalization, and treatment.

The book has 11 parts. Part I provides a historical perspective on the importance of psychosocial factors and coping processes in health and illness. The overview presents a conceptual approach that helps to understand the crisis of physical illness. It also outlines seven basic adaptive tasks and offers a new framework of nine sets of coping skills that fall into three major coping domains.

Parts II through V present information about the crisis of illness and injury. Part II covers birth defects and perinatal death and emphasizes parental reactions to the birth of a premature or unhealthy baby, the process of mourning after a stillbirth or neonatal death, and fathers' responses to sudden unanticipated infant deaths. Part III describes a systems approach to the process of coping with childhood cancer, the problems encountered by children who must have a limb amputated, and the diverse coping strategies employed by adolescents who have leukemia.

Part IV highlights the crisis of cancer among adults. The selections provide a model for psychosocial phasing in cancer and describe the adaptive coping styles used by adult leukemia patients in remission, and one patient's incisive ideas about how health care staff can facilitate coping. Part V covers chronic conditions among children and adults, including the reactions of families to children with Duchenne muscular dystrophy, family adaptation to a child's traumatic spinal cord injury, and a personal account of the process of coping with quadriplegia.

Parts VI through IX provide information on the crisis of hospitalization and treatment procedures. Part VI covers issues in the psychological care of pediatric oncology patients, special problems experienced by families of children who are being treated in a pediatric intensive care unit, and the way in which families and health care staff communicate and cope with fateful prognoses. Part VII describes the stages of bone marrow transplantation and the factors that affect coping of adolescents and their family members on reverse isolation units.

Part VIII focuses on kidney dialysis and transplantation. The articles highlight the stages of adaptation to hemodialysis, the way in which patients and spouses cope with long-term home dialysis, and the issues patients and their families face in selecting a living-related kidney donor. Part IX describes the early and later psychological and social responses of patients who are on total parenteral nutrition.

Part X examines the stress entailed in working in health care settings and how staff members cope with them. The selections describe the syndrome of caregiver's plight, the way in which mutual support and information groups can promote effective coping among staff and how hospital work environments can be improved and made less stressful for staff.

Part XI emphasizes death and the fear of dying. The selections cover the adaptive tasks faced by terminal patients and the value of mutual support groups in helping persons who have only a short time to live confront their final crisis. The last article contains a moving account of the support that can be provided for a person who wishes to die at home.

I have compiled and organized this book in collaboration

with Jeanne Schaefer, who searched through an extensive amount of information, coauthored the overview article, and helped to prepare the commentaries for each section. The work was supported in part by the John D. and Catherine T. Mac-Arthur Foundation, Grant MH28177 from the National Institute of Mental Health, Grant AA02863 from the National Institute of Alcohol Abuse and Alcoholism, and Veterans Administration medical and health services research funds. I wish to thank Janel Burnett and Adrienne Juliano for performing typing and secretarial tasks involved in the preparation of the book.

I dedicate this book to Bernice who helped me avoid and then confront an acute health crisis of my own. After handling that crisis better than I did, she tackled the more difficult task of coping with a psychologically absent husband. Fortunately for me, she is succeeding remarkably well.

RUDOLF H. MOOS

Contents

I

Overview

The Crisis of Physical Illness
An Overview and Conceptual Approach

RUDOLF H. MOOS and JEANNE A. SCHAEFER

An acute health crisis is often a key turning point in an individual's life. The vivid confrontation with a severe physical illness or injury, prolonged treatment and uncertainty, and intense personal strains can have a profound and lasting impact. Most patients cope reasonably well with such a crisis and are able to recover and resume their prior level of functioning. Some individuals, however, are utterly demoralized and suffer serious psychological consequences, whereas others emerge with a more mature outlook and a richer appreciation of life. What factors affect the ultimate psychosocial outcome of a health crisis? Why do some patients continue to struggle under the most harrowing circumstances? What are the major adaptive tasks seriously ill patients encounter? What types of coping skills do they use to promote recovery? Are there common phases or stages through which individuals progress as they negotiate a health crisis? What stressors are encountered by health care professionals and how can they nourish the psychological healing process among patients and their families? We deal with these issues here by consid-

RUDOLF H. MOOS and JEANNE A. SCHAEFER • Department of Psychiatry and Behavioral Sciences, Stanford University and Veterans Administration Medical Center, Palo Alto, California 94305.

ering physical illness as a life crisis and by describing how patients and staff cope with the stress of illness and of treatment.

Historical Overview

Current approaches to the field of coping with physical illness have been shaped by the evolution of concepts in psychosomatic and behavioral medicine, the formulation of a theory of coping, and the integration of these perspectives into a biopsychosocial orientation to health care.[11]

Psychosomatic and Behavioral Medicine

The classic psychosomatic perspective asserts that personality factors and emotions can affect bodily functions, health status, and the onset and course of physical illness. The work of Sigmund Freud, Ivan Pavlov, and Walter Cannon stimulated the growth of the field. Much of the early research in the 1930s and 1940s grew out of a psychodynamic perspective that focused on specific personality traits or underlying conflicts thought to be characteristic of individuals with particular types of disorders. Psychoanalysis or long-term dynamically oriented psychotherapy was commonly employed as a treatment to try and alter such traits or conflicts and thus alleviate the disorder.

Harold Wolff and his colleagues at Cornell took a different tack. They studied the physiological effects of experimental stress situations and evolved a theory that psychosomatic illness is an *adaptive* response to life stress. This new focus spurred attempts to link aspects of the physical and social environment (that is, the stressors) to the onset and course of diseases such as diabetes mellitus, peptic ulcer, rheumatoid arthritis, and the like. Some investigators found that such illnesses were more likely to begin and to have a stormier course in the context of interpersonal conflicts or ongoing crises such as separation and divorce or the death of a spouse or other close family member. These studies emphasized environmental or life stress factors more heavily than personality traits. They supported the idea that brief, focused counseling or psychotherapy could speed the process of recovery from illness by helping the individual cope with the stress.

Thus, the psychosomatic perspective considered the role of personal and environmental factors in the onset and course of illness. But only some ("psychosomatic") illnesses were studied, and the specific coping skills that individuals employ to adapt to stress were relatively neglected. These issues are being addressed more systematically by the evolution of behavioral medicine, in which the principles of behavior modification are being integrated with the biomedical approach.[16] By emphasizing the *active* role of the individual in the etiology and management of illness, behavioral medicine has taken a valuable step beyond the classical psychosomatic perspective. The behavioral approach has sparked new interest in an educational paradigm in which individuals are taught specific problem-solving skills that can help them to adapt and to control some of the consequences of physical illness. Moreover, by reducing the exposure to risk factors (such as overeating or smoking) and promoting healthy life-styles, such skills can reduce the incidence of relapse and perhaps even of the initial occurrence of disease.

Formulations of Coping Processes and Resources

Theoretical formulations of coping processes and resources have reflected roughly the same historical trends that shaped psychosomatic and behavioral medicine. Such formulations began with psychoanalysis and ego psychology. Freud believed that ego processes served to resolve conflicts between an individual's impulses and the constraints of external reality. Their function was to reduce tension by enabling the individual to express sexual and aggressive impulses "indirectly" without recognizing their "true" intent. Psychosomatic disorders were thought to develop when such impulses were repressed and when the energy attached to them was diverted to impel altered bodily functions. Subsequently, ego psychologists emphasized reality-oriented or primitive coping processes of the "conflict-free" ego sphere such as attention, perception, and memory.

In addition to highlighting the processes of defense and coping, psychoanalysis and ego psychology inspired the formulation of a developmental perspective on the accumulation of coping resources over an individual's life span. For instance, Erik Erikson[4] described eight life cycle stages, each of which must be negotiated successfully in order for an individual to cope adequately with the next stage. Personal coping resources (such as trust and autonomy)) "accrued" during the adolescent and young adult years are blended into the self-concept and promote the process of coping in adulthood and old age. Successful encounters with life crises lead to coping resources such as a sense of competence that can help to resolve subsequent crises.

Charles Darwin's evolutionary theory of adaptation spawned a behaviorally oriented counterpart to the psychoanalytic preoccupation with intrapsychic and cognitive factors. This orientation led to an emphasis on concrete problem-solving activities and their consequences and eventually promoted the development of behavior modification procedures and behavioral medicine. Initial applications of the "behaviorist" tradition focused on the behavioral aspects of problem solving, but more recent clinical procedures have attended to cognitive components of coping skills.

Cognitive behaviorism is consistent with ideas about coping that are derived from personality theory, in that it emphasizes the active role of the individual in self-regulation and the belief that an individual's cognitive appraisal of a crisis may be more important than its "objective" characteristics.[7] Consistent with Erikson's developmental theory, current formulations highlight the value of a sense of self-efficacy as a coping resource. Specifically, individuals must believe they can succeed in an endeavor in order for them to try to master the tasks involved actively. Successful coping promotes future expectations of self-efficacy, which, in turn, inspire more vigorous and persistent efforts to master difficult tasks and situations.

A Biopsychosocial Orientation

The biopsychosocial orientation to health care provides a holistic integration of the trends we have reviewed. This multicausal systems approach enables clinicians to consider biological, psychological, and contextual information about a patient and to make "diagnoses" and develop treatment recommendations that encompass all three domains. The framework supplies a unified approach that can inform health care staff about the determinants and effects of coping resources and processes.[9,15]

Many of these historical threads have been linked in the last decade, during which time the multifactorial nature of all illness has become more generally accepted. There has been a striking increase in research on psychological and social factors that may influence not only the etiology and onset of disease but also its course and outcome, the response to treatment, and the use of health care services. Personal and environmental factors are now seen as intimately involved in all phases of all diseases. There is also a more dynamic perspective now that emphasizes the active role of the individual in health care and the power of feedback mechanisms that help to maintain psychological as well as physiological homeostasis. After introducing crisis theory, we set forth a biopsychosocial framework that views the coping process as influenced by medical aspects of illness as well as by personal and environmental factors.

Crisis Theory as a General Perspective

Crisis theory is concerned with how people cope with major life crises and transitions. Historically, the theory has provided a conceptual framework for preventive mental health care and for understanding severe life crises such as physical illness or injury. The fundamental ideas were developed by Erich Lindemann, who described the process of grief and mourning and the role community caretakers can play in helping bereaved family members cope with the loss of their loved ones.[10] Combined with Erikson's formulation of "developmental crises" at transition points in the life cycle[4], these ideas paved the way for the outgrowth of crisis theory.[2]

In general, crisis theory deals with the impact of disruptions on established patterns of personal and social identity. Similar to the need for physiological homeostasis, individuals have a need for social and psychological equilibrium. When people encounter an event that upsets their characteristic pattern of behavior and life-style, they employ habitual problem-solving mechanisms until a balance is restored. A situation that is so novel or so major that habitual responses are inadequate is a crisis and incites a state of turbulence that is often accompanied by heightened fear, guilt, or other unpleasant feelings.

Because a person cannot remain in a state of extreme disequilibrium, a crisis is by definition self-limited. Even though it may be temporary, some resolution must be found and some equilibrium reestablished within a few days or weeks. The new balance may represent a healthy adaptation that promotes personal growth and maturation or a maladaptive response that foreshadows psychological deterioration and decline. Thus, a crisis experience may be seen as a transition—a turning point—that can have lasting implications for an individual's adaptation and ability to meet future crises.

The crisis of physical illness is almost always a serious "upset in a steady state" that may extend over a long period of time and lead to permanent changes for patients and their family members. The potency of the crisis stems from the typically sudden and unexpected onset and the ultimate threat to an individual's life and well-being. A person may face hospitalization and separation from family and friends, overwhelming feelings of pain and helplessness, permanent changes in appearance or bodily function, the loss of key roles, and an uncertain future involving the prospect of an untimely death. Moreover, even the state of tentative equilibrium that patients achieve may be shattered at any moment by unforeseen circumstances.

These problems are compounded by specific aspects of health crises that make it hard for an individual to assimilate the sudden turn of events and select appropriate coping strategies.[6] Health crises usually cannot be anticipated, clear information is lacking, definitive decisions may have to be made quickly, and the ultimate meaning for the individual is ambiguous. Moreover, a person typically has only limited prior experience in handling serious illness and thus cannot rely on previously successful coping responses. Because family members are also uncertain about what to do, they may react in ways that encourage ill-advised behavior. Given these issues, it is remarkable that most individuals cope adequately in the aftermath of a health crisis. In fact, survivors of serious illness sometimes report enhanced personal growth and maturity, a change in focus of energy from the constant pressure of work to family relationships, more realism and acceptance of life, and heightened awareness of religious and humanitarian values.

According to crisis theory, an individual is much more receptive to outside influence at a time of disequilibrium. Such accessibility offers health professionals and others who deal with patients an unusual opportunity to exert a constructive impact. In addition, the crisis of illness may extend over many months or years, presenting patients with new issues and circumstances that leave them in a constant state of provisional equilibrium. This fact expands the leverage of professional caregivers and underlines the value of learning crisis resolutions and psychological counseling techniques.

An Integrative Conceptual Framework

We have evolved a framework in which a serious physical illness or injury is understood as a life crisis. Through a cognitive appraisal of its significance, the crisis sets forth basic adaptive tasks to which varied coping skills can be applied. The individual's cognitive appraisal, definition of the adaptive tasks involved, and selection and effectiveness of coping skills are influenced by three sets of factors: demographic and personal characteristics, aspects of the illness, and features of the physical and social environment. These factors jointly affect the resolution of the initial phase of the crisis; in turn, this resolution may alter all three sets of factors and thereby change the ultimate outcome. It is important to recognize that family members and friends as well as patients are affected by the crisis, encounter many of the same or closely related adaptive tasks, and use the same types of coping skills. In the next sections, we briefly review the basic tasks and skills and the three sets of factors determining outcome.

Major Adaptive Tasks

The major tasks of adapting to a health crisis can be divided into seven categories. Three of these tasks are primarily illness related, whereas the other four are more general and apply to all types of life crises (see Table 1).

The first set of tasks involves *dealing with the discomfort, incapacitation, and other symptoms of the illness and injury*. This covers a range of disturbing symptoms such as pain, weakness, dizziness, incontinence, paralysis, loss of control (such as in convulsive disorders), the feeling of suffocation (in respiratory ailments), permanent disfigurement, and the like. Patients must learn to recognize the signs of impending medical crises and, more generally, to control their symptoms whenever possible. For instance, a person with a heart disorder must regulate his diet and daily exercise, whereas a diabetic person must be able to prevent potential crises that may be caused by complications of sugar excess or insulin shock.

A second and closely related set of tasks entails the *management of the stresses of special treatment procedures and of the hospital environment*. The increasing sophistication of medical technology has created a host of new problems for patients. Surgical procedures such as mastectomy and colostomy, debridement as a treatment for burns, radiotherapy and chemotherapy with their

Table 1. Major Sets of Adaptive Tasks

Illness-related tasks
Dealing with pain, incapacitation, and other symptoms
Dealing with the hospital environment and special treatment procedures
Developing and maintaining adequate relationships with health care staff

General tasks
Preserving a reasonable emotional balance
Preserving a satisfactory self-image and maintaining a sense of competence and mastery
Sustaining relationships with family and friends
Preparing for an uncertain future

concomitant side effects, the need to wear a cumbersome brace for certain orthopedic disorders, long-term hemodialysis and organ transplantation—all these are therapeutic measures that create adaptive tasks for patients. Specialized hospital environments such as operating and recovery rooms, intensive care units, premature baby nurseries, and even the waiting room of an oncology clinic also are significant stressors. Separated from family and exposed to unfamiliar routines and procedures, patients (especially children) find hospitalization itself to be upsetting. The "crisis of treatment" is increasingly salient in defining the tasks confronted by seriously ill patients and their families (see Parts VI, VII, VIII, and IX).

The third set of tasks consists of *developing and maintaining adequate relationships with medical and other health care staff.* Consider the questions patients may ask themselves: Can I express my anger at the nurse for taking so long to answer my call for help? How can I ask for additional pain medication when I need it? How can I cope with the condescension I sense in the nurses who care for me? How could I let my doctor know my wishes if I were to be incapacitated and near death? The frequent turnover and change in personnel, particularly among staff who come into direct contact with patients, makes this an unusually complex set of tasks. Such tasks can be difficult even for a physician-patient who is intimately familiar with hospital settings.[8]

The fourth category of tasks involves *preserving a reasonable emotional balance by managing upsetting feelings* aroused by the illness. There are many "negative" emotions associated with health crises, such as the sense of failure and self-blame at giving birth to a deformed child (see Part II), anxiety and apprehension of not knowing the outcome of an illness, a sense of alienation and isolation, and feelings of inadequacy and anger in the face of difficult demands. An important aspect of this task is for the patient to maintain some hope, even when its scope is sharply limited by circumstances.

The fifth set of tasks consists of *preserving a satisfactory self-image and maintaining a sense of competence and mastery.* Changes in physical functioning or appearance, such as permanent weakness or scarring, must be blended into a revised self-image. This "identity crisis" may require a change in personal values and life-style, as, for example, when permanently disfigured burn victims and their families learn to downplay the importance of physical attractiveness. Patients who must rely on mechanical devices like cardiac pacemakers or hemodialysis to sustain their lives must come to terms with a "half-man–half-machine" body image (see Parts VIII and IX).

Other tasks that belong in this category include defining the limits of independence and readjusting goals and expectations in light of changes wrought by the illness. It is important to find a satisfactory balance between accepting help and taking an active and responsible part in controlling the direction and activities of one's life. Resuming independent status after a long period of enforced passivity can be hard, as, for example, when a successful organ transplant patient is suddenly no longer an invalid. This conflict is complicated further among children by the normal developmental drive to gradually expand independence and self-direction to which illness-imposed dependence and parental protectiveness may represent a serious setback (see Part III).

The sixth set of tasks includes *sustaining relationships with family and friends.* The physical separation and sense of alienation occasioned by hospitalization and being labeled a *patient* or a *dying person* often disrupt normal relationships with friends and relatives. Serious illness can make it hard to keep communication lines open and to accept comfort and support at the very time when these are most essential. Close relationships with other people can help patients obtain information necessary to make wise decisions about their medical care, find emotional support for their decisions, and secure reassurance about the problems they face. Such relationships also enable family members and friends to prepare for the tasks they themselves will encounter. Problems that affect one member of a family also touch the others, as, for example, when the breadwinner is disabled by a stroke or when a child is chronically ill (see Part V).

The seventh set of tasks entails *preparing for an uncertain future* in which significant losses are threatened. The loss of sight, speech, hearing, a limb or breast by surgery, or life itself all must be acknowledged and mourned. Ironically, new medical procedures that raise hope for patients with previously incurable illnesses may make this task more difficult. Patients must prepare for permanent loss of function while preserving the belief that restoration of function may be possible. When death seems likely, patients and family members must engage in anticipatory mourning and initiate the grieving process while preserving the belief that new treatment procedures may prove beneficial (see Chapters 5 and 9).

These seven groups of tasks are generally encountered with every illness, but their relative importance varies, depending on the nature of the disease, the personality of the individual involved, and the unique set of circumstances. For the person suddenly rendered blind, the physical discomfort may be minor, whereas the difficulty of restoring social relations seems overwhelming. A bone cancer patient, on the other hand, usually must deal with severe pain. A woman who has had a mastectomy may find that accepting her new self-image is her most significant task. Someone who is physically active, like a professional athlete or a construction worker, probably will experience more difficulty adjusting to a wheelchair than will a person with a more sedentary occupation.

These tasks can be as difficult for family members and friends as for patients themselves. Family members must help patients control their symptoms and try to prevent new medical crises, assist in carrying out special treatment procedures, and develop adequate relationships with health care professionals. They must maintain a sense of inner mastery of their divergent emotions and try to preserve a satisfactory self-image (helping the patient as much as possible but not feeling overwhelmed by guilt when they cannot do everything she asks). They must maintain family integrity and their relationship with the patient and simultaneously prepare for an uncertain future. Active participation in health care procedures and decisions can help family and friends recognize and cope with these common tasks.

Major Types of Coping Skills

We now offer an overview of the major sets of coping skills that are commonly employed to deal with the adaptive tasks just described. These skills may be used individually, consecutively, or more likely, in various combinations. Specific coping strategies are not inherently adaptive or maladaptive. Skills that are effective in one situation may not be in another. Skills that may be beneficial given moderate or temporary use may be harmful if relied upon exclusively. The word *skill* underscores the positive aspects of coping and depicts coping as an ability that can be taught (as any other skill) and used flexibly as the situation demands.

Coping skills can be organized into three domains, according to their primary focus:[13] *Appraisal-focused coping* involves attempts to understand and find a pattern of meaning in a crisis. *Problem-focused coping* seeks to confront the reality of a crisis by dealing with its tangible consequences and trying to construct a more satisfying situation. *Emotion-focused coping* seeks to manage the emotions provoked by a crisis and to maintain affective equilibrium. We use this classification scheme to categorize coping responses into nine specific types (see Table 2).

Logical Analysis and Mental Preparation. This set of skills entails paying attention to one aspect of a crisis at a time, breaking a seemingly overwhelming problem into small potentially manageable bits, drawing on past experiences, and mentally rehearsing alternative actions and their probable consequences. Such skills are commonly used to allay anxiety, as, for example, when unfamiliar medical procedures are scheduled. Bolstering one's confidence by reminding oneself of previous successes in handling difficult problems fits into this category. On a broader scale, it also encompasses the anticipatory mourning process in which an expected death or other loss is acknowledged beforehand.

When life's happenings seem capricious and uncontrollable, as with the sudden onset of a serious health crisis, it often is easier to manage if one can find a general purpose or pattern of meaning in the course of events. Efforts in this direction constitute a related type of coping skill. Belief in a divine purpose or in the general beneficence of a divine spirit may serve as consolation or as encouragement to do one's best to deal with the difficulties one encounters. Cowie[3] described a process whereby patients try to "normalize" and make their heart attack intelligible, something that was not "really" unexpected but rather was building up slowly as the "obvious outcome" of a particular life-style. Putting an experience into a long-term perspective (with or without religious orientation) often makes individual events more tolerable.

Table 2. Major Types of Coping Skills

Appraisal-focused coping
Logical analysis and mental preparation
Cognitive redefinition
Cognitive avoidance or denial

Problem-focused coping
Seeking information and support
Taking problem-solving action
Identifying alternative rewards

Emotion-focused coping
Affective regulation
Emotional discharge
Resigned acceptance

Cognitive Redefinition.   This category covers cognitive strategies by which an individual accepts the basic reality of a situation but restructures it to find something favorable. Such strategies include reminding oneself that things could be worse, thinking of oneself as well off in comparison to other people, altering values and priorities in line with changing reality, and concentrating on something good that might develop from a health crisis. For instance, parents of a chronically ill child may compare him to one who has more serious problems (see Chapter 11), whereas some persons come to see the experience of cardiac arrest as having been of positive value in that it helped them redirect their life.

Cognitive Avoidance or Denial.   This category encompasses an array of skills aimed at denying or minimizing the seriousness of a crisis. These may be directed to the illness itself, as when a myocardial infarct patient maintains that "it was just severe indigestion." Or, after the diagnosis is accepted, these skills may be aimed at the significance of an illness as, for example, when the parents of a fatally ill child go from doctor to doctor looking for an alternate diagnosis (see Chapter 5). Cognitive avoidance or denial can also involve the potential consequences of an illness, such as the initial denial and bland affect that often occur after experiencing a stroke. These skills tend to be described by the term *defensive mechanisms* because they are self-protective responses to stress. This term does not convey the constructive value of these skills; they can temporarily rescue an individual from being overwhelmed or provide the time needed to garner other personal coping resources.

Seeking Information and Support. This set of skills covers obtaining information about the illness and alternate treatment procedures and their probable outcome. Parents of leukemic children seek information about their responsibility for the illness (initially blaming themselves, for example, for not having attended to the early nonspecific manifestations of the disease), about hospital procedures (questioning ward physicians and nurses and scrutinizing newspaper and magazine articles), and about ways of coming to terms with their expected loss (see Part III). Learning about the causes of birth defects can mitigate a sense of guilt or failure felt by the mother of a deformed baby. These skills are often used in combination with logical analysis, as patients try to restore a sense of control by learning about the demands that might be made on them and mentally preparing themselves to overcome expected problems by thinking through the steps involved.

A related group of coping skills entails the ability to request emotional support and reassurance from family, friends, and health care staff. Patients and others who keep their feelings "bottled up" or who withdraw from social interaction cut themselves off from help of this type. Emotional and tangible support can be an important source of strength in facing difficult times, but individuals must deal with the tension between seeking help and wanting to avoid "passive-dependent" roles. One way to obtain support is to join special groups such as national self-help organizations (like Mended Hearts for open surgery patients and Reach for Recovery for mastectomy patients) or smaller ad hoc groups for patients or relatives (such as spouses of hemodialysis patients). These groups can provide a type of support that is less available from alternate sources, such as information about how individuals in a similar situation handle their predicament (see Chapter 28).

Taking Problem-Solving Action. This group of skills involves taking concrete action to deal directly with a situation, for example, by learning specific health care procedures such as feeding and caring for a premature baby, running a home dialysis machine, or giving oneself insulin injections. These accomplishments can provide much needed confirmation of personal ability and competence at a time when opportunities for independent and meaningful action are scarce. Patients take pride in caring for themselves; relatives find relief in offering concrete help. These skills include learning how to control symptoms by such techniques as sitting in certain kinds of chairs (for sufferers of back pain), planning changes in daily regimens to minimize the appearance and/or effects of potentially painful symptoms (such as when a person who has had a heart attack chooses a level route for walking), and physically reorganizing or redesigning a home to accommodate decreased mobility (such as for the use of crutches or a wheelchair).

Identifying Alternative Rewards. These skills encompass attempts to replace the permanent losses involved in a health crisis by changing one's activities and creating new sources of satisfaction. Such coping responses entail making short-range plans to deal with uncertainty and setting concrete limited goals such as walking again or attending a special event (such as a wedding or graduation). Other examples include the decision to help fellow patients actively by sharing information or raising funds or to temporarily redirect one's energies toward work or school after the sudden death of a child (see Chapter 4). Such activities give patients and family members something to look forward to and provide a realistic chance of achieving a goal they consider meaningful.

Affective Regulation. These skills cover efforts to maintain hope and to control one's emotions when dealing with a distressing situation. This occurs when the parents of a hemophiliac child react calmly and stoically to a bleeding episode rather than showing their terror or dismay, or when patients discuss their symptoms with "clinical detachment." Other ways to regulate affect entail consciously postponing paying attention to an impulse (suppression), experiencing and working through one's feelings, trying not to be bothered by conflicting feelings, maintaining a sense of pride and keeping a "stiff upper lip," and being able to tolerate ambiguity and to withhold immediate action. The strategy of "progressive desensitization," whereby amputees or patients with severe disfiguration gradually "expose" themselves and dull their sensitivity to their own and others' reactions falls within this category (see Chapter 6).

Emotional Discharge.   This diverse array of responses includes openly venting one's feelings of anger or despair, crying or screaming in protest at news of a fateful prognosis, and using jokes and gallows humor to help allay constant strain. It also entails "acting out" by not complying with a treatment regimen as well as behavior that may temporarily reduce tension, such as when a dialysis patient goes on eating binges or masturbates while on the dialysis machine. Such behavior may involve a temporary failure of affective regulation, but we categorize it separately because many individuals alternate between emotional control and emotional discharge.

Resigned Acceptance.   This category covers coming to terms with a situation and accepting it as it is, deciding that the overall circumstances cannot be altered, and submitting to "certain" fate. When a beloved person's life is at stake, these coping responses often alternate with cognitive avoidance and denial. Sometimes physicians reach a hopeless prognosis and are resigned to a fateful outcome, but family members continue to expect an unlikely recovery (see Chapter 16). Rapid changes in a patient's condition may make it hard to strike a reasonable balance between continued hope and resignation. As death approaches, a conscious decision to accept the inevitable helps to promote disengagement and mitigate distress.

Almost any response to a health crisis may serve an adaptive function, but these nine categories cover the most common types of coping skills employed to deal with physical illness. Such skills are seldom used singly or exclusively. A patient may deny or minimize the seriousness of a crisis while talking to a family member, seek relevant information about prognosis from a physician, request reassurance and emotional support from a friend, and so on. A health crisis typically presents a variety of related tasks and requires a combination or sequence of coping skills.

General Determinants of Outcome

Why does one person respond differently from another to a life crisis such as serious illness? What factors influence the appraisal of an illness, the awareness of specific tasks, and the choice and progression of coping strategies? The relevant determinants fall into three categories: demographic and personal factors, illness-related factors, and features of the physical and social environment (see Figure 1). For example, the nature of adaptive tasks is affected by aspects of the illness (if the illness is life threatening the patient may wish to make a will), by personal factors (a heart attack patient who has not yet retired faces the task of returning to work), and by environmental factors (a quadriplegic person who lives in a residence that is not wheelchair accessible encounters physical barriers that may prevent independent living). In turn, the coping efforts stimulated by these tasks can change personal factors (a person may seek and obtain information that changes her attitude), environmental factors (a wheelchair-mobile patient may move to a barrier-free setting), and illness-related factors (learning relaxation skills can lessen the likelihood of tension-induced cigarette smoking and thus of the recurrence of a heart attack).

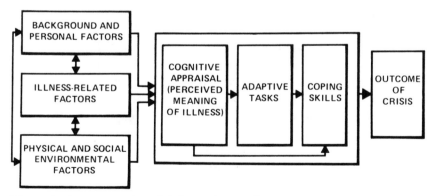

Figure 1. A conceptual model for understanding the crisis of physical illness.

Demographic and Personal Factors. Demographic and personal factors include age, gender, and socioeconomic status as well as cognitive and emotional maturity, ego strength and self-confidence, philosophical or religious beliefs, and prior illness and coping experiences. These factors influence the individual's appraisal of an illness and affect the personal and social resources available to meet the crisis. For instance, men may be especially threatened by the lack of ambition and vigor that often accompany serious illness, because, in comparison to women, they are more invested in their physical prowess and bodily functioning. The enforced dependency and passivity associated with illness is especially likely to be problematic for individuals who relish being assertive and independent.

The timing of an illness in the life cycle is particularly important. A child who has become an invalid because of rheumatic heart disease has different concerns than does an elderly patient who has been incapacitated by a heart ailment. Some adolescents have a hard time coping with physical illness because it imposes an added stress just when the tasks of gaining independence and forming personal identity and a stable body image already pose difficult challenges (see Part III). Although greater maturity and more extensive coping experience may provide middle-aged persons with richer resources on which to draw, serious illness threatens the disruption of established roles and the fulfillment of cherished life aims. These issues may be less important for elderly patients, but such patients often suffer from some cognitive impairment that reduces their coping ability.

Illness-Related Factors. Illness-related factors include the type and location of symptoms—whether painful, disfiguring, disabling, or in a body region vested with special importance such as the heart or reproductive organs. These factors are a major component in defining the exact nature of the tasks patients and others face, and consequently, their adaptive responses. Different organs and functions may have a psychological significance that has little to do with biological factors related to survival. For instance, an injury to the face or amputation of a breast can have a more profound psychological impact on a woman than severe hypertension that directly threatens her life.

The rapidity of onset and progression of a disease can affect the choice of coping strategies and their effectiveness. The parents of a leukemic child in remission may stem the process of anticipatory mourning begun when the diagnosis was first announced, only to have to resume their preparation when a relapse occurs. Localized cancer can be dealt with by seeking information and support, but once the cancer is widespread, an individual is presented with more diverse problems and tends to use different coping skills. Patients who formerly spoke openly about their medical situation and treatment may prefer to remain silent because they are afraid of provoking guilt or rejection among their friends and relatives. In advanced stages of cancer, patients often turn their feelings inward and withdraw from intimate communication to avoid confronting the grave significance of their deteriorating condition (see Part IV).

Physical and Social Environmental Factors. Aspects of the physical and social environment affect the adaptive tasks patients and their families face and the choice and outcome of the coping skills they use. The physical features of a hospital, or of special areas such as intensive care units, with their unfamiliar sights and sounds and bustle of activity, can further upset patients already burdened by a painful illness (see Part VI). The aesthetic quality of the surroundings, the amount of personal space available, and the degree of sensory stimulation all can influence a person's well-being and morale.

The human environment encompasses the relationships of patients and staff, of patients and their families, and the social supports and expectations of the wider community (such as friends, clergy, and social services). The course of an illness tends to be more benign, and recovery tends to be quicker than expected, when it occurs in the context of interpersonal understanding and empathy. Moreover, patients whose families enjoy more varied sources of support from friends and relatives are likely to experience more favorable outcomes.[12]

A patient's work setting also can play a vital role in the course of recovery. Martha Lear recounts how her husband gave up a lucrative private medical practice to fulfill his lifelong dream of pursuing a research career in a university-affiliated medical school.[8] When he sustained a serious heart attack soon after the change, he found that the problems in the university setting (such as lack of guaranteed salary support, cramped office space, minimal research funds, and the competitive pressure and relative lack of freedom) sharply exacerbated his general burden of stress. The psychologist C. Scott Moss graphically described how the intellectually harsh and competitive environment of an academic psychology department at a prestigious university hampered his recovery from aphasia following a stroke.[14]

The Therapeutic Role of Health Care Staff

Crisis theory maintains that an individual is more receptive to outside influence in a time of turbulence. This greater accessibility offers health care professionals and others who work with patients a special opportunity to exert a constructive impact. Failure to cope in a realistic and timely manner with tasks encountered in the first phases of an illness can activate a permanent pattern of impaired adjustment. This potential for disruptive psychological "side effects" renders the early detection of ineffective coping reactions as important as the early diagnosis of the disease itself.

When caregivers are aware of the major tasks and typical coping strategies involved in health crises, they can recognize and respond to the adaptive efforts their patients make. For instance, when staff members encounter a woman who has just lost a breast, a disfigured burn victim, or a patient who is terminally ill, they should know the usual responses to a given illness situation, including the probable sequence of phases in emotional processes like mourning and the inevitability and value of "negative" emotions such as anger or sadness. Understanding the need to express anger may help staff members accept the emotion, especially when it is directed at them. In practical terms, staff who must announce an impending loss should be prepared to repeat their explanations after the initial shock has subsided, because very little may be understood at the first hearing.

One of the most important ways in which health care staff can help is to provide information: to respond to patients' questions, clarify misconceptions, and prepare patients and family members by advising them of events or emotions that are likely to occur.

But staff members must also realize that patients who use avoidance or denial coping styles may not wish to hear threatening news. Moreover, there is a limit to the degree of truth even the most vigilant patients desire. Stuart Alsop found that a hospital policy that staff be completely candid made it hard for him to preserve his emotional balance and ward off despair.[1] The experience led him to formulate a rule to maintain hope: "Never tell a victim of terminal cancer the whole truth—tell him that he *may* die, even that he will *probably* die, but do not tell him that he *will* die" (1973, p. 84).

Two other coping skills that affect staff directly are individual appeals for emotional support and problem-solving efforts to maintain or rebuild a sense of personal competence. When caregivers are aware of the emotional needs of patients and family members, they can give the reassurance and understanding that is sought while recognizing at the same time that frequent repetition of such support may be necessary. Patients often deal with physical dependence by asserting their independence and testing their abilities in other areas. Family members also rely on this approach to cope with their sense of helplessness, as, for example, when parents assist in the routine care of their hospitalized child. Staff can treat such efforts as valuable ways of trying to reduce tension and regain self-confidence rather than as intrusions in their own sphere of expertise.

To be of maximum help to patients, health care professionals need to understand their own reactions to acute health crises. They need to know that they, too, face certain tasks, go through specific phases in reaction to patients, and employ similar types of coping skills. An awareness of this process can help the staff to deal with the stress inherent in the nature of their work and to keep negative feelings about a particular patient or situation from affecting the quality of care they provide (see Part X).

Professional caregivers have a special responsibility to aid those whose lives have been disrupted by illness. Beyond the realm of physical care, this includes sympathetic understanding of the coping process and recognition of their own role in nourishing that process. Sensitivity to the implications of their routine actions may evoke changes in behavior or procedure that benefit patients and their families. Golden and Davis's practical suggestions for the physician who must inform new parents that their child is defective reflect this kind of awareness:[5] The mother should be told with her husband or other close friend present, not alone; the doctor should hold the infant in her or his arms (giving a clear "message" that the child is still human and lovable); the clinical findings should be demonstrated directly on the baby; the physician should stress the similarity of the child to normal children; questions should be encouraged, and the information should be reviewed again the next day. It is hard to enumerate behavioral cues of this type for each situation, but with a general understanding of coping tasks and skills as well as of their own reaction to patients, humane health professionals can minimize the negative impact of a health crisis and promote effective coping.

References

1. Alsop, S. *Stay of execution: A sort of memoir.* Philadelphia: Lippincott, 1973.
2. Caplan, G. *Principles of preventive psychiatry.* New York: Basic Books, 1964.
3. Cowie, B. The cardiac patient's perception of his heart attack. *Social Science and Medicine,* 1976, *10,* 87–96.
4. Erikson, E. *Childhood and society* (2nd ed.). New York: Norton, 1963.
5. Golden, D., & Davis, J. Counseling parents after the birth of an infant with Down's syndrome. *Children Today,* 1974, *3,* 7–11, 35–36.
6. Haan, N. Psychosocial meanings of unfavorable medical forecasts. In G. Stone, F. Cohen, & N. Adler (Eds.), *Health psychology: A handbook.* San Francisco: Jossey-Bass, 1979.
7. Lazarus, R. The stress and coping paradigm. In C. Eisdorfer, D. Cohen, A. Kleinman, & P. Maxim (Eds.), *Theoretical bases for psychopathology.* New York: Spectrum, 1981.
8. Lear, M. *Heartsounds.* New York: Simon & Schuster, 1980.
9. Leigh, H., & Reiser, M. *The patient: Biological, psychological, and social dimensions of medical practice.* New York: Plenum Press, 1980.
10. Lindemann, E., & Lindemann, E. *Beyond grief: Studies in crisis intervention.* New York: Jason Aronson, 1979.
11. Millon, T., Green, C., & Meagher, R. (Eds.). *Handbook of health care psychology.* New York: Plenum Press, 1982.
12. Moos, R. Evaluating social resources in community and health care contexts. In P. Karoly (Ed.), *Measurement strategies in health psychology.* New York: Wiley, 1984.
13. Moos, R., & Billings, A. Conceptualizing and measuring coping resources and processes. In L. Goldberger & S. Breznitz (Eds.), *Handbook of stress: Theoretical and clinical aspects.* New York: Macmillan, 1982.
14. Moss, C. S. *Recovery with aphasia: The aftermath of my stroke.* Urbana: University of Illinois Press, 1972.

15. Schwartz, G. Testing the biopsychosocial model: The ultimate challenge facing behavioral medicine? *Journal of Consulting and Clinical Psychology,* 1982, *50,* 1040–1053.
16. Weiss, S., Herd, J. A., & Fox, B. (Eds.). *Perspectives on behavioral medicine.* New York: Academic Press, 1981.

II

The Crisis of Illness
Birth Defects and Perinatal Death

Pregnancy is usually a momentous and joyful time. In the months preceding birth, expectant parents plan for the arrival of a healthy baby and build up high hopes for the future. For a significant number of new parents, however, the anticipated joy is shattered when their child is born with a serious defect or lost through miscarriage, premature birth, or stillbirth (for a discussion of coping with the cesarean birth experience, see Lipson and Tilden[5]). After much preparation, parents of stillborn infants return home to an empty nursery, whereas parents of premature or sick infants may be caught in the life and death drama of a neonatal intensive care unit. Some parents whose hopes are fulfilled by a healthy, thriving baby experience an unexpected nightmare when their child dies of sudden infant death syndrome.

These groups of parents encounter several adaptive tasks. Such parents must come to terms with their conflicting emotions: shock and grief over the loss of the ideal child they expected, guilt because they produced an abnormal child, or ambivalence about future pregnancies. Parents of premature or defective children face the uncertainty of not knowing whether their child will live or be normal once survival is assured. They may also be confronted with the task of getting to know their child in the surrealistic technological environment of a neonatal intensive care unit (see Part VI). They must cope with a sense of helplessness and lack of control over their child's fate, and the frustration of being bystander parents while highly trained staff act both as healers and as pseudoparents to their child.[1]

In Chapter 2, Edward Goldson describes the developmental crisis of birth as a "dangerous opportunity" for parents as they restructure their relationships in order to accommodate a new person in the family system. The birth of a child who is premature, deformed, or seriously ill presents a major challenge to the adaptive capacity of new parents whose expectations and plans have suddenly gone awry. Initially, parents are shocked and may deny the severity of the child's problems. The parents' task is to prepare for the chance that their baby may die and to maintain a balance between intense involvement and avoidance of the infant. In time, the denial and shock give way to a barrage of conflicting emotions—sadness, grief, confusion, and anxiety. The parents must accept their failure to produce a normal child and confront the reality of their infant's actual medical condition. Guilt related to activities that parents believe might have contributed to a birth defect or premature birth (for example, having sexual intercourse) needs to be resolved.

As parents come to grips with their emotions, the period of adaptation begins. Acceptance of the fact that they do not have the healthy baby they wanted usually enables parents to deal with their disappointment and resolve their conflicting feelings about their child. Family reorganization constitutes the final phase when the child is accepted and integrated into the family system. At this time, the parents' tasks are to learn about the special problems and needs of their infant, put these problems in perspective, and make plans for the infant's future. Staff members can help parents with these tasks by providing them with information and teaching them to take care of their child as independently as possible.

Parental adaptation to the severe illness or loss of an infant may be harder when the parents are not in the same phase of adjustment or when their coping strategies clash. *Incongruent bonding* and *incongruent grieving*[6] contribute to these problems. Because of her intimate physical relationship with the maturing fetus, the mother may form an intense bond with the infant prior to birth. The father also develops a close emotional attachment to the baby, but the bonding process typically lags behind that of the mother. Consequently, her grief over a miscarriage or stillbirth is likely to be more severe, and to resolve itself more slowly than that of her husband. A role reversal my be created when a mother and her critically ill infant are hospitalized in separate specialized facilities. In this situation, fathers often visit the infant on a regular basis, begin caretaking activities, and generate a closer tie to the child than does the mother. Thus, the overall organization of health care services can alter the usual bonding and grieving processes.

The process of grieving after a stillbirth is especially hard due to the simultaneous birth and death of the child and the idea that a stillbirth is a nonevent in which there is guilt and shame and no tangible person to mourn.[7] In Chapter 3, Emanuel Lewis points out that staff members sometimes engage in a "conspiracy of silence" instead of acknowledging parental grief. They minimize the loss, avoid discussion of the dead child, and fail to offer the comfort and support that parents desperately need. Lewis believes that staff can affirm the "work of mourning" by helping parents create memories that will ultimately enable them to work through their grief. He recommends that bereaved parents name and obtain a photograph of their child, request an autopsy to aid in genetic counseling, help lay out the baby, and plan and attend a funeral or memorial service.

Glen Davidson describes the searching behavior of a mother who was not allowed to see her baby.[2] She yearned desperately for an object that was the exact weight and length of her infant. When she found a rolling pin that met her needs, she cradled it and imagined what her child might have been like. Some parents are able to create memories by holding and touching their dying or dead baby. For example, Lewis describes one mother who walked her dead infant on the floor and another who cradled her dying child in her arms and tried to nurse it. Although such coping behavior may be disconcerting, it generates a clear vision of the baby, helps parents affirm the reality of the child's brief existence, and aids them in assimilating their loss and in restructuring their lives.

The phenomenon of incongruent bonding mentioned earlier

also arises in the event of a stillbirth. Because the stillborn is a nonperson for everyone except the parents, family and friends have little or no investment in the infant. Consequently, other people may not understand or respond appropriately to parental grief and thus hinder parental adaptation to the crisis. Parental failure to mourn after a stillbirth or neonatal death may lead to chronic, delayed, or absent grief that may create problems of parenting subsequent children.[3] Staff members can promote the normal grieving process by recognizing the loss as a significant one, allowing parents the option of having physical contact with their dead infant and aiding them to memorialize the child's life.[5] An interdisciplinary perinatal mortality counseling team composed of an obstetrician, social worker, psychologist, and pathologist can serve to coordinate such supportive activities.[3]

The literature on perinatal death has neglected fathers' reactions. In Chapter 4, Frederick Mandell, Elizabeth McAnulty, and Robert M. Reece describe the rich array of coping styles employed by fathers to adapt to the death of their child from sudden infant death syndrome. Some fathers initially tried to deny the reality of the child's death and to avoid the pain of grief work, whereas others acknowledged weeping openly. Nearly all of the fathers quickly took on an active role; they sought an explanation for the cause of death, made funeral arrangements, controlled their own emotions, and concentrated on comforting their wives. The fathers directed their energies outward toward work, school, or hobbies in an attempt to handle their grief by seeking alternative rewards.

When fathers did express feelings, they entailed remorse about not having been more involved in the care of the child, a sense of being less of a man, and powerlessness in the face of unexpected events over which they lacked control. Fathers' emotions may be masked in expressions of grief that reflect the cultural stereotype of men as strong, silent types who do not need support. Thus, communication may break down when a grieving wife seeks comfort from a husband who is trying to control his emotions in order to fulfill his own expectations of himself. Frederick Mandell and his colleagues encourage health care professionals to be aware of the bonds between father and child and of the varying coping strategies favored by grieving men and women.

References

1. Bowie, W. K. Story of a first-born. *Omega*, 1977, *8*, 1–17.
2. Davidson, G. W. Death of the wished-for child: A case study. *Death Education*, 1977, *1*, 265–275.
3. Kellner, K., Kirkley-Best, E., Chesborough, S., Donnelly, W., & Green, M. Perinatal mortality counseling program for families who experience a stillbirth. *Death Education*, 1981, *5*, 29–35.
4. Kirkley-Best, E., & Kellner, K. R. The forgotten grief: A review of the psychology of stillbirth. *American Journal of Orthopsychiatry*, 1982, *52*, 420–429.
5. Lipson, J., & Tilden, V. P. Psychological integration of the cesarean birth experience. *American Journal of Orthopsychiatry*, 1980, *50*, 598–609.
6. Peppers, L. G., & Knapp, R. J. *Motherhood and mourning: Perinatal death.* New York: Praeger, 1980.
7. Stringham, J. G., Riley, J. H., & Ross, A. Silent birth: Mourning a stillborn baby. *Social Work*, 1982, *27*, 322–327.

2

Parents' Reactions to the Birth of a Sick Infant

EDWARD GOLDSON

The birth of any infant is a developmental crisis for the family. Parents usually anticipate the birth of an infant with excitement and respond to the event with positive growth and development. Nevertheless, even under the best of circumstances, the birth of a child, and particularly of the first in a family, means that new sets of relationships are established, relationships which alter the pre-existing family or husband–wife equilibrium.

Under normal circumstances the delivery of a healthy baby follows a natural process of conception, pregnancy, birth, and integration of the infant into the family. During this process, there has been anticipation of the birth, and a growing bond to the infant has developed. At the same time, new relationships between the mother and father have begun to be established during the 9-month period of gestation. These new relationships present a crisis, a "dangerous opportunity," which typically is a masterable challenge to the family and one that, under most circumstances, is met successfully.

The birth of a sick infant, however, be he premature, de-

Reprinted in abridged form from *Children Today*, July–August 1979, *8*, 13–17.

EDWARD GOLDSON • Director, Family Care Center, the Children's Hospital and Department of Pediatrics, University of Colorado Medical Center, Denver, Colorado 80220.

formed, or seriously ill, presents an even greater crisis in that it challenges all the goals and expectations that the parents have held prior to conception and during the pregnancy. How the parents will work through this crisis depends on what strengths they bring with them and the kind of support that is provided for them.

The birth of a sick infant, particularly that of a premature baby, is precipitous and unexpected. It interrupts the natural progression of adaptation and often postpones the establishment of a relationship with the infant. When a baby is born early, the parents do not have the anticipated opportunity to grow with their unborn child and to prepare themselves fully for his or her birth. In one sense, the premature infant has premature parents who may be ill prepared and ill equipped to nurture the baby.

The birth of a deformed or a full-term sick infant is also difficult in that parents, who hoped and expected to have a perfectly normal, healthy infant, now have a baby who may or may not live, or who may have many problems if he does survive.

How parents respond to the crisis of the birth of a sick infant is determined by many factors. How they were parented themselves and their own ability and experience in coping with stress—any stress—will influence the way they respond to their sick child. The quality and nature of the support systems available to the parents—such as the comfort and support which grandparents, other relatives and friends may offer—and the stability of the marital relationship will significantly influence how the couple will cope with the crisis and to whom they will turn for help, *if they turn to anyone.*

Finally, what the parents expect of the infant and what the pregnancy and infant mean to them can be of critical importance in the resolution of the crisis. For example, if the couple had decided to have a child in order to bolster a faltering marriage, the outlook could be grim in regard to maintaining the intactness of the marriage and the parents' ability to cope with a sick baby and his subsequent care.

Parents' Developmental Tasks

No matter what the final outcome for the infant, each parent has several developmental tasks which must be accomplished if a parent is to be able to relate to the infant to any meaningful degree. These tasks have been outlined by David Kaplan and Edward Mason.[1] As they note, the first stage that occurs after the premature birth is one of anticipatory grief and depression. The parent's task at this stage is preparation—to prepare for the fact that this much-wanted child may die.

The second task that the parent is confronted with, and one that usually involves the mother more, is that of accepting the fact that she has not produced a normal, full-term infant. In a sense, this is a failure on the mother's part, at least in her mind, and it is an issue with which she must come to grips if the third stage or task is to be approached and accomplished.

Fathers also have to accomplish the first two tasks, but there are different issues for them. Fathers often will ask if anything was wrong with them that resulted in the premature birth. They may also ask if there was anything they did or did not do to or for the mother that resulted in the premature birth. (Did having sexual intercourse precipitate the delivery, they may wonder, or did the long hike the couple took influence the onset of labor?) Fathers also must grieve for the child they did not have and accept the facts about the one who *was* born.

The third task that confronts parents, although the fantasied infant did not materialize, is that of resuming their interaction with the infant who was born. This task often presents many difficulties. Instead of the infant expected and anticipated, the parents now have one who is smaller or sick, or both, and who may require many mechanical support systems to sustain life. Some parents may also be confronted with an infant who is grotesque and malformed. In either case, the task confronting the parent is how to deal with the disappointment and then to reestablish contact with the real infant while separating symbolically from the idealized one. This task must be accomplished if a parent is to progress effectively to the final stage.

It is difficult to ascertain just how parents accomplish the tasks discussed. How individuals come to accept and cope with tragedy is truly a remarkable phenomenon. However, as the infant progresses toward improved health and parents receive the support of friends and family and the understanding of medical and allied personnel, most are able to deal with the issues described.

The fourth task that parents must accomplish follows naturally after successful completion of the previous ones. This job requires that the parents come to see the infant's special needs and that they be able to act constructively upon this understanding. They need to arrive at an intellectual comprehension of the infant's problems as well as an emotional acceptance of and commitment to the care of their child.

The working through of this task is an area in which many professionals can be of help. By providing parents with information they can understand and absorb, by offering support and being available to answer questions or listen to parents' concerns, medical and allied personnel can positively influence how parents will come to view their child and how they will be able to meet his special needs.

For example, the parents of a baby who had been quite ill were confused by the conflicting messages they received from different hospital staff members regarding their infant's status and prognosis. As a result, they had difficulty in understanding what they might be able to do for their baby and what plans to make for the future. When their frustration and anger with the staff was brought to the attention of the attending physician, he and a social worker met with the parents to discuss the infant's strengths and weaknesses. A plan for therapy was developed and an appropriate referral for later care of the baby was made. As a result of this intervention, the parents were able to put their infant's problems into an understandable perspective and could now enlist the resources needed in order to deal with the future.

The preceding description of the four tasks or developmental stages provides a framework from which to view the clinical issues. There are clinical correlates and expressions that accompany the parents' tasks. Researchers (Drotar *et al.*) have identified some definite clinical signs and symptoms manifested by parents which are associated with the birth of a malformed child.[2] I believe that they are also associated with the birth of any premature or sick infant. These also occur in phases.

Phase I.   The initial response of most parents of a sick infant is shock and questioning: "How could this happen to us?" The state of shock then progresses, over a period of time that varies for different parents, to one of denial. A parent may deny that his child has a defect or deny the severity and gravity of the infant's illness. For example, a parent might say, "No, the doctors are wrong. My child does not have Down's syndrome!" or "Oh well, it isn't so bad that my baby has had an intracerebral hemorrhage. He will be perfectly alright once he gets over this problem!"

Very often shock and denial accompany each other. As a result, the parent may withdraw from the infant while still hoping that he will survive. One often sees parents who refuse to visit or hold their infants until they are sure that they will live. Such behavior may persist for days or even weeks, during which time the parents do not allow themselves to risk establishing a further relationship with the infant. This period may be helpful in cushioning the blow of the unexpected birth, or it may be destructive in that it distances the parent from the infant in such a way that he or she will have difficulty in establishing a relationship with the baby later.

These clinical findings coincide with the first adaptive task the parent of a "sick" newborn has to master: anticipatory grief and depression, as shown in Table 1.

Phase II.   This phase involves a spectrum of emotions that includes sadness, grief, anger, and anxiety. The denial and shock are partially over and the parent is now confronted with the reality of a sick infant. Both parents experience this phase; yet it has different meanings for each one. For the mother the phase involves the second task that she must accomplish—acknowledg-

Table I. Parent's Reactions To The Birth of A Sick Infant

Stage	Kaplan and Mason[a]	Drotar et al.[b]
I	Anticipatory grief and depression	Shock Denial
II	Acceptance of the fact of the birth of a sick infant	Sadness, grief, anger, anxiety
III	Resume relationship to the child	Adaptation
IV	Parent comes to see infant's special needs and comes to act upon that understanding	Reorganization

[a]From Kaplan and Mason (1960).
[b]From Drotar et al. (1975).

ment of her biological failure in that she has not given birth to a normal, healthy infant. For the father the phase means recognition that with the birth of this child all of his expectations for parenting, growth, interaction, and development are not yet, nor may ever be, possible. During this phase the reality of their child's condition can and often does involve many ambivalent feelings for parents: a feeling of love for the infant and resentment of the fact that he is not normal, a feeling of happiness at being a parent, and feeling anger toward the infant because he is ill. Parental ambivalence must be worked through if the parent is to relate to the child. The social worker, nurse, or physician must be available to help the parent through this period of ambivalence.

For example, after Jamie was born prematurely and suffered a very difficult perinatal course, his mother felt both anger and guilt about the birth and then became quite depressed and withdrawn. She would come to the nursery to visit Jamie but could only sit and look at him—lovingly—but overwhelmed by the grief and depression which immobilized her. Recognizing her ambivalence and depression, the staff began to involve her in the day-to-day care of the infant, giving her positive reinforcement for any task she performed. Soon she began to assume almost complete care of the baby. The infant, in turn, became more alert and responsive, thereby reinforcing her efforts to relate to him. Over a period of time her depression lifted. Formerly withdrawn, self-deprecating and noncommunicative, she became more openly responsive to the staff. She also came to enjoy Jamie and to take pride and pleasure in his progress.

By being supportive and providing instruction without being condescending or intrusive, the staff was able to help Jamie's mother deal with her ambivalence and depression, thereby allowing her to come into closer contact with her infant.

Phase III.   The parents of a sick infant begin a period of adaptation to their unexpectedly altered lives and to the realities of their infant's condition. Many of the previously described feelings have already been or are in the process of being dealt with. The parents now begin their third task, which is to resume their relationship to the child, although the relationship will be an altered one. In a sense the parent is saying, "I'm through crying, now it's time to go to work!"

This process involves both parents, but it does not always proceed at the same pace for each one. When both parents can accomplish these tasks together, they can provide support for each other and grow together as they begin to relate to their infant. If there is a difference in the rate with which each resumes his or her relationship to the child, their ability to support one another and to adapt to the child can be compromised.

The differential in rates of progression through the stages is another phenomenon that the clinician must understand in order to be supportive and sensitive to the needs of each parent. The clinician must recognize that at a given time each parent has his or her own task to accomplish and that it may be different from that of the other parent.

For example, the father of Keith, a sick, hospitalized infant, was very unsure of himself as a parent, a factor that made his son's illness more difficult for him to handle. A rather uncommunicative person, he was also afraid of hospitals. In contrast, Keith's mother was an open woman who was naturally anxious about Keith but nevertheless comfortable with her role as mother. The hospital staff recognized that each parent was at a different stage of development, as reflected by the father's not visiting his son and the mother's total involvement with him. Staff members then were able to help the mother understand her husband's behavior, which had distressed her. They were also able to support the father and to allow him to air his feelings and deal with his insecurity.

Phase IV. The final family process one may observe is that of reorganization, which involves a positive acceptance of the child, his incorporation into the family, and the parents' support of one another. This phase coincides with the parents coming to see their infant's special needs and their being able to act realistically upon that understanding. In the case of a sick or deformed child, this reorganization is critical if any progress in rehabilitative therapy is to be made. Furthermore, it is essential if the parents are to come to accept the child as an individual who has special needs that they can and must meet.

How long do these phases last? There is no simple answer. The reactions of individual parents vary and each phase may well overlap with the one preceding and the one following it. . . . Recognition of this overall process and of how it varies with individual parents is necessary if we—pediatricians, nurses, psychologists, and social workers—are to work with stressed parents effectively.

All the characteristics and past experiences of parents influence the accomplishment of these tasks and their clinical correlates. All these tasks are not usually completed during the child's hospitalization. Some are begun in the hospital, and some begin once the child goes home. Often there may seem to be regression on the part of a parent, who may actually be adapting to the sick infant. With each crisis associated with an infant's illness, a parent may return to an earlier stage—expression of anger—by confronting the medical and nursing staff or by being very demanding and openly critical. On the other hand, a parent may withdraw and/or refuse to visit his child. Moreover, as a child's condition varies, so will a parent's response and ability to relate to the child.

The characteristics of the child also influence the way in which parents' work through the various phases of grief. If an infant is unable to elicit responses from and relate to his environment, his parent will find it difficult to adapt to and include the child in his world. For example, if an infant is very passive, feeds poorly, and does not respond to the parent, the parent may well have difficulty in trying to relate to him, stimulate him, or even love him!

Other Factors

Several other factors can influence the working through of the various issues, tasks, and phases that parents are confronted with after the birth of a sick and/or handicapped infant. The degree of the infant's illness or handicap will influence how well his parents resolve some of these conflicts. The period of separation that is necessary before the child can be returned to the parents exacerbates some of these conflicts and can have a profound effect on the parent–child relationship. Sicker children require longer hospitalization, and the longer the separation, the more difficult is the adaptation to the child. In such cases, parents may return to their older pattern of interacting only with one another and their environment, without really involving the infant. Earlier anticipation of bringing an infant home and acknowledgment of impending reorganization in their lives diminishes with the length of the infant's hospitalization, factors which may hinder the inclusion of the infant into the family once he or she finally does go home.

The messages that medical and other personnel give parents can profoundly influence how they will work through their grief at having a sick or deformed infant. When hospital staff members are judgmental or accusatory, the work that a parent has to perform is increased. It is essential that medical staff members offer support to parents, even after the child's condition is stable and he is recovering from his illness.

Parents can be expected to ask such questions as: "Can I manage this baby?"; "What will others say about the baby and about me?" and "How will the other children feel about the baby?" How staff members respond to these spoken and unspoken concerns is of vital importance when it is time for the infant to go home and be cared for by his parents. A parent's self-confidence can be immeasurably enhanced by the nonjudgmental, positive input and support that staff members, particularly the nursing staff, can provide.

However, although the staff must be supportive, it should be particularly careful not to compete with the parent in the care of the child. By and large, parents whose infants have been sick feel guilt about the illness and incompetent to care for the infant. If nursing or other staff members convey a message, even nonverbally, that they too feel the parent is incompetent, the parental task becomes enormous. Staff members must never forget that an infant is in their specialized care for only a brief period. They must always remember that one of their most important tasks and goals is to return an infant to his parents.

All of these issues must be balanced in trying to understand how parents respond to a sick infant, what these responses mean, and how we, as clinicians, can help support them. We must learn to interpret parental responses, since they determine the degree to which we can effectively relate to parents. We should observe more than the superficial behaviors of parents. We must be able to stand back and look at the emotional content and at the adaptational effects reflected by the parents' responses. Parents' behaviors may have much deeper meanings to which we must be sensitive. Finally, we must never forget that the birth of a sick infant is a unique, phenomenal stress. As clinicians we must learn how to support parents through this crisis and to remain a continued source of support.

References

1. Kaplan, D. M., & Mason, E. A. Maternal reactions to premature birth viewed as an acute emotional disorder, *American Journal of Orthopsychiatry*, 1960, *30*, 539–547.
2. Drotar, D., Baskiewicz, A., Irvin, N., Kennell, J., & Klaus, M. The adaptation of parents to the birth of an infant with a congenital malformation: A hypothetical model, *Pediatrics*, 1975, *56*, 710–717.

3

Mourning by the Family after a Stillbirth or Neonatal Death

EMANUEL LEWIS

Stillbirth is a common tragedy occurring in about one in 100 deliveries. Yet, after a stillbirth everyone tends to behave as if it had not happened. In hospitals bereaved women are usually isolated and avoided and then discharged as soon as possible. Although this is meant kindly, to protect the mothers from the painful awareness of live babies, it also means that the hospital staff do not have to face their own anxiety about stillbirth. Back at home, the family, friends, and professionals continue to avoid talking to the bereaved mother, depriving her of the talk that would help her mourn. There is silence. Statistical evidence shows that family doctors are astonishingly reluctant to know or remember anything about the patient who has a stillbirth.[1] This avoidance by the helping professionals extends into neglect of the study of the effect of stillbirth on the mother and the family. There is a conspiracy of silence. We seem unwilling to come to terms with the fact that it is a tragedy which can seriously affect

Reprinted from the *Archives of Disease in Childhood*, 1979, *54*, 303–306, by permission of the *British Medical Journal*.

EMANUEL LEWIS • Consultant Psychotherapist, the Tavistock Clinic and Consultant Psychiatrist, Department of Child and Family Psychiatry, Charing Cross Hospital, London, England NW3 5BA.

the mental health of a bereaved mother and her family. After the failure to mourn a stillbirth, mothers can have psychotic breakdowns, or there can be severe marital difficulties. Children born before or after a stillbirth where there has been a failure to mourn the stillbirth can have severe emotional difficulties. Many mothers have mothering difficulties with the child born subsequently.[2] The surviving twin of a stillbirth faces profound difficulties in life.

The psychoanalytical view of mourning is of an ongoing process during which the conscious and unconscious mind works on coming to an understanding of the memories, thoughts, and feelings about the dead person. The dead person is unconsciously imagined as being taken inside our mind and our body. The dead can be felt as dead inside us. We identify with the dead person. Doctors meet this phenomenon when a bereaved person develops imaginary symptoms related to the illness of the dead person. During the work of mourning we digest our memories and feelings about the dead and free ourselves from the identification. With incomplete or failed mourning, the identification can persist and result, for instance, in a depressive illness with somatic symptoms. Or a failure to come to terms with our inevitably mixed feelings for the dead can lead to a denial of negative feelings and an overemphasis of positive feelings. A potentially dangerous idealization of the dead person can result. When a mother idealizes her dead child there can be dire consequences for the mothering of her subsequent children.

It is the nature of stillbirth that leads us all to avoid the subject. Bourne[1] described stillbirth as a nonevent in which there is guilt and shame with no tangible person to mourn. A stillborn is someone who did not exist, a nonperson, often with no name. It is an empty tragedy, and a painful emptiness is difficult to talk about. After a stillbirth there is a double sense of loss for the bereaved mother who now has a void where there was so evidently a fullness. Even with a live birth the mother feels a sense of loss, but the consolation of a surviving "outside baby" helps the mother to overcome her puzzling and bewildering sadness at losing her "inside baby".[3] With a stillbirth, the mother has to cope with an outer as well as an inner void. There is an even more puzzling sense of nothingness for a mother who is anaesthetized at delivery—for example with a cesarean section.

Memory facilitates the normal mourning processes essential for recovery. With other bereavements there is much to remember. These memories can be shared and cried over with family and friends. Not so with stillbirth—there is no one to talk about and no one to talk to about it. The bereaved mother may herself avoid contact with people because of unconscious feelings of shame and guilt. Her shame is associated with the sense of having failed as a woman. She may feel that there is something wrong with her womb. Her guilt has to do with fantasies that her thoughts or actions have caused the death—for example, by having considered a termination of pregnancy or by having sexual intercourse late in pregnancy. If we allow mothers to isolate themselves we may seem to be confirming that their shame and guilt are justified. Many bereaved mothers keep their distress to themselves, not only to avoid too intense an awareness of their loss, but to protect others from distress. By so protecting others they deprive themselves of the talk which would aid mourning. And, of course, husbands and children also have their guilt about a stillbirth because of their mixed feelings about the pregnancy. This impedes their mourning.

To facilitate mourning I recommend that a stillbirth be managed by making the most of what is available and can be remembered. The aim is to fill the emptiness that impedes mourning.[4] Bereaved parents should be encouraged to help lay out their dead baby. A postmortem photograph, examination, and x-ray will assist genetic counseling. Parents should also be persuaded to take an active part in the certification of stillbirth, to name the baby, and to make the funeral memorable. The practice of burial in a common and nameless grave should be avoided. The family should be encouraged to attend the funeral or cremation and to know of a marked place or grave. Other children in the family find the idea of a stillbirth incomprehensible and frightening. Yet it is they, in particular, who tend to be left in the dark about the stillbirth, left without help with their grief.

It is my impression that if a stillbirth has been a real experience for the family in the ways that I have described, mourning will have been facilitated. This leads to fewer psychological problems for the mother and her family. When a stillbirth is managed in the way that I have suggested, I believe that it is a helpful experience for staff and patients. However, there is a need to be prepared for some upsetting and crazy experiences. The management of stillbirth causes considerable anxiety, particularly if the child is macerated as a result of intrauterine death or is malformed.[5] For this reason it is helpful if those managing such a painful happening as a stillbirth can have discussions with staff who have had experience with it. The reaction of parents and staff themselves to stillbirth and neonatal death can be disconcerting. The normal reactions to bereavement *are* disconcerting. Freud[6] said of normal mourning that it would seem like an illness were we not aware of the bereavement. Most people know little of the natural history of the normal reactions of parents handling their dead babies.

With stillbirth or neonatal death, it is partly the loss of what might have been, the loss of experience in the future, which makes them such heart-rending and deeply frustrating experiences.

A baby of 27 weeks' gestation was resuscitated several times in the 10 days it survived. The mother had seen the baby collapse and thought it dead, but it was resuscitated to live a short time. With difficulty, the ward sister was able to arrange a funeral and cremation for this baby, even though it was under 28 weeks' gestation. The baby was laid out in the incubator. The mother was encouraged first to touch and then to hold him. She became frenzied, clutching her baby, and then stripping the clothes off. She kissed his navel and his penis. She forcibly opened his mouth and said, "That's where his teeth would have been." Then she "walked" her baby on the floor. Soon the mother calmed down and gave the baby back to the sister. The sister was distressed, but when the parents came to see her later, her impression was that this mother was coping better than many bereaved mothers.

The detailed study of the natural history of bereavement has shown that many seemingly crazy ideas and actions are within the normal range of responses to loss[7]. Although this mother's behavior appears mad, if we examine it more closely we can see the sense in her behavior. She was attempting to come to terms with the baby's lost future. In her mind she maintained the continuity of the cycle of life. By kissing the umbilicus she was remembering her creative link with the baby *in utero;* kissing the mouth may be linked to the kiss of life, to the resuscitation. The mother longed for her son to grow teeth and learn to walk, and kissing his penis could be considered a wish to restore her dead son's potential capacity to create life. Creating memories about her baby in this way facilitated mourning.

A nurse, a senior sister, suggested that the parents of a dying, severely brain-damaged "prem" look at and touch their baby. Knowing that the mother had wanted to breast-feed her baby, the nurse suggested that the mother might take off her blouse and hold her baby close to her skin. This suggestion by the nurse seems to ignore the critical state of the infant and may have been provoked by her wish that this virutally dead baby might live. To the nurse's consternation the mother put the dying "prem" to her breast, expressed milk into the infant's mouth, and then moved its mouth to encourage swallowing. When the baby died the parents washed and dressed him in the baby clothes that the nurse had suggested they bring with them. In her next pregnancy this mother's memory of her dead baby was of cradling him in her arms. So far, although at times tearful when remembering her dead child, she is making a good job of the mothering of her new baby. While the nurse went further than I would have advised out of my concern for the physical management of the admittedly moribund baby, nevertheless she may have helped the mother when the baby was beyond medical help.

A 28-week premature baby died at 3 days. The mother telephoned the nurse who suggested that the parents come to see their dead baby son. The mother asked if she could bring baby clothes, and the nurse agreed. The nurse took the parents to the viewing room by the mortuary. They dressed their baby and told the nurse the baby's name. After this sort of experience with their dead baby, many parents, because they find it helpful, keep in touch with the staff. The mother later visited the unit and asked the nurse whether she considered blue a morbid color to paint their living room. She also said that she was learning to crochet. It seems to me that this mother was thinking about the blues and perhaps associating blue with boys and her dead son. She may also have been asking permission to go on living, to improve her living room, which unconsciously was probably symbolic of her womb, just as learning to crochet may have been symbolic of her making a new baby. She seemed to be asking the nurse if she could be considered the sort of woman who could be trusted with another baby. Unconscious destructive feelings to a lesser or greater extent are always present as part of the normal mixed feelings that a mother has about her pregnancies. After the baby died this mother feared that her unconscious destructive feelings were a reason for the child's death. Because of this she seemed to need the nurse's reassurance about her baby-making ability versus her destructiveness.

I am loath for parents to rush into pregnancy after a stillbirth until they feel that they have adequately mourned their dead baby. They need time to think through and come to terms with the stillbirth and to understand how to avoid the idealization of a dead baby that so often bedevils the life of subsequent children.

A premature baby died. The father gave away the baby clothes, etc. The mother went home, took out a small bundle of baby clothes that she had hidden away, guessing that her husband might give the baby things away, and cried over the clothes.

The wife of a medical student studying anatomy had a stillbirth. He remarked to a fellow student that he wanted to get hold of his stillbirth to dissect it. His colleague was amazed but now understands the father's need to have some tangible experience of his stillborn child, so as to facilitate mourning. This story seems upsetting but is an example of how bereaved parents will seek of themselves to get an experience of their stillborn, sensing that this will help them to mourn. Obviously, this father would have benefited from other help.

Similarly, many mothers seem to know that it would be helpful to look at their dead baby, although they are usually put off when they ask hospital staff whether they should do so. One mother, in trying to get an experience of her stillborn child, made the most of what she had seen—a cot and a wisp of black hair on the top of his head. This is now a dear memory for her.

A photograph of a dead baby can help parents who have been unable to see their stillborn child. Or other eyes that have seen can tell the parents. A husband carefully described to his wife how his stillborn daughter had looked, described her face and hair, her delicate normal body and limbs, and also the dark-stained blotches on one side.

A woman house surgeon did something like this for the parents of an anencephalic baby which her consultant had refused to allow her to show the parents. She described to the mother and father the normal body, the normal delicate hands and fingers, legs, feet, and toes of the anencephalic baby. The doctor also encouraged the father who had wanted to protect his wife by leaving her out of the funeral, to take her along. The doctor said it was also the mother's baby and so the father did take his wife to the funeral.

It is necessary to make recommendations about the management of stillbirths in hospitals. I believe that parents left to themselves, and this is particularly so with domiciliary delivery, would do things better. You may feel that my suggestions about the management of stillbirth and neonatal death are silly. But I suggest that the normal "rugby pass" management of stillbirth in hospital is rather more bizarre. I refer to the catching of a stillbirth after delivery, the quick accurate back-pass through the labor room door to someone who catches the baby and rapidly covers it and hides it from the parents and everyone. Our hospital culture tends to impede the normal healing process of mourning. We do this even by asking the mother whether she wishes to see her dead baby. Really, what could be more natural? It heartens me when I hear of a father describing the baby in detail to his wife, of the mother who hid the baby clothes to cry over, or of the father who wished to dissect his baby, or of the mother who kissed and walked her dead baby. Sometimes people know how to help themselves. It is difficult in hospital. A senior midwife was encouraged by the obstetrician to show a stillbirth to the parents. She took the macerated stillbirth out of the labor room saying, with the irony of the unconscious, that "to show them the baby would put them off stillbirth for life." Fortunately this midwife recovered, brought the baby back to the parents and, with great sensitivity, showed them the normal limbs, fingers, and toes, and asked them the name of the baby.

In the Far East there is a cactus with white fragrant flowers that blooms briefly only every few years. Each bud opens and dies visibly in front of one's eyes within a few hours. A family may sit together and watch the birth and death of the flower, for it brings good luck. A Far Eastern couple buried their stillborn in a little grave with a small headstone inscribed with the name of this cactus given to their child. An act of creative poetic self-healing.

References

1. Bourne, S. The psychological effects of stillbirths on women and their doctors. *Journal of the Royal College of General Practitioners*, 1968, *16*, 103–112.
2. Lewis, E., & Page, A. Failure to mourn a stillbirth: An overlooked catastrophe. *British Journal of Medical Psychology*, 1978, *51*, 237–241.
3. Lewis, E. The atmosphere in the labor ward. *Journal of Child Psychotherapy*, 1976, *4*, 89–92. (a)
4. Lewis, E. The management of stillbirth: Coping with an unreality. *Lancet*, 1976, *2*, 619–620. (b)
5. Lewis, E. Psychological dilemmas confronting the physician and the parents of a malformed abortus, stillborn, and deceased newborn. *Proceedings of the National Birth Defects Conference*. New York: National Foundation March of Dimes, 1978.
6. Freud, S. Mourning and melancholia. In *Complete psychological works*, (Standard Edition, Volume 14). London: Hogarth Press, 1957.
7. Parkes, C. M. *Bereavement: Studies of grief in adult life*. London: Tavistock Publications, 1972.

4

Observations of Paternal Response to Sudden Unanticipated Infant Death

FREDERICK MANDELL, ELIZABETH McANULTY, and
ROBERT M. REECE

Should we begin to challenge the stereotyped role of the father who loses a child? Mothers have traditionally been the primary caregivers for most infants, and research on the early development of involvement and investment has focused on the mother–infant interaction. Professional support provided to families experiencing the loss of an infant to sudden infant death syndrome (SIDS) has concentrated on understanding the effects of the disruption of bonding and its consequences on the mother's sense of self. However, fathers also form significant relationships with their infants. Studies of father–neonate relationships are beginning to emerge.[1-6] The sudden infant death syndrome brings a drastic and abrupt end to that relationship. Manifestations of grief are seemingly influenced by the traditional expectations of

Reprinted from *Pediatrics,* February 1980, *65,* No. 2, 221–225. Copyright American Academy of Pediatrics 1980.

FREDERICK MANDELL, ELIZABETH McANULTY, and ROBERT M. REECE • Children's Hospital Medical Center and the Massachusetts Sudden Infant Death Syndrome Center, Boston, Massachusetts 02115.

masculine behavior. In Western societies we are only just beginning to observe the emotional importance of father–infant tenderness and loyalty. The behavior of the father in response to the loss of his child is the subject of this report.

Background and Description

Forty-six families who lost infants to SIDS during a period of several months were visited at home by a community health nurse. Fathers were present and participated in 28 of those visits. The interviewer, who was aware of the specific circumstances of the deaths, assessed the parental reactions to the tragedy. The results reported are observations on patterns of paternal grief.

Age and Race

Eighteen of the 28 infants died between the ages of 4 weeks and 4 months, four died between ages 4 months and 6 months, and four between 6 months and 1 year. One infant was older than 1 year, and one infant was younger than 1 month. Twenty-four of the infants were white, two were black, and two were Hispanic. Of the fathers, 12 were between 22 and 30 years of age, seven were between 18 and 21 years, and eight were over 30. One father was under 18 years of age.

Observations

Denial of Loss

In well over half of the families, it appeared that fathers were attempting to deny the reality of their child's death and avoid the pain of grief work. Denial was implicity evident in a variety of observed behaviors which included accomodation to a manager-like role and intellectualization of distress. Fathers who used denial also exhibited increased involvement outside the home, had strong feelings about subsequent children, and avoided professional support.

Managerial Role

All of the fathers in this sample, except one, assumed a manager-like role during the first several days after the baby's death. Characteristics of this role included forced control of emotional expression and preoccupation with the emotional support of the wife. There also appeared to be a distinct tendency to find an explanation for the cause of death and to become directly involved in funeral arrangements and other details. A frequently heard comment during the days immediately after the infant's death was:

> Things like this happen. I don't want S. to blame herself—she was a perfect mother . . . I have to stay strong for everyone else.

Intellectualizing of Grief and Blame

In several instances the fathers were able to discuss their own grief, but frequently even this appeared to be intellectualized:

> It is much harder for S. [wife], she was with him all the time . . . It has affected me, but I am accepting J.'s death . . . I don't expect or want people at work to ask me about it. No one can bring J. back . . . we have to go on living.

The behaviors of these fathers were often in direct contrast to those of their wives, who were, in almost every instance, tearful and frequently incoherent. Most of the fathers acknowledged that they had cried, but none of the fathers in this sample cried during the home visit. All of the mothers cried during the home visit and described their own behavior as far more expressive.

This group of fathers directed their energies and attentions outward while mothers appeared to withdraw. Many of the mothers were very much self-absorbed in grief and seemed to notice very little around them, while frequently the fathers seemed almost awed by the responses from relatives, friends, and the community.

> I'm telling you, this is beautiful. The whole office came to the funeral. People are just coming out of nowhere . . . I never thought anyone would care.

In some instances it appeared as if the parents had not previously discussed their feelings with each other. In other instances fathers appeared to devote great energy in assuring the mothers of their blamelessness. There was some denial of anger toward the wife for "letting" the baby die and also denial of anger toward the wife's grieving behavior.

> It was really hard for her . . . after all she spent the whole day with the baby.

Increased Involvement Outside Home

In this study mothers identified verbalizing of feelings as important and were almost always able to identify a female relative, usually their mother, or a friend with whom they could talk. This was generally not the pattern for fathers. The most predominant coping mechanism identified by fathers was "to keep busy." For many fathers this meant taking an additional job, taking graduate school courses, accepting additional workload responsibilities, or seeking energy-absorbing hobbies. Few of the fathers could articulate the emotional pain which promoted a desire for concrete escape. One father commented:

> I shouldn't go, but I may have to leave . . . it is too much—I want to hit out on someone. The crib, seeing it hurts too much. When I am here it reminds me of how everything is wrong. She [his wife] keeps talking about G.—I don't want to hear it.

Feelings about Subsequent Children

A denial of the irreversibility of the loss seemed implicit in several of the fathers' thoughts about future children. These fathers appeared to have attitudes different from those of their spouses. During the first four months after the sudden infant death, many of the mothers describe a tremendous fear of a subsequent pregnancy. None of the fathers in this sample verbalized this fear, and there was even a predominant expression of urgency to have another child as soon as possible. In the months following the infant's death, the mothers frequently mentioned the issue of a subsequent pregnancy as a source of conflict between the parents.

Avoidance of Professional Support

In 18 of the 46 families, fathers seemed to very purposely avoid being home when the nurse visited. The mothers frequently said that the fathers felt that talking to someone else about the baby's death accomplished nothing, and in some cases the mothers were somewhat secretive about their contacts with the community health nurse.

> He doesn't want me to talk about our private problems. If I tell him that you were here he would say 'I don't want to know about it.' When I call you I need to wait until he is out of the house.

In this sample, 14 of the 28 mothers requested crisis support regarding particular situations after initial contact with the nurse. None of the fathers initiated a request. Seven of these mothers (50%) identified as the presenting problem their concerns about the fathers. These difficulties centered around communication or specific concerns about the father's behavior. Several fathers in this group were able to verbalize some of their feelings after encouragement. They often repeated the comment of one of the fathers who said:

> I can't talk to anyone. I just can't tell anyone about my problems. It doesn't help to talk about it. It won't bring the baby back.

Expressions of Grief

Although there was a tendency for fathers to deny the loss, a few talked about obstacles to catharsis:

> After the funeral we came back to the house . . . seeing the emptiness . . . I really broke down and cried. It was like everyone backed off . . . was embarrassed for me. No one would hold me then, although they had been doing this for her [wife] for three days.

Feelings which tended to be acknowledged by some fathers included self-reproach over a lack of involvement with the infant and a decreased sense of self-esteem and powerlessness.

Involvement with Infant's Care

During the interviews only nine of the fathers spontaneously discussed their involvement with the baby who died. Three of these infants were the firstborn. The fathers who spoke of feeling comfortable with the infant's care tended to be in those families in which there were other children. One father was able to discuss his enjoyment in caring for the baby quite fully. He spoke of how he was grateful for this time and that "at least he didn't feel that he had not known the baby."

More frequently, fathers expressed remorse over a lack of involvement in infant care:

> I just kept thinking that when he got older I would have time. It doesn't make sense, but I almost wonder if he thought I wasn't a good father.

Another father learning of his fourth child's death wondered "if maybe we didn't love her enough."

Decreased Self-Esteem

Frequently fathers talked of feeling inadequate and that a part of them had died with the baby:

> To tell you the truth, this may sound crazy, but losing the baby makes me feel less like a man.

Feelings of diminished self-worth were also expressed by other fathers more indirectly. One father, who immediately after the baby's death became engrossed in funeral arrangements, demonstrated this. He said:

> Everyone took over. No one really listened to what I wanted. It was like I was a kid all over again.

This statement expressed a feeling of powerlessness which was repeated by both fathers and mothers in almost every encounter.

> When M. was born everything seemed like it was golden. I felt like I was on top of the world . . . I felt like a real man. Like I had a family and I could take care of them.

Special feelings of helplessness and frustration were expressed by fathers who initially tried to resuscitate the baby.

Marital Stability

The dissolution of marriages and families following SIDS has frequently been a source of concern. In this sample we know of six fragmented relationships over a one-year period of follow-up. Four of these were situations in which the parents were young (under 21 years of age), and in all six families the deceased child was the firstborn. Frequently, parents said that their marriage was rushed by the pregnancy that resulted in the child who died.

Discussion

Behavioral scientists have had disproportionally little to say about the impact of the father on very early child development. Some child care professionals have considered fathers to be good to have around, the best babysitters, and certainly an important emotional support for the mother, but without a critical emotional involvement in the infant. The maternal-infant relationship is considered so exclusive that the medical profession continues to offer services labeled "maternal-child" clinics or departments.[4] It is thus not surprising to witness a devaluation of the father's role at the time of the death of an infant.

Recent research has provided evidence that fathers do form significant relationships with their infants.[7,8] While mothers begin to sense a baby's rhythms prenatally and usually provide much of the caretaking in the early weeks, fathers also engage in mutually regulated interchange with their babies.[5]

Fathers present in the delivery room were observed to develop a bond with their infants by the first three days after birth and often earlier. This "engrossment" was also observed to have a discernible influence upon the father.[1] Studies of infant attachment demonstrate that fathers are an attachment figure for infants and that this interaction can be just as sensitive to infants' needs as that between mothers and infants.[9] Moreover, the father and the mother may play qualitatively different roles in their relationship with infants and family. As infants become older the development of attachment becomes more defined. The father's interaction is not limited to caretaking functions, but appears to be broader based and extends over more playful activities.[5,8]

While we learn about the adaptive mechanisms of the infant–father relationship, we must also realize the harshness of the sudden termination of fatherhood. In a study of families with Down's syndrome, Gath[10] found marital tension, which may have resulted from the father's grieving and mourning after having produced a defective offspring.

Fathers have been sons and the complexity and consequences of fatherhood are drawn from a stock of experiences with their fathers and mothers.[9,11,12] A new father accommodates to the experience of fatherhood. Sometimes it reshapes his world, altering his images of himself, his wife, and his parents. A new father is influenced and will be affected by the development of his child. Between the two there transpires communications from the deepest parts of both participants. The adult crisis provoked by infant death, then, must be profound.

When sudden death is due to a known cause, the concrete character of the event can be incorporated into the normal rationalization of mourning. When, however, death is due to an unknown and unanticipated mechanism, the immediate effect is even more overpowering. Fathers generally have less insight into the mechanics of child rearing and child health risks and may be less prepared to accept the fragility of life and the constraints on their own control over their children's environment or destiny. In this small sample there were many thinly disguised statements of blame toward the mother who is traditionally designated as the primary caretaker.

In general the observed men seemed to be more angry and aggressive, while the women were more depressed and withdrawn. In this report the majority of fathers assumed the role of manager. These concrete ceremonies reinforce the reality of the death and provide an outlet for expression of final offerings. Although the role of manager may have been a natural tendency for fathers reeling from the shock of the infant's death, there may also have been familial and societal expectations which forced this.

As a group, the fathers in this experience seemed to indicate that men also have the need to grieve but require different kinds of outlets. Even those fathers who sensed their own need for help seemed to limit their requests for it or, more significantly, their requests were not recognized. Directly associated with the father's reluctance to seek help or to discuss emotional pain may be the experience of a diminished sense of masculine power provoked by the infant's death. Verbalizing or exposing helplessness may further exacerbate an already painful assault on self-esteem. Our own experiences suggest that if fathers are given an opportunity to express feelings and a validation of their feelings, they will constructively utilize support.

A difference in attitude between men and women regarding the urgency of subsequent pregnancy appeared within the study group. The men seemed rather quick to focus on having another child. These attempts to regain the lost child and provide evidence of virility are active modes of dealing with stress. This may also serve as a method of eluding the work of mourning. In either case, under psychological conditions of mourning and guilt, women who do attempt to quickly conceive a "replacement child" appear to have a higher rate of infertility and spontaneous abortion in the first year after SIDS loss.[12]

This study group offered a reflection of cultural subtyping: that men should be tough and stoic and that one need not be concerned with reactions or general well-being of the fathers. These paternal behaviors, which emerge at a time of crisis and which obstruct full expression of grief, may unwittingly be promoted by medical and health care providers who are anxious to help fathers fulfill societal expectations of masculine strength.

The long-term effects of these personal and societal attitudes are difficult to estimate, and broad conclusions should not be drawn from this small, short-term observational sample. However, it is important for health professionals caring for families who lose a child suddenly to be aware of affectional bonding between infants and fathers and to be sensitive to the effects of the sudden, unexpected shattering of that linkage.

References

1. Greenberg, M., & Morris, N. Engrossment: The newborn's impact upon the father. *American Journal of Orthopsychiatry*, 1974, *44*, 520–531.
2. Abelin, E. L. Some further observations and comments on the earliest role of the father. *International Journal of Psychoanalysis*, 1975, *56*, 293–302.
3. Brazelton, T. B., Yogman, M. W., Als, H., & Tronick, E. The infant as a focus for family reciprocity. In M. Lewis & L. Rosenblum (Eds.), *The child and its family*. New York: Plenum Press, 1979.

4. Yogman, M. W. *The goals and structure of face-to-face interaction between infants and fathers.* Paper presented at the meeting of the Society for Research in Child Development, New Orleans, 1957.

5. Earls, F., & Yogman, M. The father–infant relationship. In J. Howells (Ed.), *Modern perspectives in the psychiatry of infancy.* New York: Brunner/Mazel, 1980.

6. Klaus, M., & Kennell, J. *Maternal-infant bonding.* St. Louis: C. V. Mosby, 1976.

7. Yogman, M. W., Dixon, S., & Tronick, E. *Father–infant interaction.* Paper presented at the meeting of the American Pediatric Society for Pediatric Research. St. Louis, 1976.

8. Lamb, M. Forgotton contributors to child development. *Human Development,* 1975, *18,* 245–266.

9. Parke, R. D., O'Leary, S. E., & West, S. Mother–father–newborn interaction: Effects of maternal medication, labor, and sex of infant. *Proceedings of the American Psychological Association.* Yellow Springs, Ohio: Fels Research Institute, 1972.

10. Gath, A. The impact of an abnormal child upon the parents. *British Journal of Psychiatry,* 1974, *125,* 568–582.

11. Ross, J. M. *Paternal identity.* Paper presented at the Seminar for the Development of Infants and Parents, Boston, May 1978.

12. Mandell, F., & Wolfe, L. C. Sudden infant death syndrome and subsequent pregnancy. *Pediatrics,* 1975, *56,* 774–776.

III

The Crisis of Illness
Childhood Cancer

Recent treatment advances in childhood cancer have turned an almost certain killer into a chronic life-threatening illness. As a result, children and parents may face years of uncertainty in which the chance of remission or cure is juxtaposed against potential relapse and eventual death. Parents must come to terms with the shock of diagnosis and support their child's efforts to cope with treatment. They must mourn in anticipation of losing their child while maintaining hope for a cure. Other tasks entail establishing a working alliance with health care staff, obtaining information about the disease, and making hard decisions about treatments that may be experimental or involve disfiguring surgery.

Parents also encounter additional problems as the impact of childhood cancer reverberates throughout the family. They face the challenge of sustaining more than a semblance of a normal home life and preserving a good relationship with each other and their healthy children.[6] These are especially difficult tasks to master, given the constant disruptions and financial burdens that accompany childhood cancer. Frequent trips to outpatient clinics play havoc with daily routines. When specialized treatment centers are distantly located, family finances can be strained by the expense of motel rooms, restaurant meals, long distance telephone calls, and baby-sitters for children at home. Moreover, family income may decrease when parents switch to part-time jobs in order to spend more time with their sick child.[3,4]

Remissions bring family members welcome respite from their

struggle. However, when a child relapses, parents must expand their coping repertoire. They may be faced with agonizing decisions about further treatment that offers a chance of increasing their child's life span at the price of renewed pain and suffering. They may have to learn basic nursing skills in order to care for their dying child at home. Ultimately, parents encounter the task of communicating honestly with their dying child about impending death.[5]

In Chapter 5, Yehuda Nir and Bonnie Maslin describe the interdependent stages of emotional response and coping mechanisms of parents, children, and health care staff during the course of childhood cancer. The stage of optimism occurs early in the disease process as children and parents use denial to cope with the fear and helplessness aroused by the diagnosis. Because they wish to allay the fear cancer provokes, physicians' own coping strategies may promote optimism by providing reassurance and the promise of potential cure. During this time, some parents aggressively pursue a cure by shopping around for the best treatment or by reading the latest cancer research and closely monitoring their child's progress. Staff may resent these parental coping styles and respond by practicing "defensive medicine" (that is, an overly cautious approach oriented toward avoiding mistakes).

When the initial treatment fails and the child relapses, optimism quickly turns to disappointment. At this stage, parents may cope with the threat of death by increased denial and by continuing to seek alternate opinions. A stage of disillusionment sets in if subsequent treatment fails to achieve a remission. Faith in the physician is shattered, and hope for a cure is lost. If parents are unable to accept the impending death of their child, the troublesome stage of abandonment may occur. Parents cling to denial and search for miracle cures, whereas physicians may cope with their own vulnerability to rejection by withdrawing from the child or ordering more tests and treatment primarily to appease angry parents. The stage of rapprochement begins once parents and physicians confront the inevitability of the child's death. At this time, parents engage in anticipatory grieving and unite around the child for a last farewell. In the final stage of reconciliation, parents and physicians try to accept the fact that the child has died.

Health care professionals and families cannot spare children the torment and suffering that accompany some cancer treatment. Children must cope with the pain of illness, disfiguring surgery, and the side effects of treatment, such as nausea, hair loss, and possible sterility. Given all these assaults, children need to maintain their self-esteem and negotiate normal developmental tasks.[6] Finally, when children return home, they are confronted with problems of reentry, such as returning to school and facing peers who may stare at their flawed body[2] or tease them about the wig that covers their baldness.

In Chapter 6, Judith A. Ritchie describes the concerns and coping patterns of children who experienced a radical, disfiguring treatment—limb amputation. The children responded to news of the need for an amputation with both denial and anger. Prior to surgery, some children showed a lack of concern or withdrawal, whereas others asked detailed questions about the operation and the artificial leg or tried to reduce their tension by crying and screaming in protest. Nearly all of the children were worried about the ugliness of their stump and the appearance of the artificial leg. Cognitive coping strategies included trying to anticipate what the new leg would be like and how it would function.

Postoperatively, the children employed remarkably resilient and flexible coping strategies. They dealt with the initial shock at the sight of their stump by refusing to look at it but then gradually exposed it to themselves and to other people. Similarly, some children actively sought information but then "dosed themselves" by withdrawing temporarily to avoid feeling overwhelmed. The children expressed anger and disappointment when they saw their artificial leg, but their mood improved dramatically when they began physiotherapy and found they could learn to walk again. Moreover, the children showed unusual sensitivity in that they tended to express their grief and anger primarily to persons who were able to accept such emotions. Ritchie recommends that staff promote children's adjustment by encouraging the expression of emotions, providing honest answers to questions, showing the child an artificial limb, or having the child meet with an amputee. After surgery, firm reassurance helps children to begin self-care of the stump and to incorporate it into their body image.

Cancer does not excuse children from negotiating the hurdles posed by normal developmental tasks. These tasks are especially challenging for sick adolescents. Some adolescents respond to their uncertainty and the ever-present threat of relapse by being unable to plan for the future. An adolescent's fragile self-concept, need for peer relationships, and emerging sexuality may be threatened by treatment that makes him or her physically unattractive or isolates him or her from friends. Some adolescents relish the attention and care that comes with being a patient and are reluctant to regain their independence when they are in remission. Others cope with feelings of lack of control over their lives by taking risks, using drugs, or avoiding treatment.[1]

In Chapter 7, Dianne Fochtman describes how a humane staff responded to the developmental needs and diverse coping strategies to two adolescents who were terminally ill with leukemia. Beginning with diagnosis, staff worked to establish an alliance with Ann and John based on open sharing of information about the disease and treatment. Ann wrote to her close friends and told them of her illness, requested their acceptance of the physical changes she had experienced, and asked them to help her maintain their friendship. John chose a different approach by avoiding any discussion of his illness with his friends.

Staff provided both adolescents with an opportunity to maintain some control by allowing them to make decisions about their care and treatment. Ann chose the sites for her intravenous injections, and John came unaccompanied to the clinic for treatment. When John could no longer tolerate the side effects of chemotherapy, he decided to stop treatment. Staff members and his parents supported this decision. John tried to shield his family from pain by limiting his discussions of his illness and his approaching death with them. Ann openly expressed her feelings and made an effort to say a special goodbye to the staff a few days before her death. John and Ann were involved in making decisions about where they would die; both decided to die at home. Staff also encouraged them to make plans about their funeral and burial. By responding flexibly to diverse coping styles and sustaining independence and participation in treatment, staff can help adolescents meet even the most difficult developmental tasks.

References

1. Dunlop, J. G. Critical problems facing young adults with cancer. *Oncology Nursing Forum*, 1982, *3*, 33–38.
2. Kagen-Goodheart, L. Reentry: Living with childhood cancer. *American Journal of Orthopsychiatry*, 1977, *47*, 651–658.
3. Kalnins, I. V., Churchill, M. P., & Terry, G. E. Concurrent stress in families with a leukemic child. *Journal of Pediatric Psychology*, 1980, *5*, 81–92.
4. Koocher, G. P., & O'Malley, J. E. *The Damocles syndrome: Psychosocial consequences of surviving childhood cancer.* New York: McGraw-Hill, 1981.
5. Krulik, T. Helping parents of children with cancer during the midstage of illness. *Cancer Nursing*, 1982, *5*, 441–445.
6. Spinetta, J. J. Behavioral and psychological research in childhood cancer: An overview. *Cancer*, 1982, *50*, 1939–1943.

5

Psychological Stages in Childhood Cancer

YEHUDA NIR and BONNIE MASLIN

Medical advances in pediatric hematology and oncology during the past few decades have significantly influenced the survival and cure rate for leukemias and other forms of cancer. Though a child may ultimately die from the disease, new therapeutic interventions have greatly extended the time a child can expect to live once the diagnosis of a fatal illness has been made.

Survival or an extended life span is a result of prolonged and aggressive treatment with chemotherapy, radiotherapy, and surgery, either separately or in combination. On a daily basis this treatment may include lumbar punctures, bone marrow aspirations, and painful venipunctures that occasionally result in infiltrations. Loss of appetite, nausea, painful mucosal ulcerations, total loss of hair, and weakness (necessitating prolonged bed rest) are the grave consequences of cancer treatment that confront the child. In addition, chemotherapy may produce severe neu-

Reprinted from *Psychiatric Clinics of North America,* 1982, *5,* 379–386. This article was originally entitled "Liaison Psychiatry in Childhood Cancer—A Systems Approach."

YEHUDA NIR • Director of Pediatric Psychiatry, Memorial Sloan-Kettering Cancer Center and Associate Clinical Professor of Psychiatry, Cornell Medical College, New York, New York 10021. BONNIE MASLIN • Consultant in Occupational Mental Health, New York, New York.

tropenia, requiring periods of isolation and, consequently, sensory and emotional deprivation. Ironically, all of the above (and this is an incomplete list) are the consequences of the procedures and side effects of treatment and not of the disease itself.

This new medical reality creates a series of overwhelming problems for the young patient, his family, the physician-in-charge, nurses, and other health caretakers. These problems are both physical and psychological and tend to interdigitate in the course of the child's illness, particularly as the disease progresses.[7]

In working with children, families, and staff as they negotiate the various milestones on the disease continuum (diagnosis, remission, relapse, or death), we have observed qualitatively different coping strategies that emerge as the disease takes its course. We regard these various shifts as occurring in stages.

The notion of stages through which a terminally ill individual proceeds is not new. The work of Kubler-Ross,[4] while currently questioned by clinicians,[1] delineates an invariant series of stages (denial, anger, bargaining, depression, acceptance) that describe the intrapsychic experience of the dying person. More recently, Weisman[12] has provided an important model of psychosocial phasing in cancer that focuses on assessment of patient vulnerability during the various stresses encountered as the disease progresses (see Chapter 8). His aim is to integrate typical problems, concerns, and distresses of cancer patients with clinical staging, treatment, and disease progression.[13] These stages and assessment processes, while valuable, focus primarily on the individual patient. In his more recent work, Weisman has directed attention to the vulnerability of the oncologic caregiver and has detailed "therapeutic suggestions for identifying and correcting caregivers plight" (see Chapter 24).

Due to the crisis-ridden nature of oncologic diseases and the long-term and arduous course of treatment that often ensues, patient, family, and health care professionals enter into a complex interdependent system. Therefore, an assessment and intervention must address itself to the interactive nature of this intricate system. Such a model is in keeping with the general system theory. Developed by von Bertalanffy,[11] Miller,[6] and others, this approach perceives man and his environment as interacting wholes with integrated sets of properties and relationships. Applying this concept to childhood cancer means that everyone in contact with the patient has to be seen as an interdependent part of the larger therapeutic network. A less comprehensive model can offer a skewed view of the biopsychosocial problems that may arise.

This notion of a systems model is nowhere more important than in childhood cancer. Factors such as the child's dependence on the adult world, the untimeliness of the disease,[5] the pathos of a suffering child, the reversal of the natural order of life (child's death preceding parental death) create an intense community of concern—a compelling interdependency of patient, family, and health care professional.

The concept of stages as suggested in this article is an initial attempt to consider the phase-specific psychologic issues that emerge as the disease progresses and the nature of the interactions among the individuals within the system. We have designated these stages as optimism, disappointment, disillusionment, abandonment, rapprochement, and reconciliation. This sequence does not seem to be invariant, rather it appears dependent upon the vagaries of the disease process. All the stages will not be encountered, for example, if the child is cured. This article will attempt to explore the psychological meaning of these stages and address itself to the way the child, his family, and the pediatric oncologist cope and negotiate the vicissitudes of childhood cancer.

Optimism

This stage is characterized by faith in the physician's power to effect a cure and seems to emerge as a response to the potentially overwhelming impact of diagnosis, which at Sloan-Kettering is communicated frankly to child and family. In our view optimism is generally adaptive—enabling staff and patient to forge a working alliance against the disease. Optimism is often fostered by the physician, who, in response to the fear that cancer evokes, may resort to reassurance and promises of potential cure. During this period patient and family use denial and blocking to ward off feelings of helplessness, panic, and confusion. Frequently they fail to comprehend the details of the physician's statements as if to prevent the input of additional anxiety-provoking material. Even families who have been told about the diagnosis by a referring physician behave as if they have heard the news for the first time—disbelief in the service of denial, a defense mechanism that fosters the emergence of hope.

Studies on informed consent given during the initial phase of treatment have demonstrated how little the average cancer patient comprehends about the nature of the disease, the treatment, and its side effects.[11] Perhaps such findings may indeed reflect the patient's unconscious need to replace knowledge with a binding trust in the physician—a prerequisite for optimism.

In this atmosphere of optimism, both children and adolescents, if offered proper support, seem to adjust to the diagnosis of cancer and react with relatively minor complaints about the disease, the side effects of chemotherapy, or surgical intervention (such as limb amputation). However, such adjustment may not be forthcoming if psychopathology in child or family members that predates the cancer prevents optimism from emerging.

> From the time he was diagnosed as having acute lymphoblastic leukemia, John, nine years old, refused to cooperate with treatment. He was referred with his mother to the liaison psychiatrist. It became apparent that his mother's narcissistic preoccupation with her pain and her feeling that John would die prevented her from providing the much needed reassurance and support. Mother's inability to respond to the child's need was highlighted on one occasion when the two drove past a cemetery on the way home from the hospital. The boy, noting the tombstones, said, "When I die I would like to have a statue of Superman on my grave." His mother answered, "Oh no, this would look silly."

The patient's question clearly indicated concern about his own vulnerability and mortality. It could have been dealt with by a reassuring statement pointing to the hope for a remission, which was, in fact, to follow; yet the mother's inability to identify her son's feelings resulted in a statement that conveyed a morbid, pessimistic message: "Yes, you will have a tombstone—which one remains only a technicality." Such messages and others repeated in more direct ways—for example, associating the child's illness to a grandfather's death from cancer—preclude optimism.

Another important factor that generally becomes evident in the stage of optimism is the style with which parents pursue medical care for their sick child and the way in which they relate to the health care personnel. Successful treatment is aided if the staff is aware of these factors.[2] To facilitate this awareness we attempt to classify families along this parameter.

A large segment of our parent population may be characterized as "aggressive pursuers." The seemingly disproportionate representation of this group is probably due to the international reputation of our center. The parents have usually "shopped" around and have chosen the center (often coming from as far away as Pakistan, Aden, or Argentina, or within the United States from the Midwest, Texas, or Florida). They want the best and are in quest of, and expect to find, a "cure." This attitude can evoke a mixture of resentment and excessive compliance in the health care professional, perhaps in response to the underlying aggression.

At the other end of the spectrum are parents we have designated as "silent sufferers." (More often than not they are referred by local physicians.) They are characterized by a sense of equanimity and acceptance of fate often tied to religious beliefs. They are generally cooperative—in the "best interest of the child." Their attitude with its concomitant passivity and helplessness evokes very positive reactions from the staff, who often rally to support them.

Another, smaller group is characterized as "intellectual" in their approach. Usually professionals whose obsessive compulsive character encourages the pursuit of information as a way of coping with anxiety and helplessness, they may present a threat to the medical establishment. They strive to become up to date on the latest research studies, check and recheck every blood count, and point out mistakes and discrepancies in the administration of medication and treatment. This continued surveillance may force the health care professional into defensive medicine as a protection against what is experienced as a parental assault.

While these examples do not exhaust our categories, they suggest how a particular style can have a decisive role in establishing the tone of this first stage and all others that follow. For example, the aggressive style suggests the possibility of limited parental tolerance for staff who do not provide unqualified assurances about a cure. This information, in the hands of the liaison psychiatrist, oncologist, nurses, and so on, may help keep a parent from taking angry flight if such assurances are neither possible nor appropriate.

In addition to parental attitudes, the particular nature of the medical intervention, and its actual or symbolic meaning is often critical to the formation of optimism. Radical interventions, such as limb amputation, particularly in young boys, is a crisis that can have a powerful impact on this stage. It may compel some parents—fathers in particular—into an extreme form of denial (a kind of "wild optimism"). One father of an 11-year-old with osteosarcoma wrote on his son's cast, following below the knee amputation, "Bitten off by a shark" and planned a fishing trip two days after discharge. Such massive denial may engender treatment noncompliance, since a child, in order to maintain this emotional climate, may feel obliged to act as if he is not ill at all.

Personal and family stressors have a significant impact on the biopsychosocial system of childhood cancer. In particular, families in which the marriage is on the verge of collapse and for whom the death of the child might precipitate the final breakup are among the most difficult to handle. Threats of suicide, divorce, and abandonment may overshadow concern about the sick child. On one occasion, a nine-year-old leukemic girl whose parents were separated insisted that the mother get pregnant to have a child to replace her in case she died. She admitted to the psychiatrist that she thought this would get her parents back together. Such anxieties may prevent family and child from focusing on treatment-related goals. An effective oncologist recognizes the overlap between the existing family system and the one that develops around the disease.

These are only a few of the many factors that come to bear on the formation of a therapeutic alliance and emergence of optimism. If remission does occur, the majority of children and their families show amazing resilience and ability to recover from the emotional crisis and upheaval. Koocher and O'Malley[1] in a study of 117 cancer survivors found 62, or 53 percent, to have no evidence of psychological impairment. An additional 25.6 percent functioned adequately, and only 2.7 percent had severe impairment.

Though a sense of vulnerability continues, the disease in remission permits the continuation of the stage of optimism.

Disappointment

The occurrence of a relapse ushers in the next stage—disappointment. For most patients this is more traumatic than the initial diagnosis. Holland[4] has stated that with the increase in the cancer survival rate for many patients only a relapse is perceived as a true indication of the gravity of their condition and the threat of death. During this period there is still hope, but "promise" of a cure has been broken and the trust in the medical establishment is shaken. It is often during this stage that the child and family contemplate or seek second opinions. In many there is initial resistance to a renewed and often more drastic chemotherapeutic regimen. It is not uncommon to hear from an adolescent patient, "I'd rather die than lose my hair again." This resistance may be overcome with proper support. In our experience, treatment usually proceeds with the same vigor that accompanied the first induction. One can often observe increased denial, which compensates for the diminished chances for a good outcome.

Disillusionment

If cancer is not arrested at this stage and a new relapse follows, there is a dramatic change: the threat of imminent death and with it the stage of disillusionment. The patient and his parents realize that there is no hope for cure, that death is inevitable, and that it is only a question of time. The oncologist may dramatically lose his importance or become peripheral. This may, in fact, be as much the physician's response to his own feelings of helplessness and impotence as the family's reaction to shattered faith in his powers. Many families opt at this point to have their child die at home. Perhaps they recognize that medicine does not offer a solution and that new treatments are futile. The focus shifts from illness to child. The child, during this period, is usually angry with both parents and physician, feeling, however, dependent on both. He does not display his anger overtly but often turns it against himself. Unless the health care professionals are aware of it and intervene, what can follow is withdrawal, depression, anorexia, and increased dependence on pain-killing medication. The appearance of these symptoms is frequently the time when either the social service or psychiatry is called for assistance.

Abandonment

Many oncologists and other medical specialists are highly vulnerable to the pain of the dying child and the rejection they experience from the disillusioned patient. This might lead to an often unconscious withdrawal from the patient, with the physician becoming less available and less responsive, cutting down the number of visits. These observations are supported by studies that indicate that the number of visits to the patient drops dramatically during the last period of illness. This stage of abandonment is not inevitable but it is nonetheless common. When this stage occurs, the children become acutely aware of the abandonment. Some die within a very short period of time, in an almost predictable fashion—following the conclusion of a hallmark in their life (for example, immediately after a birthdate, an important wedding, or completion of a project). Others become panicked, hypervigilant, and refuse to go to sleep—for fear of not waking up. In our judgment this represents a highly undesirable development and one that can be avoided.

Abandonment often pitches parents into a desperate denial of reality. This is illustrated by a wealthy father of a three-year-old girl with an incurable hepatoma. During a two week interval he traveled with his wife and daughter to a cancer research center in Switzerland, to Lourdes with hope for a miracle, to a faith healing group in the Philippines, and a Laetrile clinic in Jamaica, only to have the child die a week after their return. By and large these actions seem to be attempts to contain this overwhelming anxiety and reverse helplessness into activity.

Requests for experimental drugs are frequent at this stage. Participation in an experimental protocol may in fact restore a relationship with the physician, reengaging him as a resource of hope. Often a physician unable to contend with his own loss of control over the situation responds favorably to this request. We do not regard this interaction as true optimism, since it does not come in the first stage of treatment when a tried protocol is available and a cure possible.

If experimental drugs fail, they may be followed by what can be considered pseudomedical interaction—tests and treatment ordered without sound medical justification, seemingly to give more hope but more often to appease angry, distraught parents. Many physicians resort, at this stage, to communication that, while seemingly scientific, is at best ambiguous. More often than not they are confusing or unintentionally misleading. Some expressions we have noted are "She is sicker than we think"; "There is a modicum of hope"; "Unless we come up with something new" (knowing that there is nothing new to offer). For a patient who has lost bladder and bowel control, "His bowel and urinary controls aren't what they used to be"; "There is no hope but we should continue treatment."

At this stage the child needs an advocate to protect him from his despairing parents who may not be able to face reality and the well-meaning but occasionally overzealous physician. This is particularly important, since the informed consent is given by the parents, and the child has little or no say about his treatment. An ethics committee, such as the one at Memorial Sloan-Kettering Cancer Center in the Department of Pediatrics, can serve as a forum where the hospital staff can obtain guidance and assistance in making decisions that would ensure the best interest of the child.

The stage of abandonment can be avoided altogether when both parents and physicians are capable and willing to confront the realities as they appear during disillusionment, accept the fact that the child is terminal, and help him to die as comfortably as possible. To achieve this the physician has to resort to what are primarily psychotherapeutic tools—namely, understanding of transference and countertransference, insight, empathy, and dispassionate objectivity.

Rapprochement

A successfully negotiated stage of disillusionment can lead directly to rapprochement, bypassing the stage of abandonment.

The child, usually exhausted and physically in acute discomfort, experiences death as a relief from prolonged suffering. Having his parents and his physician appreciate his plight renders a child less afraid of dying—fully aware of their concern and love. There is a joint anticipatory grieving, which reunites and strengthens the family before the final tragedy. Parents who do not go through anticipatory grieving, who do not go through the rapprochement and whose child dies suddenly in the midst of treatment (never having moved beyond abandonment), describe themselves as cheated out of saying goodbye. The relationship lacks closure, intensifying the loss.[9]

Reconciliation

A successfully negotiated rapprochement leads to the last stage, that of reconciliation. It represents, after death, the mutual acknowledgement by parents and physician that all that was possible was attempted. If achieved at the time of the child's death, parents may express their gratitude symbolically. The "thank you" can, for example, take the form of permission for autopsy, as if to say "You have done a good job, we're going to respond by supporting your scientific pursuit of a cure." It may be expressed by an invitation to the funeral, wake, or shiva. Another expression of reconciliation by parents is the creation of a research fund in the name of the deceased child, where control of the fund is given to the physician in charge of their child's treatment. This act epitomizes the optimal end of a difficult relationship—the pursuit of the conquest of cancer is seen as the joint goal of the bereaved parent and the committed physician/scientist.

References

1. Holland, J. C. personal communication, n.d.
2. Kimball, C. *The biopsychosocial approach to the patient.* Baltimore: Williams & Wilkins, 1981.
3. Koocher, G. P., & O'Malley, J. E. *The Damocles syndrome.* New York: McGraw-Hill, 1981.
4. Kübler-Ross, E. *On death and dying.* New York: Macmillan, 1969.

5. Levy, A. M., & Nir, Y. Chronic illness. In J. R. Bemporad (Ed.), *Child development as normality and psychopathology*. New York: Brunner/Mazel, 1980.
6. Miller, J. G. Living systems: Basic concepts. In W. Gray, F. J. Duhl, & N. D. Risso (Eds.), *General systems theory and psychiatry*. Boston: Little, Brown, 1969.
7. Nir, Y. Psychological support for children with soft tissue and bone sarcomas. *National Cancer Institute monograph*, 1981, *56*, 145–148.
8. Nir, Y., & Maslin, H. Psychological adjustment of children with cancer. In J. Goldberg (Ed.), *Psychotherapeutic treatment of cancer patients*. New York: Free Press, 1981.
9. Nir, Y., Pynoos, R. S., & Holland, J. C. Cancer in a parent: The impact of mother and child—A consultation–liaison clinical case conference. *General Hospital Psychiatry*, 1981, *3*, 337–342.
10. Penman, D., Bohna, G., & Holland, J. C. Patient's perception of giving informed consent for investigation chemotherapy. Abstracts AACR, May 1980.
11. von Bertalanffy, L. *General systems theory*. New York: Braziller, 1968.
12. Weisman, A. D. A model for psychosocial phasing in cancer. *General Hospital Psychiatry*, 1979, *79*, 187–195.
13. Weisman, A. D. Understanding the cancer patient: The syndrome of caregiver's plight. *Psychiatry*, 1981, *44*, 161–168.

6

Coping by Children Undergoing Limb Amputation

JUDITH A. RITCHIE

Literature on the child amputee's behavioral responses is relatively sparse, and except for occasional case studies, most papers about children's reactions to amputation are fragmented and incomplete. However, the reviewed literature does reveal some consistent behaviors.

A period of grief and mourning has been observed in children aged 3 to 16 years following limb amputation. They have expressed their feelings by talking about their grief, crying, regression, somatic symptoms, anger, and hostility. Faced with amputation, children lose self-esteem, expect nonacceptance by society, and fear further loss or mutilation. Several authors have described individual children's concerns and fantasies about the appearance of the stump and the appearance, fit, and function of the artificial limb.[1-9] Child amputees also often respond to their situations by using the defense mechanism of denial, which may

JUDITH A. RITCHIE • Associate Professor, Graduate Program of the Dalhousie University School of Nursing, Halifax, Nova Scotia B3H 3J5, Canada.

take the form of anxiety marked by increasing uncom-municativeness.[3,4,10] Reports of the phantom limb phenomenon vary; some authors describe it as transient—coming and going—and some say the phantoms are not painful. On the other hand, many children experience vivid and persistent phantoms.[1,3–6,8,11]

Furthermore, over a 2-year period of involvement in the nursing care of 12 children undergoing limb amputation, I observed that these children stimulated considerable anxiety among surgical and nursing personnel. Both nursing staff and orthopedic surgical residents repeatedly verbalized feelings that I experienced on the afternoon the first child facing amputation was referred to me. I asked myself: "How will she react?; "What should I say?"; "What should I do?"

This is a report of the primary areas of concern and patterns of behavior of the five girls and two boys, aged 9 to 14 years, with whom I was most intensively involved (see Table 1). I knew the children and their parents for periods ranging from 18 hours to 5½ months prior to surgery and gave complete nursing care to each child for from one to seven hours daily throughout their hospitalizations for surgery. Afterward, we maintained contact on an outpatient basis through telephone calls, letters, and clinic and prosthetist visits for periods ranging from three months to two years.

Preoperative Reactions

During the interval between being told about the surgery and going to the operating room the children's behavior varied wide-

Table 1. Study Subjects

Name	Age (yr)	Type of amputation	Reason for amputation
Tony	8¾	Hip disarticulation	Osteogenic sarcoma (femur)
Mary	10	Hip disarticulation	Osteogenic sarcoma (femur)
Michelle	11	Hip disarticulation	Chrondroblastic sarcoma (femur)
Michael	12	Knee disarticulation	Trauma (femoral artery laceration)
Jane	13	Above-knee amputation	Osteogenic sarcoma (tibia)
Kim	13	Above-knee amputation	Osteogenic sarcoma (tibia)
Carole	14	Above-knee amputation	Osteogenic sarcoma (tibia)

ly—from quiet activities and apparent lack of concern with the amputation to generalized grief and active exploration of facts related to the amputee state and anesthesia. However, all the children protested with anger and denial when first they were told an amputation was necessary. For example, Carole screamed hysterically, "No! I don't want my leg off!" Yet most of the children told us they suspected their legs would be amputated. Two highly anxious children blurted out, "Are they gonna cut my leg off?" Three of the children cried for up to half an hour, then spent several hours asking detailed questions about the operation.

The two youngest children—Tony who was not yet nine and Mary who was ten—cried briefly, then refused to discuss the amputation further. Mary, who earlier had been taken to a faith healer by her mother, refused to discuss surgery during the preoperative period, telling us: "I'm going to be healed." Despite staff efforts to encourage her to face the reality of an impending amputation and our suggestions that perhaps her "healing" meant the tumor would not spread to any other area of her body, Mary stood firm. As she was wheeled into the operating room, she said, "It's not so. I will be healed—you'll see!" Except for a limited exploration of feelings and questions about how he would be able to walk and the nature of his artificial limb, Tony spent most of the preoperative period aggressively playing with his toys—his actions were hyperactive and he was unable to complete quiet tasks such as drawing. Tony's parents also had great difficulty accepting the diagnosis and then coping with the amputation.

Anticipation and Concerns

Between being told about the amputation and actually going to surgery, the children's grief responses varied to some extent. Both boys directed their attention toward games or other activities or withdrew into sleep. Mary, the youngest girl, also slept frequently as a withdrawal mechanism. The other girls for the most part interacted quietly with parents, roommates, and staff, or they engaged in making crafts.

When alone with their parents or with me, Michelle, Jane, Kim, and Carole (the older girls) frequently cried. They said they did not want surgery and asked why this had happened to them, expressing anger that it had. I encouraged the children to cry as an outlet for grief, because a child facing limb amputation has a right to feel sad and angry. When the children asked, "Why me?" I said, "No one can answer that question," and assured them nothing they had done had caused the tumor; the reason for such tumors is still unknown.

Except for Mary, all the children expressed concern about the appearance of the stump and expected it to be ugly. The five oldest children frequently questioned us about the exact level of their amputations and were shocked and angry when told. Sometimes, they sought reassurance that the surgeon would not amputate more than he said he would. Anger subsided somewhat after detailed and technical explanations were given. The children said they wanted the artificial limb to be identical to their own leg in appearance and function. They asked repeatedly: "Is the leg soft?"; "What is it made of?"; "Exactly what color is it?"; "Is it exactly the same?"; "Can anybody tell?"; "Does it bend at the knee?"; "Does it have toes?"; "Does it have hair and toenails?" When the appearance of an artificial limb was described to them, they became angry and agitated. We noticed their anger was considerably more marked if the surgeon had told them the prosthesis would look "just like real."

All the children asked what they could do once they had an artificial limb. Could they walk without crutches? Climb trees, swim, dance, and "slide into base" in a baseball game? They wondered if the limb would feel pain or bleed. Some children verbalized fantasies that they would receive a leg transplant, a bionic leg, or an artificial leg that could be sewed on and would stay on all the time.

Fears

The four oldest girls feared how people would react to them as amputees. At times they said they would "never go out" and "never go to school" after their legs had been removed. The girls expected to be objects of staring and ridicule, so I told them their concerns were understandable and other children who faced amputations worried as they did. However, I reminded them that "never is a long time" and they *might* feel differently once they had recovered. One girl's friend helped when she bluntly said, "It won't make no difference. You'll still be Jane."

Other concerns of the children included fear of death during surgery, of wakening during surgery, and of *not* wakening after surgery. However, I found the child amputees I cared for had less fear of anesthesia than children who faced other types of operations. Concerns directly related to the loss of a limb were most dominant. Nevertheless, I discussed each child's fear of anesthesia frankly and assured him I would be in the recovery room to waken him.

Postoperative Reactions

After the operation each child spent time grieving the loss of a limb and identifying the reality of being an amputee. Each attempted to come to grips with the situation of an altered body image. The pattern was one of seeking out information, then preventing herself from receiving too much by withdrawing into denial and refusal to discuss the subject. Such behavior usually decreased after the fifth postoperative day, when adaptive planning and self-care behaviors increased.

All the children were depressed and withdrawn. The girls, however, were more able to express their grief than the boys. Frequently, Mary, Carole, Michelle, Jane, and Kim went through periods of weeping and talking about their amputations. By the third day, the behavior patterns had changed from long periods of sleeping to increased interest and active participation in ward activities. Sporadically, periods of weeping continued throughout hospitalization and during the first two weeks following discharge. Verbal expressions of grief continued during hospitalization, and for as long as I kept in touch with the children—a period of about 2 years.

The children continued to wish their legs would somehow be returned to them and to question, "Why did this have to happen to me?" Some sought information about the disposal of the amputated limb, and they all expressed a desire to escape from the situation—"I just want to go home and be normal." Eventually they acknowledged that the loss of the limb was terrible and difficult but it was their only chance to live. Kim and Jane each wondered aloud if it wouldn't be better to die from the malignancy than to live without a leg.

The boys did not cry as readily but frequently withdrew into sleep. They asked for "sleeping shots" during the day and had difficulty sleeping at night. They made more run and fetch requests of the nurses than did the girls. Tony, Michael, and Mary exhibited dependent behavior and showed outbursts of anger when they were asked to do anything, such as walk or bathe themselves, as the following examples illustrate:

> Tony was unwilling to do any self-care throughout the first ten post operative days. He became angry when asked to help himself and was uncooperative at physiotherapy; frequently he refused to get out of bed. He ordered his mother to feed him when he ate at all. Folding his arms across his chest, he would order her to lift his head and hold the cup for him whenever he wanted to drink. On the eleventh day, his mother decided not to remain in his room to sleep at night; thereafter Tony's behavior improved. He began asking questions about and discussing the amputation, the phantom limb, the artificial limb, and the activities that were possible with and without the limb. These discussions took place with me when his mother left his room and with the nursing staff after his mother left in the evening.

Both Tony and Mary denied vehemently that the loss of their legs disturbed them, saying, "It saved my life, so it's good" or "It was God's will. I'll have my leg back in heaven anyway."

Six of the seven children developed somatic symptoms of fever, nausea and vomiting, and pains of unknown origin. We felt this to be related to their unresolved and unexpressed grief. Symptoms often abated once the child was able to cry and talk about feelings of depression, anger, and fear.

> Jane had been depressed and withdrawn, complaining of phantom pain, when suddenly she developed pain in the remaining leg. She cried hysterically and complained loudly of pain and paralysis in the unaffected limb. Calmly I soothed her, explaining this was probably happening because she was afraid something would happen to her remaining leg and she would not be able to walk at all. I assured her there was nothing wrong with her leg. Jane quickly regained control, the symptoms went away, and she was able to talk openly of her fears.

The two boys and Mary expressed much more pain in their stumps and in the phantom limbs and requested more "pain shots" than the children who were able to vent their grief by crying and talking.

First Reactions

In the beginning, all the children refused to look at their bodies and kept the bedcovers over their lower bodies. When finally they looked at the bandaged or casted stump, saying, "They took so much!" Most of them abhorred the word "stump" and felt, as Kim said, "They should call it a leg. That's what it is or at least what's left of it."

We found the children needed continued support and frequent urging to look at and touch the bandaged or casted stump. They often ordered: "Keep that covered! I don't want to look at it!" Generally, by the third day, however, they were looking at and handling the stump fairly easily. Next, slowly and blatantly they would begin to expose the stump to patients and other visiting parents. But even then it took firm encouragement from the nursing personnel before they would walk in the hall or go to the hospital school. Once they were able to accomplish this, however, the desire to hide themselves disappeared. Upon discharge, all the children walked comfortably on public streets, went shopping, and visited friends.

The Stump

There were fantasies about the stump that centered around the number and location of sutures: The children feared the stump might "bleed all out" or that it was "all just hanging open down there." Many feared the stump was not healing. They expected it would be "ugly," "shriveled up," or "like an old lady's arm—all loose and hanging." Despite efforts to give them realistic descriptions of the stump, when it came time for the initial dressing change, all the children showed high levels of anxiety and were not able to maintain control during the procedure. Many refused to look at the stump when the dressing was removed because this just confirmed the reality of the amputation for them. As the cast was removed, Kim screamed, "But it just ends! It ends right there!" After her initial dressing change, crying, Jane said, "It looks worse than I thought—ugly. It just ends there."

Once the pressure dressing or cast and the sutures were removed, the medical and nursing staff wanted self-care of the stump to begin immediately. However, this was accomplished only gradually. It required a great deal of nursing encouragement and assurance to the children that the stump was well healed, and that to health care personnel it looked good. Repeatedly we reminded all of them that the stump was part of their bodies and it was essential they take proper care of it themselves.

> *Following the biopsy of her tumor, Carole refused to look at her scar. In the intervening six months, she insisted her mother wash the leg; she would not touch it herself. When her cast and sutures were removed, the resident expected Carole to assume responsibility for her own stump care immediately. However, she hysterically refused to even look at the uncovered stump. I talked to her about the importance of caring for the stump, acknowledging that while she did not yet feel ready to do it, she would be able to do so soon. Twenty-four hours later, Carole only weakly protested when it was suggested that a stump-wrapping lesson be held later in the day. When the appointed hour arrived, Carole was very apprehensive and blurted out, "I'm not looking at it!" I reassured Carole about her fear but explained again, "We'll do it slowly, but we'll do it now." Carole nodded her head yes, but said, "But I ain't gonna look at the stitches."*
>
> *As I worked very slowly and shielded the suture line from her sight, Carole said, "OK, I'll just peek." After she had visually examined the anterior aspect of the stump, she agreed to look at the suture line using a mirror. I changed the position of the mirror very slowly until Carole could see the suture line. During all this time I continued to encourage Carole, touching and rubbing her stump, and telling her that it was well-healed and looked good. Quietly, but firmly and repeatedly, I acknowledged that she was frightened but that she absolutely had to look at and touch the stump on that day. At the end of 45 minutes, Carole began examining the stump in detail, first visually, then with her fingertips. She talked freely about it and then had it washed and wrapped. The next day she was using her whole hand in handling the stump. Upon discharge from the hospital unit, two days later, Carole performed all of the stump care by herself.*

The Phantom Limb

Only three of the children were told preoperatively about the possibility of the occurrence of a phantom limb, but all seven experienced the phantom as they recovered from anesthesia. Typical comments were: "It's still there," or "I can feel my leg." They became agitated when they felt the phantom limb, and in the recovery room three of the children insisted they be given a pillow for the amputated leg because they said, "My leg's floating."

The phantom limb experience was vivid and disturbing. We explained that the sensation was normal, expected, and always happened, which relieved the children to some extent. The three who had been prepared said they had not believed the preoperative explanation. All children except Tony eventually accepted the phantom limb as a normal experience and over time discussed it in detail. They talked easily to me about the feelings of anger and frustration that the phantom aroused. Tony was more disturbed than the rest by the phenomenon and would discuss it briefly only when I urged him.

The phantom limb seemed to interfere with the children accepting the fact of their amputations. Following surgery, Kim said, "It really feels like it's still there." Jane told me she fell because "I forgot my leg wasn't there and I tried to walk on it."

When the phantom limb was nonpainful it was described as being "just there": numb, tingling, and itching. All the children experienced sensations of the phantom limb moving—"going through" the bed or wall; the distal portion of the limb was felt most vividly. Most of the children described the toes telescoping to mid calf level within three weeks. Two, whose legs had been amputated at the hip, reported the phantom toes had moved up to the level of the amputation within one month of surgery.

When the phantom was painful it was described as "burning," "jagging," or "like a razor cutting"; this was experienced by all children by the fourth post operative day. Frequently, after they had cried and verbalized their feelings, the phantom spontaneously became less painful. All the children continued to experience a phantom limb even after the pain subsided; with Michael still reporting a painful phantom beyond the fifth postoperative week. He never told any member of his family about the phantom limb, had a large area of slough at the surgical site, and continued to complain of severe phantom pain when discharged to a rehabilitation center three months after surgery.

The Artificial Limb

Most children did not mention the artificial limb within the first few days after surgery, but questions from all the girls were abundant by the end of the first week. Neither boy discussed the artificial limb until the third postoperative week; even then their questions were less frequent and less specific. The children expressed anger at the length of time it took to prepare the artificial limb. The exact appearance and the functional ability of the leg were what interested them most. When they understood the limb would not be "just like real," they were angry and disappointed.

Kim and Carole were provided with an immediate prosthesis and their reactions to the temporary limb were shock and dismay. They considered it ugly and told us to put it away where they could not see it. However, both came to regard the "ugly old pipe leg" as a useful temporary device soon after they found they could walk on it in physiotherapy. Both girls accepted the permanent prosthesis easily.

Kim rejected the temporary limb during the first four postoperative days. She spoke angrily about it and attempted to avoid looking at or touching it. She hid the limb under her bed, and when she wore it to her first physiotherapy session on the fourth day, she put on slacks in order to cover it. She frequently verbally rejected the limb and the idea of walking on it, saying, "I don't want it. I don't want to walk on it. I won't go anywhere. It's just an ugly old pipe."

By the sixth day, Kim no longer wore slacks to cover the limb, saying, "I pull the knee sock up over the pipe and it doesn't look so bad." She first identified the temporary limb as "my pipe" on the sixth day. The limb became more acceptable as she saw it helped her walk again. By the eleventh day, she was handling the limb freely, "It's not so bad. It's not bad at all," she said.

Throughout hospitalization, Kim asked many questions about the permanent artificial limb. She wanted it to be "just like real," with a knee and ankle that were the "exact same as my own leg" and with toes. When she received the permanent limb ten weeks after surgery, she accepted it readily and showed no indication of being reluctant to circulate socially. Indeed, she had accepted a date for the prom, which was to be held two weeks later.

Mary, Michelle, and Tony had not had temporary prostheses and were angry at the appearance of the permanent limbs. However, they accepted it better once they learned to use it fairly well. In contrast, four months later, Jane continued to say she hated the leg.

The children freely explored the nature of their functional capacity with an artificial limb. They discussed whether and in what manner their usual activities and future career options would be altered now that they required a prosthesis. Their questions were answered truthfully, and, in areas where no clear answer was possible, the children were told, "You won't know if you can do it unless you try or until you try to relearn."

Michelle was fitted with a Canadian bucket prosthesis; she asked whether she would be able to ride her bicycle. I told her it might be very difficult to learn, but there was no reason she could not try. Eighteen months later she triumphantly reported that after several months of hard work she had mastered riding her bicycle.

To the children, walking again represented partial restoration of their loss. Spirits markedly improved after their initial visit to physiotherapy, and they became more interested in exploring the realities of the amputee state. All of the children, except Tony (who developed a wound infection early in the postoperative period) participated in their exercise programs with great determination. The girls appeared to have much greater pain tolerance at physiotherapy. Michael, after he developed complications at the surgical site two weeks after surgery, and Tony did not cooperate with the physiotherapy program as satisfactorily. They both frequently refused to do exercises, complained more often of fatigue, and were more easily distracted. Even after their surgical complications cleared up such behavior continued.

The children reacted in a pattern of struggle, attempting to master their grief over the loss of a limb and at the same time beginning to reformulate an image of their body as it was after surgery. They were forced to adjust to a new self-concept. Most importantly, their behavior pattern of grieving occurred at the same time as their effort to obtain realistic information about themselves as amputees. The children quickly learned who could tolerate their explorations of what it would be like to be an amputee and their expressions of grief, anger, and fear related to the amputation and underlying illness. When it happened that their parents, surgeons, or members of the nursing staff could not tolerate such expressions, the children altered their behavior. They would change the subject and not talk about their feelings and worries until they were alone with a staff member who was more tolerant or in some instances discuss it with their parents.

An Approach

I approached nursing all of these children by:

- encouraging their verbal and nonverbal expression of emotions and concerns; particularly by letting them cry and express their anger. At the same time I acknowledged such feelings were reasonable and expected.
- providing factual answers to questions and using verbal explanations, models, pictures, and drawings. In some instances, I was able to arrange for the child to meet another amputee. This was most helpful during the second postoperative week. I believe it would also have been helpful to show the child an actual artifical limb.
- permitting the child to set her own pace for expressing emotions and for seeking out information. This included respecting the child's need to limit such information through periodic use of denial and withdrawal.
- setting firm goals in the child's gradual progression to independence. Each child was expected to do his own care, to participate in ward activities, to go to the hospital school, and to carry out physiotherapy programs as soon as he was physically able. When the child felt unable to do this, I firmly stated what was expected and when.
- establishing that the stump is an acceptable part of the body

by referring to it, touching it, and encouraging the child to care for it. This process began on the day of surgery, when the child and parents were firmly encouraged to look at the bandaged stump as soon as she had recovered from anesthesia.

- reassuring the child that the experience of a phantom limb is a universal phenomenon and it gradually will decrease or disappear over time.
- encouraging exploration of concerns about the future and by helping the child to plan how to respond to social activities and society's reactions.

Because Tony and Michael (and other boys followed during the period) had great difficulty telling me about their feelings and concerns, I wondered if perhaps they saw such expressions to a female as a threat to their masculinity. However, it was found that they were even less able to talk about their feelings with a male child psychiatrist.

Nursing the child undergoing limb amputation is a difficult challenge. But it is an assignment that becomes more manageable once the similar patterns of behavior in each child amputee are recognized. The nursing approaches I have described here were effective with the 12 children I was involved with during the two years I nursed Tony, Mary, Michelle, Kim, Michael, Jane, and Carole and with all the child amputees I have worked with since then.

References

1. Easson, W. M. Body image and self-image in children. Phantom phenomenon in a 3-year-old child. *Archives of General Psychiatry,* 1961, *4*, 619–621.
2. Geist, R. A. Onset of chronic illness in children and adolescents: Psychotherapeutic and consultative intervention. *American Journal of Orthopsychiatry,* 1979, *49*, 4–23.
3. Kikuchi, June. A preadolescent boy's adaptation to the traumatic loss of both hands. *Maternal-Child Nursing Journal,* 1972, *1*, 19–31.
4. Kyllonen, R. R. Body image and reaction to amputation. *Connecticut Medicine,* 1964, *28*, 19–23.
5. Plank, E. N., & Horwood, C. Leg amputation in a 4-year-old child. *Psychoanalytic Study of the Child,* 1961, *16*, 405, 522.
6. Ritchie, J. A. Body image changes following amputation in an adolescent girl. *Maternal-Child Nursing Journal,* 1972, *1*, 136–146.

7. Ritchie, J. A. *Adjustive and affective responses of school-aged children to a leg amputation.* Unpublished doctoral, dissertation, University of Pittsburg, 1975.

8. Ritchie, J. A. Children's adjustive and affective responses in the process of reformulating a body image following limb amputation. *Maternal-Child Nursing Journal,* 1977, *6,* 25–35.

9. Watson, E. J., & Johnson, A. M. The emotional significance of acquired physical disfigurement in children. *American Journal of Orthopsychiatry,* 1958, *28,* 85–97.

10. Spring, J. M., & Epps, C. H. Jr. The juvenile amputee. Some observations and considerations. *Clinical Pediatrics,* 1968, *7,* 76–79.

11. Weinstein, S., & Sersen, E. A. Phantoms in case of congenital absence of limbs. *Neurology,* 1961, *11,* 909–911.

7

How Adolescents Live with Leukemia

DIANNE FOCHTMAN

Adolescence is a time of tremendous change, characterized by conflicting high and low periods as the individual seeks to find his own unique identity, establish his autonomy, and determine his place in the world. The adolescent is no longer a child and not yet an adult. The feelings generated by this unique position in the life cycle create conflicts between the dependency needs of his childhood past and the natural striving for the independence of his adult future.

As the adolescent strives for independence and seeks to establish his identity, he is often inconsistent, uncertain, and rebellious. He vacillates between being childish one minute and grown-up the next, and experiments with many different roles, philosophies, values, standards, and beliefs. Confusion often results from the many internal and external demands on the adolescent, his search for a definition of who he is and what he will become, and also his awakening sexual identity. Rebellion may occur as the adolescent attempts to find ways in which he is differ-

Reprinted in abridged form from *Cancer Nursing*, 1979, *2*, 27–31. Copyright Masson Publishing USA, Inc., New York.

DIANNE FOCHTMAN, • Clinical Specialist in Pediatric Oncology, the Children's Memorial Hospital, Chicago, Illinois 60614.

ent from his parents and society. Rebellion may also reflect his fear of loss of control as he strives for independence.

To receive support in his efforts toward autonomy, the adolescent most often turns to his peers. Peer groups and relationships become an important component of his life. The opinions and attitudes of his peers often become more significant than those of adults. Peer acceptance is important to the adolescent's sense of self-confidence and worth.

In conjunction with peer acceptance and identity problems, the adolescent is also concerned with what he appears to be in the eyes of others. This concern may lead him to regard even minor blemishes as serious defects. If minor blemishes alone can cause feelings of doubt in the adolescent, one can imagine how much more serious are the problems faced by the adolescent with a chronic illness. Such an illness may isolate him from meaningful peer relationships, deprive him of control over himself or his environment, foster dependence and apathy, and impede the transition to responsible, self-actualizing maturity.

However, these outcomes do not inevitably result from chronic, even life-threatening illness in the adolescent. As the following discussion indicates, some teenagers with potentially fatal illness can complete many of the developmental tasks of adolescence, gain a sense of control and mastery over their own lives, and establish their own identity and self-esteem.

Anne was diagnosed with acute monomyelogenous leukemia (AMML) at the age of 13 years. She received chemotherapy and remained in remission for 6 months. After much difficulty, she managed to achieve a second remission which lasted only a few weeks. She then had a progressively downhill course and died at 14 years of age, 13 months after she had been diagnosed.

John was diagnosed with acute lymphocytic leukemia (ALL) at 13 years of age. He remained in his first remission on chemotherapy for 3 years when a relapse occurred. With further chemotherapy he again achieved remission. Several more relapses were also successfully treated. However, the length of remissions shortened, and the drugs used caused increasing nausea and vomiting. Because of this, John chose to discontinue therapy while in remission. He relapsed in 6 months, refused further therapy, and died 2 weeks later at age 17.

The problems and concerns we encountered in working with Anne and John are not unique to these two individuals; they are shared by many adolescents with similar diseases. Because they both could verbalize their feelings and reactions relatively well, they had much to teach the staff about the unique and universal problems of the adolescent living with leukemia. They also helped us to understand the adolescent's ability to cope with a life-threatening illness and some methods by which we can provide support and encouragement to other teenagers.

Helping the teenager to find appropriate methods of coping and adaptation begins at the time of diagnosis. The adolescent demands honest and accurate information and tends to lose trust in the adult who he believes is telling him less than the truth. From the time of diagnosis, both Anne and John were fully informed by compassionate, caring staff about their disease and the planned method of treatment. Anne was aware of the potentially poor prognosis in children with AMML. John's prognosis, on the other hand, was less clear-cut, since many long-term remissions are being achieved in children with ALL. Both teenagers later indicated that this was the time when the development of their trust in staff began. Because their questions were answered honestly in the beginning, with stress on the hopeful aspects of treatment, and some of the more painful facts were not withheld, they felt they could believe and trust the staff in the future.

Both Anne and John were able to cry when they learned about the diagnosis. They were supported in their efforts to accept the disease, the treatment, and the possibility of death. Within a relatively short period of time, they began to focus their attention on the issues of peer acceptance. The entirely different methods employed by these two adolescents illustrate the need for allowing each teenager to approach the problem in a way which seems most comfortable for him.

As these two approaches demonstrate, the adolescent may choose to tell everyone about his disease, only a few close friends, or none of his peers. During her initial hospitalization, Anne wrote letters to several of her close friends describing her illness and her hopes of achieving a long-term remission. She stressed that at times, though she might appear different, she would still really be herself. She asked that her close friends inform others and assist in her acceptance into the larger group when she was able to return. This letter was an inspiration to her peers and to those of us who worked with her. In Anne's case, her basic outgoing personality combined with the support of her friends facilitated her reentry into her peer group.

Such acceptance, however, may not always occur, since adolescents may reject those who appear different. With the strong emphasis in adolescence on conformity to peer group standards, the teenager himself may strive to avoid being different from the others in any way. If he is aware of such differences in himself, he may attempt to conceal this from the others. Often, however, changes in appearance, particularly hair loss, may force the adolescent to devise some explanation for his being "different." The adolescent may still choose not to inform peers of the cause. Attractive wigs are available, particularly for girls. Boys may choose to define their baldness as "a new fad."

John chose not to inform his peers about his disease. The fact that a vacation period covered most of his hospitalization and he did not lose his hair facilitated his concealment. Although we felt that it would have been easier to deal with the problem and receive support if John was open and honest with his friends, we accepted his decision to do otherwise. It was his right to make that decision, and we had to respect it. As John later related, interference with his decision would have caused anger, resentment, and loss of trust. Adolescents like John who choose not to share with their peers need additional support from parents and staff. All teenagers need an atmosphere that encourages them to express their fears and concerns, but this is especially true for the adolescent who is unable to share these feelings with his friends.

All efforts in the realm of peer acceptance must be directed toward preventing withdrawal, rejection, and isolation of the adolescent. Anne and John were encouraged to return to school as soon as possible after the diagnosis had been made. Because of her chemotherapy schedule and the side effects of therapy, Anne was not initially able to consistently attend school for the entire day. However, she was able to attend some classes and thus maintain peer relationships. Social and extracurricular activities are also important. Although she could not play basketball with her team, within a week after her diagnosis Anne enjoyed attending a game and cheering the team on. Because the Christmas vacation period started shortly after he was diagnosed, John missed very little school. He was soon back with his peers in their favorite activity, making and racing go-carts.

In our efforts to support the adolescent, we are often assisted by the strengths which he may possess or develop. One of these strengths is his use of denial. Too often we tend to label denial as maladaptive, when in fact it can be a normal coping mechanism, particularly during periods of remission. Denial can help to reduce anxiety, decrease stress, and conserve energy. Although the adolescent with leukemia faces the possibility of an early death, he does not need to dwell on this eventuality all the time. Both Anne and John asked some questions about death when the initial diagnosis was made, but once remission was achieved those questions stopped. Although their thoughts may at times have turned to death, these instances were probably relatively few during the period of remission. Once relapse has occurred, the intensity of denial tends to decrease, though the adolescent may not yet be able to discuss his own death. If subsequent remissions are easily achieved, the teenager may appropriately continue to use denial in his efforts to cope with day-to-day living.

Individual differences and methods of coping must be respected. After her first relapse, Anne began to discuss her death more frequently. She openly expressed her realistic fears and concerns to her parents, her physician, and several of the nurses. Once she had dealt with a particular problem or reaction to the possibility of dying, she tended to close the subject. Especially on days, or even weeks, when she felt well, she went on with the business of living.

John, on the other hand, did not begin to discuss death very much until he asked to stop therapy because he could not tolerate the side effects (primarily nausea and vomiting) and he knew there was no hope of any prolonged remission. Although he could discuss his impending death with his parents and his physician, he chose to express his fears and concerns primarily to one nurse who had provided him with support throughout the course of his illness. Thus, it can be seen that denial can be one of the strengths of adolescents that enables them to live with leukemia on a day-to-day basis.

Another strength which must be encouraged in the teenager with leukemia is the striving for independence. Achieving emancipation from parents and developing the ability to make decisions about one's life are some of the developmental tasks of the adolescent period. Completion of these tasks is always difficult but becomes even more complicated in the teenager with leukemia. Illness itself may increase dependence. Parents may be fearful of allowing independence and choices for the teenager. Staff, often accustomed to dealing with younger children, may forget the adolescent's need for autonomy and his ability to make decisions about himself and his care. Although for some of these adolescents death will occur before the tasks of emancipation and independence are attained, appropriate steps toward this goal can be achieved with adequate guidance and support.

Knowledge of the disease and treatment can strengthen the adolescent's sense of self-reliance. Parents must be encouraged to allow as much independence as possible, even when the teenager is debilitated by the disease or the side effects of therapy. Although she became physically dependent on her parents in the last few months of her illness, Anne did maintain a degree of control throughout her illness. For example, during her hospitalizations, she chose the sites for intravenous placement and often regulated the electronic intravenous pump when a nurse was not there promptly to do it. She planned and later greatly enjoyed a trip with her mother. She wrote a newspaper article expressing some of her feelings and encouraging other teens with cancer.

John maintained his physical autonomy until the last 2 days of his life. He also had a strong sense of psychological independence which his parents and the staff encouraged. He often came by himself for clinic visits. Although we maintained communication with his parents, he made the majority of decisions about his care himself. His realistic choice to stop therapy was accepted by his parents and staff. Both Anne and John chose to die at home.

Strength in the adolescent can also be found in their care and concern for others. Anne worried about how her parents and her brother would cope with her death. At a time when she needed and wanted her mother, she encouraged her instead to spend time with her brother who also needed his mother's attention. She openly expressed to both her parents her love and concern for them. She also cared about other patients, helped and encouraged many of them, and grieved when some of them died.

John, sensing the grief of those close to him, tried to protect his parents and siblings by seldom discussing his illness or death with them. One of his major concerns as he approached the terminal stage of his disease was an earlier argument with an older brother. He managed to greatly improve this relationship before his death. He, too, was concerned about other patients, and he often became a "big brother" to younger roommates during his hospitalizations.

These strengths of the adolescent must be fostered by the staff throughout the course of his illness. All efforts must be directed toward helping and supporting the adolescent as he attempts to cope with his life and his disease. He cannot cope adequately unless he is able to recognize and acknowledge his own feelings and reactions. The staff can often help him to identify his feelings by discussing some of the reactions expressed by other patients.

In order to truly support the adolescent in his efforts to cope with the changing aspects of his life, one must maintain a consistent level of involvement. Mutual trust and respect must be established early in the course of therapy. The adolescent must be fully informed, and he must feel he has a part in the decisions which must be made about his care. The supportive relationship is greatly fostered when he can share with those he trusts aspects of his life which are not related to his illness. John could talk for hours about his accomplishments in rebuilding cars. Anne liked to write. Listening and responding to such discussions with interest will enable the staff to see the teenager as a person and will help him to establish his individuality.

If the teenager with leukemia becomes terminally ill, this supportive bond becomes particularly important. The continued availability of those he trusts becomes critical. He needs reassurance that the staff will make his death as comfortable as possible. Once he accepts the inevitability of death, his greatest fear often is that the dying process will be painful.

He also needs the opportunity to express some last wishes. Unless the staff openly encourages this, he may not even recognize his right to do so. Anne planned her own funeral, and John chose the spot where he was to be buried.

Termination is often difficult, particularly when one has been emotionally involved with a teenager. In the process of termination one must recognize the needs of the adolescent and of the staff. The teenager may need reassurance that he will not be forgotten. The week before she died, Anne came for an outpatient visit. Knowing what little time she had left and how much the staff loved her, I asked if she wished to say good-bye to them. She asked if I would say the words for her if her voice faltered from crying but that was not necessary. Simply and lovingly, she said a good-bye to each person on the unit. It was difficult for her and for the staff, but it had a great deal of meaning. It terminated in a very special way a loving relationship with a unique individual. It met her needs and ours. Three days later she died at home.

Anne eloquently defined the philosophy which should be adopted by both the teenager and those who interact with him. "I am living with, not dying of, cancer. Nobody knows what the future will be, but if I think of myself as dying, how can I go on living?" Our approach to the adolescent with a life-threatening disease must be, "What are you going to do with the here and now, and how can we support and help you?"

References

1. Giuffra, M. J. Demystifying adolescent behavior. *American Journal of Nursing*, 1975, 75, 1724–1727.
2. Lacasse, C. M. A dying adolescent. *American Journal of Nursing*, 1975, 75, 433–434.
3. Lore, A. Adolescents: People not problems. *American Journal of Nursing*, 1973, 73, 1232–1234.
4. Maier, H. W. *Three decades of child development.* New York: Harper & Row, 1969.

IV

The Crisis of Illness

Cancer among Adults

Most adults envision cancer as a uniquely frightening illness. Cancer is associated with progressive physical debilitation, passive submission to protracted treatment that may involve pain and mutilation, and a capricious course that creates a pervasive sense of uncertainty.[6] Adults who develop cancer must accept the diagnosis and their altered status, deal with the discomfort of physical symptoms and treatment procedures, and cope with the increased dependency and loss of personal dignity that are often entailed in becoming a patient.

Patients' personal accounts highlight the value of active coping strategies in managing the stress of cancer. Ann O'Connell read as much as she could about her disease and obtained a sense of control over it by learning its pathophysiology.[5] The knowledge she acquired countered some of her hopelessness in that she became more optimistic when she discovered that she had a slow-growing tumor. Ann also dealt with her illness actively by using mental imagery to try to strengthen her body's immune system. Another patient, Neil Fiore, systematically acquired information about the precise prognostic indicators of his disease and about the particular treatment recommended by his physician.[2] He also found that mental imagery provided some sense of mastery over the illness and enabled him to fight the cancer actively rather than relying solely on the therapy his doctor advocated. More generally, positive adaptation depends on the characteristics of the disease (such as the extent of spread and need for surgery and adju-

101

vant therapy), the psychological resources of the patient, and the supportiveness of the social context.[3,8]

In the first article, Avery D. Weisman outlines four psychosocial phases that cancer patients may experience during the course of their illness. His aim is to identify high-risk periods and promote appropriate interventions by making typical problems more expectable. The first phase, existential plight, begins with diagnosis and may continue for up to four months. Patients are unusually vulnerable during this phase, and their major concern is whether they will live or die. They may respond to the threat posed by their illness with anxiety, sadness, and temporary denial. But this is also a time of optimism, as patients seek information, share their concerns, and hope for an eventual cure.

Part of the uncertainty patients experience in this phase is due to their worry about the potency of treatment. David Nerenz and his associates suggest that staff can decrease patients' distress by providing them with the information and skills necessary to appraise the state of their health accurately and track the effectiveness of treatment.[4] For example, they recommend that patients be taught to monitor symptoms, such as feelings of pressure or pain from tumors or decreases in the size of lymph nodes. Patients can also be shown their x-rays or lymphangiograms to enable them to see the extent of the cancer and note improvements as treatment progresses. Moreover, graphic presentations of specific cancer sites might dispel patients' visions of wildly growing cancer cells invading their entire body.

In the second phase, patients cope by trying to accommodate to the illness and to mitigate their distress. They return to customary activities and resume the business of normal living. At this time patients must come to grips with the residual effects of the cancer and its treatment, such as decreased energy and morale and loss of body function or disfigurement. Patients adopt a "wait-and-see" attitude to deal with the fact that resurgence of the cancer may necessitate more treatment. Phase three, which begins when there is a recurrence or relapse, marks the end of optimism and the formation of a grimmer outlook. Patients and their families may shy away from additional treatment because they are disenchanted with the physician or are afraid of the agony of another course of therapy.

Eventually, when a cure or reprieve is no longer possible, the patient enters the fourth and final phase, deterioration and decline. At this point, the patient has fewer options and limited time. Acceptance of the inevitable may promote some disengagement and therby mitigate distress. In general, patients cope better with the vicissitudes of cancer when they seek information and confront problems directly, redefine salient issues in solvable terms, flexibly alter their behavior as circumstances permit, and are cooperative but not overly compliant. Patients who are able to communicate their distress and express their anger openly may survive longer than those who cannot.[1]

Remission is one of the few bright spots in the cancer experience. Hope abounds. But remission has its own special problems. One problem is the underlying dread that the cancer has not been totally eliminated and may reappear. In the second article, Judith B. Sanders and Carl G. Kardinal describe some adaptive coping patterns of leukemia patients in remission. Denial proved effective for patients receiving outpatient therapy. These patients had no physical symptoms and thus could try to forget about being ill, maintain their self-image, and resume normal activities. Because the hospital vividly reminded patients of their precarious physical state, returning to the clinic for chemotherapy was hard. One patient avoided facing the reality of his illness by not showing up on scheduled days for treatment.

When patients reentered the hospital for maintenance therapy, they identified with other patients and the camaraderie of the "hospital family." Patients compared treatments, discussed recent cancer research, and speculated about their chances for survival based on the number and length of remissions experienced by their peers. These exchanges helped patients to cope by enabling them to predict their likelihood of recovery, though anxiety about the future surfaced when fellow patients died. In the ensuing process of mourning for their peers, patients were able to grieve for themselves. Mutual support and psychotherapy groups can facilitate anticipatory grieving and provide a "desensitizing experience" in which patients share their fears about death and acquire some mastery of them (see Chapter 28). Such groups also contribute to patients' well-being by teaching them active ways of managing stress and reducing their reliance on indirect and less adaptive coping styles.[7]

The cancer patient must try to maintain a satisfying life while confronting a potential untimely death. The final article is an eloquent personal statement about living with the threat of death. Alice S. Trillin, a victim of lung cancer, reflects on the fear of dying, the way we try to deny our mortality, and most important-ly, how she and other cancer patients come to live with the shadow of death that has been cast over them.

Trillin describes the talismans (coping mechanisms) cancer patients use to gain a sense of control over their fear and ennui. Some patients are sustained by faith in the physician's power to keep them well. Others are calmed and derive a sense of mastery from their physician's explanations about the disease process. The talisman of will plays an important part in helping cancer patients to cope. The author's own will to live was strong. She found hav-ing cancer unacceptable and delighted in hearing about people who refused to succumb to their illness. Trillin also notes how cancer patients put on a "brave act" to convince themselves and people around them that they are well. Cheerfulness, optimism, and tales of successful cures help patients face the uncertain fu-ture. Another way to cope with the threat of death is by being involved in everyday life—people and work. Following a course of chemotherapy, the author relished her ability to concentrate on such mundane activities as the care of her garden peas instead of having to worry about symptoms and how her body was function-ing. Like other cancer patients (see Chapter 28), Trillin speaks of living a richer life because she has confronted death and not been destroyed by it.

References

1. Derogatis, L., Abeloff, M., & Melisaratos, N. Psychological coping mechanisms and survival time in metastatic breast cancer. *Journal of the American Medical Association*, 1979, *242*, 1504–1508.
2. Fiore, N. Fighting cancer—One patient's perspective. *The New England Journal of Medi-cine*, 1979, *300*, 284–289.
3. Holland, J. C., & Mastrovito, R. Psychologic adaptation to breast cancer. *Cancer*, 1980, *46*, 1045–1052.
4. Nerenz, D. R., Leventhal, H., & Love, R. R. Factors contributing to emotional distress during cancer chemotherapy. *Cancer*, 1982, *50*, 1020–1027.
5. O'Connell, A. L. Death sentence: An invitation to life. *American Journal of Nursing*, 1980, *80*, 1646–1649.

6. Silberfarb, P., & Greer, S. Psychological concomitants of cancer: Clinical aspects. *American Journal of Psychotherapy*, 1982, *36*, 470–478.
7. Spiegel, D., Bloom, J., & Yalom, I. Group support for patients with metastatic cancer: A randomized prospective outcome study. *Archives of General Psychiatry*, 1981, *38*, 527–533.
8. Weisman, A. D. *Coping with cancer*. New York: McGraw-Hill, 1979.

8

A Model for Psychosocial Phasing in Cancer

AVERY D. WEISMAN

Few oncology professionals would argue the contention that cancer often creates problems beyond those of the tumor itself. From the patient's viewpoint, the human context of cancer encompasses more than a chronic disease of unknown origin, erratic course, unpredictable treatment, and uncertain outcome. For some patients, treatment offers an immediate solution; that is, they are cured. But for others, the diagnosis and original treatment are only the beginning of what may be an arduous and periodically distressing course that affects other aspects of life.

Psychosocial problems and emotional vulnerability are far from constant, even in the same individual. People vary widely in their capacity to cope with problems, and cancer-related concerns are apt to fluctuate. At times distress is minimal. But at other times, turmoil may put excessive demands on any patient as well as on everyone else involved, including the professionals[1].

As a rule, unless a patient makes inordinate demands, be-

Reprinted in abridged form by permission of the publisher from *General Hospital Psychiatry*, 1979, *1*, 187–195. Copyright 1979 by Elsevier Science Publishing Co., Inc.

AVERY D. WEISMAN • Project Omega and Department of Psychiatry, Massachusetts General Hospital and Harvard Medical School, Boston, Massachusetts 02114.

comes very depressed, anxious, agitated, or obstreperous, or shows other indications of deep emotional trouble, psychologic issues and problems derived from failure to cope effectively are thought to be somewhat peripheral. The main business is managing cancer. Vulnerability and psychosocial effectiveness are not primary considerations nor is episodic emotional distress deemed typical. Nevertheless, it is not uncommon to discover that successful cancer treatment has exacted a price that damages a patient's quality of life and therefore undermines the concept of comprehensive cancer care.[2]

Key questions in understanding psychosocial issues in cancer management and doing something about them are: (a) which patients are most vulnerable or at risk to begin with; (b) when are cancer patients as a group likely to become distressed; and (c) what kinds of problems do cancer patients tend to find most difficult to cope with?

Anatomic and clinical staging, a controversial topic[3] in itself, certainly cannot answer psychosocial questions like these. Physical symptoms can only account in part for emotional distress and concomitant social problems.[4] Psychosocial assessment, therefore, is relatively independent of deciding about anatomic changes and stages, but their measurements are not totally unrelated. The major obstacle to linking psychosocial factors with clinical and anatomic findings is the lack of a conceptualization broad enough to take all three dimensions into account.

The purpose of this paper is to propose a hypothetical model for relating psychosocial events in cancer to their clinical and therapeutic counterparts. As used here, the term "phases" refers to expectable problems and concerns, accompanied by distress, which are closely related to staging, treatment, responsiveness, and progression of cancer itself. This unfinished concept is presented in summary form. If it proves useful to clinicians, then psychosocial phasing will alert physicians and others to those periods and transitions when many cancer patients find it most difficult to cope. As a result, relevant interventions and research efforts can be matched to patients in a specific phase, instead of being unsystematically distributed or grouped only according to somatic criteria.

Background

The hypothesis of expectable psychosocial crises and phases is the outcome of studies about how cancer patients at various stages of illness cope and fail to cope with ramifications and repercussions beyond the disease itself. Although this paper is largely an outline, the data on which the supposition of phasing is founded have been presented in several recent publications.[4-7]

Our first project was designed to compare psychosocial concomitants of terminal cancer patients with patients admitted to the hospital after a suicide attempt or for kidney transplant evaluation. Information was obtained by a multidisciplinary unit comprised of psychiatrists, psychologists, social worker, and nurse clinician. Data from interviews, tests, clinical records, and other observations were brought together using the format of the psychological autopsy, a retrospective synthesis.[8]

It was found that psychosocial factors not only changed a dying patient's quality of life but could even lengthen it.[9] Cancer patients who lived longer than expected also had good relationships with others who supported and sustained them. Patients with fewer significant and supportive others tended to withdraw into seclusion, isolating themselves emotionally and antagonizing the people looking after them. They were dejected, morose, hopeless, and apathetic to the fate that soon overtook them. Those who had "better" deaths interacted with others, seemed less depressed and anxious, and did not openly express a wish to die. Patients who complained a great deal while experiencing turmoil, blame, and anxiety did not survive as well as those who could openly ask for help and receive it.

Although much was learned about the psychology of death and dying, it became obvious that the terminal period is, after all, only the distal segment of life, a brief sample drawn from the mainstream of existence. What were these patients like at the onset of the illness, during early treatment, remission, recurrence, before hope for cure turned into a struggle for existence?

To answer these and still other questions, focus was shifted away from the dying patient in order to investigate how newly diagnosed cancer patients cope with various problems and concerns. The staff now included a psychiatrist, psychologists, and social workers. Using methods and specific criteria for selecting patients (described below), we also found that, although most newly diagnosed patients coped well over the follow-up period, everyone reported current concerns of varying severity. These concerns were not always severe enough to be called "problems," but could, however, be classified into preoccupations with: existence ("Will I live or die?"); health care ("Is this treatment going to cure me?"); delivery of services ("Can I rely on what I'm told? Will someone be available if I need anything more? What will now happen to me?"); work and finances ("If I can't work, how will I support my family or do the things I'm expected to?"); or symptom control ("Am I going to suffer a lot?"). Family concerns were much more prominent than worries about friends, religion, or, at times, personal well-being. Self-regard, a more indefinite idea, was no less a real concern. It referred to problems about autonomy, control over the future, and competence as well as to cosmetic issues. No group of cancer patients was exempt from existential or self-regard concerns.

It was essential to identify types and levels of distress at various intervals. Consequently, an index of vulnerability was developed; this is a scale consisting of 13 variables rated on a 4-point continuum. More recently, this has been expanded for future use into a 16-variable scale of existential vulnerability (Table 1).

Methods and Material

In devising appropriate instruments to evaluate cancer patients, it is necessary to realize that these people are often too sick or disinclined to take part in procedures that ask too much or seem irrelevant to the primary task of getting home again. A semistructured interview was developed which social workers administered at the time of diagnosis and at 4- to 6-week intervals thereafter for about 6 months. The interview was supplemented by special scales and inventories developed for the project. In addition to vulnerability, we principally tried to identify general coping strategies, resolution of current concerns, and prevailing moods.

Table 1. Existential Vulnerability

Annihilation
  Anxiety
    Closed time perspective
    Hopelessness
    Fears and dreads
Alienation
  Depression
    Apathy
    Abandonment
    Repudiation of self or others
Endangerment
  Anger
    Self-rebuke
    Vengeful and truculent
    Helplessness
Denial
  Falsification of facts
    Superoptimism
    Dissociations
    Inflated self-image

Patients were selected on the basis of first diagnosis of cancer. Types of cancer included carcinoma of breast, colon, or lung, malignant melanoma, and Hodgkin's disease. Emotional problems were not a criterion, although about one-third of all patients evaluated fell into a category called "higher emotional distress" (HED), while the remainder belonged to a group called "lower emotional distress" (LED).

Psychosocial Phases

Psychosocial phases are outlined in Table 2, and show variations in vulnerability levels during each phase for HED and LED patients. Vulnerability, especially as indicated by the rubric "existential vulnerability," is a comprehensive enough indicator for comparing changes in distress levels.

In the ensuing descriptions of each phase, only those outstanding characteristics that are consistent with successive expec-

Table 2. Psychosocial Phases of Cancer

Phase I. Existential plight
  Diagnostic impact
  Plight proper
Phase II. Accommodation and mitigation
  Original treatment only
    Responsive (+)
    Resistive (−)
  Follow-up treatment
    Responsive (+)
    Resistive (−)
Phase III. Recurrence and relapse
  Relapse during phase II treatment
    Responsive (+)
    Resistive (−)
  Recurrence after phase II treatment
    Responsive (+)
    Resistive (−)
  Limbo (no active treatment)
Phase IV. Deterioration and decline
  Palliative treatment
  Supportive measures only
  Death watch—Terminality

tations are presented (Table 3). Just as some patients report different physical symptoms, one can hardly expect identical changes in current concerns and vulnerability. Vulnerability tends to be associated with numerous problems, but many LED patients also have problems which they manage well. The typical nondistressed patient reports fewer problems, while the distressed patient has more problems and concerns. Furthermore, the site, stage, type of treatment, socioeconomic status, and a host of other less tangible considerations can also impinge upon overall adaptation and alter adaptation at a particular phase. Some LED patients may, at recurrence, respond with vulnerability increases up to the level of HED patients, while recurrence is not so distressing to others.

The concept of psychosocial phasing does require a few assumptions:

1. Cancer has ramifications and repercussions in aspects of life beyond the physical.

Table 3. Expectations at Successive Psychosocial Phases

	Existential plight	Accommodation and mitigation	Recurrence and relapse	Deterioration and decline
Aims	Cure	Surveillance	Control	Care
Impairment	Transient	Variable	Increased	Nearly total
Quality of life	Same or slight change	Variable	Definite limitation	Drastic revision
Goals	No more disease	No more concerns	Respite and reprieve	Relief
Attitude	Optimistic	Optimistic	Guarded	Pessimistic or resigned
Time perspective	Ambiguous or open	Open	Cautious or restricted	Closed
Denial	Temporary	Mixed	Slight	Seldom
Coping	Active	Active	Mixed	Passive

2. The most effective treatment is usually given first, when a patient is least impaired.*
3. Psychosocial considerations are apt to become increasingly important with the passage of time, especially if the original treatment plan is not effective.
4. No cancer patient can be kept uninformed indefinitely.
5. Treatment is given or withheld only for a good reason, namely, to control spread and to relieve symptoms, and not for social, emotional, or experimental purposes.

Phase I. Existential Plight

The impact of being a cancer patient, with its dire implications, should, theoretically, begin before the definite diagnosis. Some patients even have "preclinical" premonitions about what is wrong. For practical purposes, however, it is appropriate that the phase called "existential plight" begin at the time of initial evaluation by a physician because the diagnosis is dated from that point.

Existential plight may be divided into early impact distress, followed by more protracted plight proper.[10] The latter usually ends during early convalescence when a patient goes home and attempts to resume regular duties. Impact has been compared to an acute fever that subsides quickly, leaving no aftermath. But higher levels of vulnerability may only decrease gradually, so that many weeks are required before a relatively quiescent state is reached. Impact distress is almost synonymous with life and death concerns. Worries about getting and paying for the right treatment or concerns about working again are secondary to the private dread that comes when one realizes his or her mortality.

Plight proper may last as long as 4 months after diagnosis and treatment, but the usual period is shorter. Patients with higher emotional distress are much concerned about the future and less

---

*There are two seeming exceptions. Sometimes, radiation is used in order to shrink a tumor before an operation. In such cases, surgery is the most effective treatment, and radiation is simply preparatory. The other apparent exception is a cancer patient who, for example, has an intestinal obstruction at the time of diagnosis but later returns with an asymptomatic recurrence or metastasis. Despite severe initial symptoms, such a patient is less impaired at diagnosis than one with metastasis, and, in any case, the best treatment is given first.

inclined to be optimistic. Patients living alone as a result of widowhood or divorce show higher vulnerability levels because, in truth, they expect little or no genuine support from others. Evidently, patients who were never married have acquired a self-sufficiency that carries them along. Advanced staging at diagnosis often means more emotional distress, but not necessarily. Other complications, treatment, many symptoms, prolonged disability, unemployment, and family trouble conspire to prolong existential plight proper.

Clinically, existential plight is not often expressed dramatically. More typical is a subdued anxiety, followed by sadness and lack of customary interests. Patients may also deny their plight, but denial tends to be transient, gradually yielding to the realities of treatment and the perception of others.[11] Very few patients are able to deny their diagnosis beyond plight proper.[12] Conversely, existential plight proper is shortened and made less painful by sharing private concerns with others and by being given adequate information that does not pretend to be prophetic.

Phase II. Accommodation and Mitigation

The existential plight may have a ripple effect, causing non-medical problems which are seldom reported to the physician. Obstacles occur and concerns multiply unexpectedly. For example, a patient may feel useless when he or she cannot return to work and resume activities with the same vigor as before. Impaired parenting, householding, sexuality, socializing, intellectual interests, and many other activities that require adequate performance can undermine self-confidence. Patients who do return to work often find that energy, morale, endurance, and capacity to confront everyday decisions are reduced.

Convalescence is typified by one's feeling neither sick nor well. Moreover, patients must adapt to the insistent reminder that cancer might come back or that additional treatment could be required. On the whole, however, most cancer patients who make a good physical recovery do well in other respects, even though in some instances drastic psychosocial changes occur. For example, a man may be cured of bladder cancer but rendered impotent. Patients do become depressed at times during phase II, but it is an unusual person whose depression is as profound as that found among psychiatric outpatients. Cope we must, and, for the most part, the majority does a reasonably good job.

Phase II begins when a patient returns to a routine, regardless of secondary psychosocial concerns. Some patients, of course, are cured; their treatment over, they put the cancer behind them. Others, however, must permanently contend with doubts and reminders, disabilities and revisions in their way of life.

The phrase "accommodation and mitigation" is perhaps the most comprehensive expression available to convey the broad range of adaptive efforts and tactics for alleviating or coming to quiescence and equilibrium with the residual effects of cancer. It is only reasonable to expect patients to differ enormously. Nevertheless, someone who receives only original treatment will almost certainly have a different phase II than another patient who gets supplementary or adjuvant therapy for a protracted period. Side effects of secondary treatment are sometimes feared more than the original surgery, and often with good reason. These patients ask, "How long must I go on like this?" But for other patients, postoperative radiation or chemotherapy is like a promise or guarantee. ("My doctor just wants to make sure that all the cancer's gone.")

Very little is known about psychosocial effects of recovery. "Cured cancer clubs," however, would not exist unless there were a need for information and mutual support. A small group of patients, followed without recurrence for periods of over 6 months, revealed that those who were treated surgically are more confident that cancer has been extirpated than are patients who receive additional therapy. The hiatus can last indefinitely. Still, many patients adopt a "wait and see" strategy as they return to customary activities, resume familiar roles, and go on with the business of living. Nevertheless, phase II, regardless of disability, is a time of comparative quiescence.

Phase III. Recurrence and Relapse

For many, cancer returns either during treatment (relapse) or long after treatment (recurrence). The cancer has only been dormant, not dead. Why cancer undergoes a resurgence is a major medical mystery.[13] As a rule, more treatment is given, but with a grimmer outlook. For a patient, comforting thoughts about an unlimited free period are gone, and reassurance is difficult. Optimism, high morale, and even denial are scarcely possible. But the most alarming challenge to accommodation and mitigation is that, in a sense, earlier treatment has failed.

Phase III is a secondary existential plight, although another remission may seem likely. Pessimism is somewhat justified. Vulnerability levels rise, even among LED patients. Strangely, little psychosocial investigation into this phase has been done, although it may be the most discouraging and difficult period that a patient has to face.[14,15] Later, during deterioration and decline, recovery is not expected; disappointment with earlier treatment is therefore less acute. Under the best of circumstances, at the end of phase III, limbo may still be merely a pause. There are other more moderate expectations besides cure and surveillance; respite, control, and reprieve are bonuses. Patients who were once very recalcitrant and resistant about follow-up become more cooperative; this in itself is a benefit.

Phase IV. Deterioration and Decline

During limbo, patients are inclined to become more passive and compliant, as if realizing that there are fewer options and less time. With the advent of better therapy, however, cancer patients can be expected to have fewer relapses and briefer recurrences before entering another remission. This also means that with greater rescue potential of new treatments, patients who might have died at one time will now live to have additional recurrences and may be in limbo for many years. Even the most optimistic cancer therapists ultimately expect only a gradual decline in deaths, not an abrupt cure for everyone. Hence, the prospect for many patients, regardless of treatment, is a recurrence—or perhaps several—before limbo ends.

Factors that suddenly release a cancer from forces that have restrained its spread are as enigmatic as the reasons why some tumors metastasize earlier than others. Deterioration and decline may be insidious or abrupt; no sharp delineation exists except for the professional opinion that the purpose of further treatment is palliative, not curative. Palliation, however, may call upon all available treatment modalities, because during the first subphase of deterioration and decline, relief and some degree of respite are still possible. Mere symptomatic measures are more typical of the later subphase called preterminality.

Psychosocial problems seem to become more apparent as deterioration progresses, at least in the sense that unfinished business needs to be completed. On the other hand, certain very pressing problems start to recede, as if acceptance of outcome provides a sense of distance which reduces distress. For example, worries about returning to work or resolving chronic family problems are central only when a patient can actually do something about them. Ultimately, physical changes coalesce; impairment of one organ inevitably compromises all. Patients become exhausted, somnolent, somewhat confused, episodically depressed (or at least observers think so), and, of course, very sick.[16] A rapidly declining patient shows a wide range of emotional and communicative responses, from anger and confusion to a more serene acquiescence, mingled with apathy and, on occasion, lucidity and traces of denial. The main task is to help bring about an appropriate death, since some deaths are, no doubt, better than others. Alsop[17] has said that a dying man needs to die, as a sleepy man needs to sleep, and there comes a time when it is wrong as well as useless to resist.

Many people have taken the Kübler-Ross stages[18] of dying quite literally, as if each successive step (denial, anger, bargaining, depression, and acceptance) were immutable. Actually, few clinicians really accept the Kübler-Ross sequence; not only are there too many exceptions, but also the phenomena that accompany the dying process are not that simple. Kastenbaum[19] has cogently and comprehensively discussed various objections to the Kübler-Ross concept. Much more is to be learned about dying than is currently known. If, for example, investigators in other specialties were to study when dying begins, and did not give so much attention to the precise moment when it ends, we might learn how to recognize and relieve expectable, salient physical and psychosocial problems.

Discussion

Significance of Psychosocial Phases

Social, emotional, and personality factors have long been postulated for cancer incidence, as Fox[20] demonstrated in his comprehensive review. The relation between cancer and such a straightforward factor as socioeconomic status, which is well documented[21], has not, however, been incorporated into oncology practice or evaluations. A similar fate applies to practically every other psychosocial observation pertaining to cancer. Therefore, it is virtually impossible to answer pertinent questions such as whether cancer patients from SES I and II really do better than those at the bottom of the socioeconomic scale. How much does it matter if an unemployed father with cancer of the lung is deeply discouraged? Will his plight have an effect on survival? What is the relation of recurrence to diminished morale? Some of these and other questions yet to be formulated might be answerable if psychosocial phasing were to be correlated with cancer diagnosis, treatment, recurrence, and survival. Although it is unlikely that a direct relation exists between emotional problems and vicissitudes of cancer[22], perhaps intervening variables might be revealed.

Distinct differences between early and late psychosocial phases can be recognized (Table 3), which suggests that problems differ from phase to phase. With further investigation, it is reasonable to expect other descriptive variables characterizing phase-specific problems. At this time, as Gilbert and Kagan[23] indicate, there is no recognized staging system that combines treatment responses, prognostic factors, quality of survival, progression of illness, and changes in a patient's social and personal network.

The severity, or even the incidence, of problems, depends to some degree on what is done for, as well as to, a patient. Not everyone is expected to be the same, and psychosocial evaluation and screening require a measure of training and experience. The potential significance for cancer management using psychosocial phasing would become clear if one were merely to surmise when nonmedical problems are most likely to occur. Periods of high problem expectancy would roughly correspond to transitions in the course, as modified by internal and external factors:

1. Emotional impact of diagnosis
2. Early convalescence
3. Impairment of regular activity
4. Episodes of relapse or recurrence
5. Limbo, or extended uncertainty, after treatment ends
6. Progressive decline, deterioration, and the search for relief until death.

In general, patients undergo distress when they surrender remnants of earlier autonomy. The principal aim or purpose in postulating psychosocial phases, therefore, is to identify high-risk periods, to render typical problems more expectable, to compare patients at the same clinical stage but in different psychosocial phases. In a word, we want to do for the ability to cope with cancer what clinicoanatomical staging does for its treatment.[24]

Phase-Specific Problems and Appropriate Interventions

Cancer patients seem to do better emotionally when they confront principal problems, armed with ample information offered by a compassionate physician; they are then able to act appropriately to bring about a resolution.[25] Coping, after all, is what one does, or refrains from doing, in order to bring about relief, reward, quiescence, and equilibrium; and it is a never-ending process. Perception of a problem is followed by preliminary action, then correction, repeated action, redefinition in terms of results, and so on, with successive decisions about further direction, correction, and action.[26] Appropriate interventions, which may be very modest indeed, are more effective when aimed at helping patients with specific problems, using their available resources.

For example, the very impact of diagnosis increases vulnerability. But specific distress can usually be relieved by supplying as much accurate information as a patient can use. For a newly diagnosed patient, the only genuine question is how much truth that patient can deal with in coping with immediate concerns. An optimistic attitude, conveyed compassionately and with candor and consistent with facts as presently known, is to be encouraged.

As one shifts to phase II, plans for surveillance are made. This includes watchfulness, encouragement, interest, and availability in case of emergency or simply to answer a question. Obviously, when no problems exist, no special interventions or timetables are required, because coping proceeds spontaneously. Phase III is difficult for both physician and patient. Regardless of earlier gains, recurrence represents failure. Appropriate interventions must be designed for the specific problems, not the reverse. Kiesler[27] has wisely pointed out the "uniformity myth" in psychotherapy and other interventions, which tends to force problems and concerns into Procrustean categories. Phase IV, decline until death, has been a somewhat trendy topic in recent years. Many people believe that dying patients as a group have been largely neglected, and a vast literature has sprung up around this issue. Fortunately, out of this discussion have come principles that tend to correct misconceptions and improve management of terminal illness.[28]

Physicians are mistaken if they believe that after all treatment has been given, nothing else can be done. They are also mistaken, although not so conspicuously, if they believe that physical treatment is ever enough, or can even take place without an implicit set of psychosocial interventions.

Phase-specific problems are sought in order to be met more effectively. Patients ask for care as well as cure, and when cure is out of the question, appropriate intervention signifying care is a reasonable expectation. A little goes a long way. Prompt intervention for known or expected concerns should help both patients and doctors with emerging difficulties, and may even prevent future complications.

References

1. Holland, J. Psychologic aspects of cancer. In J. Holland & E. Frei (Eds.), *Cancer medicine*. Philadelphia: Lea & Febiger, 1973.
2. Cullen, J., Fox, B., & Ison, R. (Eds.). *Cancer: The behavioral dimensions*. New York: Raven Press, 1976.
3. Day, S. B., Laird, W. P., Stansly, P., Garattini, S., & Lewis, M. G. (Eds.). Cancer invasion and metastasis: Biological mechanisms and therapy. In *Progress in cancer research and therapy* (Vol. 5). New York: Raven Press, 1977.
4. Weisman, A. D., & Worden, J. W. *Coping and vulnerability in cancer patients: A research report*. Cambridge: Shea, 1977.

5. Weisman, A. D., & Worden, J. W. The existential plight in cancer: Significance of the first 100 days. *International Journal of Psychiatry in Medicine,* 1976, *7,* 1–15.
6. Weisman, A. D. Early diagnosis of vulnerability in cancer patients. *American Journal of the Medical Sciences,* 1976, *271,* 187–196.
7. Worden, J. W., & Sobel, H. J. Ego strength and psychosocial adaptation to cancer. *Psychosomatic Medicine,* 1973, *40,* 585–592.
8. Weisman, A. D. *The realization of death: A guide for the psychological autopsy.* New York: Aronson, 1974.
9. Weisman, A. D., & Worden, J. W. Psychosocial analysis of cancer deaths. *Omega,* 1975, *6,* 61–75.
10. Weisman, A. D. *Coping with cancer.* New York: McGraw-Hill, 1979.
11. Weisman, A. D., & Hackett, T. P. Denial as a social act. In S. Levin & R. Kahana (Eds.), *Geriatric psychiatry: Creativity, reminiscing, and dying.* New York: International Universities Press, 1967.
12. Weisman, A. D.. *On dying and denying: A psychiatric study of terminality.* New York: Behavioral Publications, 1972.
13. Staquet, M. (Ed.). *Cancer therapy: Prognostic factors and criteria of response.* New York: Raven Press, 1975.
14. Holland, J. Psychological aspects of oncology. *Medical Clinics of North America,* 1977, *6,* 737–748.
15. Schmale, A. H. Psychological reactions to recurrences, metastases, or disseminated cancer. *International Journal of Radiation Oncology,* 1976, *1,* 515–520.
16. Hinton, J. *Dying.* Baltimore: Penguin Books, 1967.
17. Alsop, S. *Stay of execution: A sort of memoir.* New York: J. B. Lippincott, 1973.
18. Kübler-Ross, E. *On death and dying.* New York: Macmillan, 1969.
19. Kastenbaum, R. *Death, society and human experience.* St. Louis: C. V. Mosby, 1977.
20. Fox, B. Premorbid psychological factors as related to incidence of cancer. *Journal of Behavioral Medicine,* 1978, *1,* 45–133.
21. Linden, G. The influence of social class in the survival of cancer patients. *American Journal of Public Health,* 1969, *59,* 267–274.
22. LeShan, L. *You can fight for your life: Emotional factors in the causation of cancer.* New York: M. Evans, 1977.
23. Gilbert, H. A., & Kagan, A. R. Introduction. *Seminar in oncology,* 1977, *4,* 1–3.
24. Feinstein, A. R. A new staging system for cancer and reappraisal of "early" treatment and "cure" by radical surgery. *New England Journal of Medicine,* 1968, *249,* 747–753.
25. Weisman, A. D. Coping with illness. In T. P. Hackett, & N. H. Cassem (Eds.), *Handbook of general psychiatry.* St. Louis: C. V. Mosby, 1978.
26. Lazarus, R., Averill, J., & Opton, E. The psychology of coping: Issues of research and assessment. In G. Coelho, D. Hamburg, & J. Adams (Eds.), *Coping and adaptation.* New York: Basic Books, 1974.
27. Kiesler, D. Experimental design in psychotherapy research. In A. Bergin & S. Garfield (Eds.), *Handbook of psychotherapy and behavior change.* New York: Wiley, 1971.
28. Garfield, C. (Ed.). *Psychosocial care of the dying patient.* New York: McGraw-Hill, 1978.

9

Adaptive Coping Mechanisms in Adult Acute Leukemia Patients in Remission

JUDITH B. SANDERS and CARL G. KARDINAL

The adult patient with [a] life-threatening disease such as acute leukemia uses coping behaviors or mechanisms that serve the purpose of adjustment to illness and disability. The patient in a drug-induced remission possesses a unique set of circumstances as he adjusts to an altered life-style. Physically, he is asymptomatic; there is no clinical evidence of disease. Emotionally, he must adjust to learning how to deal with the always present underlying fear and anxiety that the disease will recur and become uncontrollable. Socially, he must adjust to a new role and altered life-style.

A person's response to remission is influenced by a number of psychosocial factors. His perception of the disease, of remission, of the threat to his life and former life-style, and his understanding of his treatment determine his repertoire of behavioral

Reprinted from the *Journal of the American Medical Association*, August 29, 1977, *238*, 952–954. Copyright 1977 American Medical Association.

JUDITH B. SANDERS • Director of Nursing, Fulton State Mental Hospital, Fulton, Missouri 65251. **CARL G. KARDINAL** • Department of Internal Medicine, Ellis Fischel State Cancer Hospital, Columbia, Missouri 65201.

123

responses. The manner in which the patient copes or fails to cope with disease may influence the outcome of his illness. For the patient with a life-threatening disease such as leukemia, adaptive coping behaviors serve the purpose of adjustment to illness and disability. Solving problems, gathering information, attempting to readjust life-style, and actively participating in and cooperating with the therapeutic treatment program are examples of adaptive coping mechanisms. Maladaptive coping behaviors are those that limit the patient's adjustment to the illness and environment, such as withdrawal, passive surrender to the illness, excessive dependence on the professional team, and self-destructive behaviors such as alcoholism or suicide.[1] Such maladaptive behaviors may lead to a form of psychological invalidism, hampering the patient's maximal potential to "live" whatever remaining life he may have.

Assessment and management of the patient's coping behavior should be routine parts of medical and nursing practice. Growth-promoting behavior and healthy adaptation can result if the professional identifies and reinforces specific coping behaviors that are adaptive. What are the adaptive coping behaviors of adult leukemia patients in remission? Does he maintain the sick role with all of the obligations and expectations that society has accrued to this role, or can he adopt a reasonable normal life-style?

Methods and Materials

Data were gathered from six adult, acute leukemia patients who were in clinical remission. These patients were asymptomatic at the time of the study. The remission duration ranged from a few weeks to two years at the time of the initial interview. The patients ranged in age from 24 to 62 years; there were four men and two women. All patients were being treated with monthly cycles of maintenance chemotherapy. A nonstructured assessment interview was used to determine the general themes and trends of the adjustment styles.

The interview was designed to determine (1) how the patient perceives or experiences his present condition, (2) how he perceives his present life-style and changes related to the illness, (3) what specific coping patterns he has used in the past, and (4) what his expectations are for the future. He was also asked to state his expectations for his professional caregivers (physicians and nurses), family, and friends. The assessment interviews were administered over a six-month period, usually at one-month intervals, to determine patterns in coping behavior. Additional information was obtained from the nursing assessment and medical history about such factors as life history, current social situation, and environmental factors that affect his ability to cope in an adaptive or maladaptive manner.

Results

One of the primary factors influencing the patient's behavioral response to the disease and remission state is the uncertainty of the outcome, i.e., the prospect of dying. This uncertainty evolves around maintaining the state of remission: "Will the drugs continue to work; will my 'counts' be OK?" How to deal with this underlying fear and anxiety is a prime factor in the patient's behavioral response.

Several adjustment styles to remission were identified as common to all persons in the study. They were (1) denial of being sick, (2) identification with fellow patients to form a "hospital family," and (3) anticipatory grief of one's own losses by participation and involvement in grieving another patient's death.

Denial

This became manifest in several ways. All patients expressed the need to remain in a "well" role during remission even though family members had a tendency to want them to be sick and referred to them in this manner. Activities of family members indicated to the patient that he was "sick," and he received special privileges for this role. The families' behaviors ranged from suggesting that the patient seek another physician to attempting to guide the patient to health fads and quack cures. One patient said that her family treated her like an invalid when she was home, and she had difficulty convincing them she could carry out her activities of daily living independently.

Even though the families' nonverbal behavior indicated an

obligation for the patients to remain sick, all patients indicated that little open, verbal communication occurred at home between family members and themselves about the illness, diagnosis, and outcome. Patient response and denial of illness were best described by one patient who succinctly stated, "When I'm home I feel like I'm well. I don't feel sick and I don't need treatment— I'm over it." Another patient expressed denial in this manner: "Once I leave here [the hospital], it never crosses my mind—no hospital, no sickness, no nothing." Remaining in the work world assured another patient of a well role, and much fear and concern were expressed about staying well enough to be able to work.

The stress of the anticipated return to the hospital for monthly chemotherapy maintenance treatment resulted in efforts to avoid the emotional impact of the reality of the situation and to avoid giving up the denial mechanism. Tiedt[2] cites inappropriate independent behavior as an adjustment mechanism used by patients who perceive themselves as losing control. One patient reacted so strongly to the loss of control over his life during his maintenance therapy that he would delay his return to the hospital for treatment by several days. When questioned about this behavior, his response was, "As long as I'm not in the hospital, I'm not sick." Several patients reported experiencing physical symptoms similar to the side effects of chemotherapy prior to the scheduled return visit.

Identification

The emotional impact of the illness on the patient could not be denied because of the stress each experienced in anticipating the return for the next series of maintenance treatments. Identification, or the process of seeing oneself as similar to or like another, was a mechanism of adaptation that appeared on the patient's return to the hospital for treatment. As the patient returned to the ward for one week each month, group membership appeared to influence adaptation. Once a person became an inpatient, it became necessary to learn role behavior in relation to hospitalization and that particular group membership. One means of adjustment was to adapt to the "hospital family" and benefit from the therapeutic milieu established on the ward.

A patient subculture became apparent, with high status and recognition accrued according to the number of months or years in remission. Much informal discussion among the patients focused on the types of treatment; patients compared and discussed protocols and expressed optimism about ongoing research in the hope that medical science would find a cure or a means to increase the patients' life spans. "I think I've got five years, but if they found something, it would look a lot better." Patients spend much emotional energy in helping new members (patients) cope with a similar situation, i.e., adjust to the need to return for treatment and to the uncertainty of the length of remission.

Survival rates of the group members were discussed in detail, and individual status within the group was achieved by those experiencing the longest remission periods. Members would compare and quote survival periods and numbers of subsequent remissions of other members. These data became a "yardstick" by which patients would measure their own progress and anticipated life span. Group members frequently made observations such as "Patient A has been out of remission twice; you usually don't get a third chance," or "Patient C has been coming here for two years, and his counts are still OK." Patients showed less interest in statistical success rates than personal knowledge of fellow patient survival rates.

When a death occurred among the patient group, the impact was profound. Conventional grief reactions were observed, followed by expression of feelings of insecurity and uncertainty about their futures. At the same time, group members would compare their survival periods with that of the deceased group member.

Anticipatory Grieving

By participation and involvement in grieving other patients' deaths, the group manifested this adaptive mechanism. By mourning the loss of another, a patient may further the work of mourning his own life and losses experienced by the illness, both indirectly and at a level he can tolerate more easily.[3] Greene[4] has termed the process by which the grieved person becomes involved in another's similar loss "proxy mechanisms." Proxy mechanisms appear to be adaptive in anticipatory mourning and serve the purpose of helping the patient maintain some autonomy and control over what appears to be a helpless situation.

Comment

How the patient handles the prospect of dying when he is faced with a potentially fatal long-term illness such as leukemia is influenced by a number of factors. The person's response to his disability is influenced greatly by his perception of the illness and the perceived threat to his life and present life-style. He must come to terms with how to deal with the underlying fear and anxiety of the uncertain outcome. Since the uncertainty of outcome is the paramount factor influencing the patient's behavioral response, coping responses are mainly an effort to reduce fear and anxiety.[2]

Exploratory studies[5] have recently suggested that the behavior of nonterminal patients with life-threatening illness differs substantially from the behavior reported by Kübler-Ross[6] of terminally ill patients. Gullo *et al.*[5] found that these patients resolve their grief and resume their previous life-style but with limitations. This is difficult, at best, for the leukemia patient in remission. In an asymptomatic state he is faced with (1) continuing treatment to maintain the remission, (2) reliving unfinished grief work, which is an unresolved loss that has occurred in his life, and (c) participating in anticipatory grieving for his future.

Three adaptive coping behaviors have been identified that serve the purpose of adjustment to illness and remission. Denial of the illness is adaptive when it permits the maintenance of the self-image and helps the patient minimize the probability that the potential danger will actually materialize.[7] However, the use of denial was not supported by the patient's family, and denial became less effective as the return to the hospital for continued treatment approached. Denial becomes maladaptive when the patient disregards clear-cut evidence of recurrent disease. In these cases denial appeared to be an adaptive temporary mechanism that allowed the person time to work through his loss of a previous role and adapt to a new role adjustment within the family setting.

During a clinical remission of leukemia, is the patient experiencing illness? Does he assume a "sick role"? Parsons[8,9] maintains that being sick constitutes a distinct role in society with certain expectations and responsibilities. In the patients studied, the state of remission provided a discrepancy among role expectations of the hospital staff, the patient, and the family. The patient expressed the desire and attempted to continue or resume normal behavior within the limits of his disability; family members encouraged relinquishing these behaviors for the sick role. The coping behavior of denial served to help the patient maintain some equilibrium within the family structure and to work toward the definition of a new role. Kasl and Cobb[10] view hospitalization as another barrier to the already difficult process of socialization into and out of the sick role. Both adaptive coping mechanisms, identification and anticipatory grieving, must be supported in the hospital environment in an attempt to help the patient adjust to the uncertainty of the disease outcome.

Assessment and management of the patient's coping behavior should be a routine part of medical and nursing practice if psychological invalidism is not to occur and if the patient and family are to obtain the optimum level of adaptation to the illness. Total patient management must include an assessment and evaluation of how the patient experiences his illness and how he copes with it. Ways of identifying and reinforcing specific coping behaviors that are adaptive should be identified by the health team. The patient's total response to remission in acute leukemia may be positively influenced by appropriate intervention based on an assessment of his previous and present patterns of coping. Then the patient can reach his maximal potential to "live" whatever remaining life he may have.

References

1. Lipowski, Z. J. Psychosocial aspects of disease. *Annals of Internal Medicine,* 1969, *71,* 1197–1206.
2. Tiedt, E. The psychodynamic process of the oncological experience. *Nursing Forum,* 1975, *14,* 264–277.

3. Hoffman, I., & Futterman, E. H. Coping with waiting: Psychiatric intervention and study in the waiting room of a pediatric oncology clinic. *Comparative Psychiatry*, 1971, *12*, 67–81.

4. Greene, W. A. Role of a vicarious object in the adaptation to object loss. I. Use of a vicarious object as means of adjustment to separation from a significant person. *Psychosomatic Medicine*, 1968, *20*, 344–350.

5. Gullo, S. V., Cherico, D. J., & Shadirk, R. Suggested stages and response styles in life-threatening illness: A focus on the cancer patient. In A. H. Kutscher, B. Schoenberg, A. C. Carr, D. Peretz, & I. K. Goldberg (Eds.), *Anticipatory grief*. New York: Columbia University Press, 1974.

6. Kübler-Ross, E. *On death and dying*. New York: Macmillan, 1969.

7. Wu, R. Illness behavior. In *Behavior and illness*. Englewood Cliffs, N.J.: Prentice-Hall, 1973.

8. Parsons, T. Illness and the role of the physician: A sociological perspective. *American Journal of Orthopsychiatry*, 1951, *21*, 452–460.

9. Parsons, T. Social structure and dynamic process. The case of modern medical practice. In *The social system*. Glencoe, Ill.: Free Press, 1951.

10. Kasl, S. V., & Cobb, S. Health behavior, illness behavior, and sick-role behavior. *Archives of Environmental Health*, 1966, *12*, 531–541.

10

Of Dragons and Garden Peas
A Cancer Patient Talks to Doctors

ALICE STEWART TRILLIN

When I first realized that I might have cancer, I felt immediately that I had entered a special place, a place I came to call "The Land of the Sick People." The most disconcerting thing, however, was not that I found that place terrifying and unfamiliar, but that I found it so ordinary, so banal. I didn't feel different, didn't feel that my life had radically changed at the moment the word *cancer* became attached to it. The same rules still held. What had changed, however, was other people's perceptions of me. Unconsciously, even with a certain amount of kindness, everyone—with the single rather extraordinary exception of my husband—regarded me as someone who had been altered irrevocably. I don't want to exaggerate my feeling of alienation or to give the impression that it was in any way dramatic. I have no horror stories of the kind I read a few years ago in the *New York Times;* people didn't move their desks away from me at the office or refuse to let

Reprinted by permission of the *New England Journal of Medicine*, 1981, *304*, 699–701.

ALICE STEWART TRILLIN • Formerly a college English teacher and currently an educational consultant for a public television station, Mrs. Trillin had a pulmonary lobectomy for adenocarcinoma of the lung at the age of 38, which was followed by immunotherapy and chemotherapy. She wrote this article four years later. She lives in New York City with her husband and two daughters.

their children play with my children at school because they thought that cancer was catching. My friends are all too sophisticated and too sensitive for that kind of behavior. Their distance from me was marked most of all by their inability to understand the ordinariness, the banality of what was happening to me. They marveled at how well I was "coping with cancer." I had become special, no longer like them. Their genuine concern for what had happened to me and their complete separateness from it expressed exactly what I had felt all my life about anyone I had ever known who had experienced tragedy.

When asked to speak to a group of doctors and medical students about what it was like to be a cancer patient, I worried for a long time about what I should say. It was a perfect opportunity—every patient's fantasy—to complain about doctors' insensitivity, nurses who couldn't draw blood properly, and perhaps even the awful food in hospitals. Or, instead, I could present myself as the good patient, full of uplifting thoughts about how much I had learned from having cancer. But, unlike many people, I had had very good experiences with doctors and hospitals. And the role of the brave patient troubled me, because I was afraid that all the brave things I said might no longer hold if I got sick again. I had to think about this a great deal during the first two years after my operation as I watched my best friend live out my own worst nightmares. She discovered that she had cancer several months after I did. Several months after that, she discovered that it had metastasized; she underwent eight operations during the next year and a half before she died. All my brave talk was tested by her illness as it has not yet been tested by mine.

And so I decided not to talk about the things that separate those of us who have cancer from those who do not. I decided that the only relevant thing for me to talk about was the one thing that we all have most in common. We are all afraid of dying.

Our fear of death makes it essential to maintain a distance between ourselves and anyone who is threatened by death. Denying our connection to the precariousness of others' lives is a way of pretending that we are immortal. We need this deception—it is one of the ways we stay sane—but we also need to be prepared for the times when it doesn't work. For doctors, who confront death when they go to work in the morning as routinely as other people deal with balance sheets and computer printouts, and for me, to whom a chest x-ray or a blood test will never again be a simple, routine procedure, it is particularly important to face the fact of death squarely, to talk about it with one another.

Cancer connects us to one another because having cancer is an embodiment of the existential paradox that we all experience: we feel that we are immortal, yet we know that we will die. To Tolstoy's Ivan Ilyich, the syllogism he had learned as a child, "'Caius is a man, men are mortal, therefore Caius is mortal,' had always seemed . . . correct as applied to Caius but certainly not as applied to himself." Like Ivan Ilyich, we all construct an elaborate set of defense mechanisms to separate ourselves from Caius. To anyone who has had cancer, these defense mechanisms become talismans that we invest with a kind of magic. These talismans are essential to our sanity, and yet they need to be examined.

First of all, we believe in the magic of doctors and medicine. The purpose of a talisman is to give us control over the things we are afraid of. Doctors and patients are accomplices in staging a kind of drama in which we pretend that doctors have the power to keep us well. The very best doctors—and I have had the very best—share their power with their patients and try to give us the information that we need to control our own treatment. Whenever I am threatened by panic, my doctor sits me down and tells me something concrete. He draws a picture of my lung, or my lymph nodes; he explains as well as he can how cancer cells work and what might be happening in my body. Together, we approach my disease intelligently and rationally, as a problem to be solved, an exercise in logic to be worked out. Of course, through knowledge, through medicine, through intelligence, we do have some control. But at best this control is limited, and there is always the danger that the disease I have won't behave rationally and respond to the intelligent argument we have constructed. Cancer cells, more than anything else in nature, are likely to behave irrationally. If we think that doctors and medicine can always protect us, we are in danger of losing faith in doctors and medicine when their magic doesn't work. The physician who fails to keep us well is like an unsuccessful witch doctor; we have to drive him out of the tribe and look for a more powerful kind of magic.

The reverse of this, of course, is that the patient becomes a kind of talisman for the doctor. Doctors defy death by keeping people alive. To a patient, it becomes immediately clear that the best way to please a doctor is to be healthy. If you can't manage that, the next best thing is to be well-behaved. (Sometimes the difference between being healthy and being well-behaved becomes blurred in a hospital, so that it almost seems as if being sick were being badly behaved.) If we get well, we help our doctors succeed; if we are sick, we have failed. Patients often say that their doctors seem angry with them when they don't respond to treatment. I think that this phenomenon is more than patients' paranoia or the result of overdeveloped medical egos. It is the fear of death again. It is necessary for doctors to become a bit angry with patients who are dying, if only as a way of separating themselves from someone in whom they have invested a good bit of time and probably a good bit of caring. We all do this to people who are sick. I can remember being terribly angry with my mother, who was prematurely senile, for a long time. Somehow I needed to think that it was her fault that she was sick, because her illness frightened me so much. I was also angry with my friend who died of cancer. I felt that she had let me down, that perhaps she hadn't fought hard enough. It was important for me to find reasons for her death, to find things that she might have done to cause it, as a way of separating myself from her and as a way of thinking that I would somehow have behaved differently, that I would somehow have been able to stay alive.

So, once we have recognized the limitations of the magic of doctors and medicine, where are we? We have to turn to our own magic, to our ability to "control" our bodies. For people who don't have cancer, this often takes the form of jogging and exotic diets and transcendental meditation. For people who have cancer, it takes the form of conscious development of the will to live. For a long time after I found out that I had cancer, I loved hearing stories about people who had simply decided that they would not be sick. I remember one story about a man who had a lung tumor and a wife with breast cancer and several children to support; he said, "I simply can't afford to be sick." Somehow the tumor went away. I think I suspected that there was a missing part to this story when I heard it, but there was also something that sounded right to me. I knew what he meant. I also found the fact that I had cancer unacceptable; the thought that my children might grow up without me was as ridiculous as the thought that I might forget to make appointments for their dental checkups and polio shots. I simply had to be there. Of course, doctors give a lot of credence to the power of the will over illness, but I have always suspected that the stories in medical books about this power might also have missing parts. My friend who died wanted to live more than anyone I have ever known. The talisman of will didn't work for her.

The need to exert some kind of control over the irrational forces that we imagine are loose in our bodies also results in what I have come to recognize as the "brave act" put on by people who have cancer. We all do it. The blood-count line at Memorial Hospital can be one of the cheeriest places in New York on certain mornings. It was on this line, during my first visit to Memorial, that a young leukemia patient in remission told me, "They treat lung cancer like the common cold around here." (Believe me, that was the cheeriest thing anyone had said to me in months.) While waiting for blood counts, I have heard stories from people with lymphoma who were given up for dead in other hospitals and who are feeling terrific. The atmosphere in that line suggests a gathering of knights who have just slain a bunch of dragons. But there are always people in the line who don't say anything at all, and I always wonder if they have at other times felt the exhilaration felt by those of us who are well. We all know, at least, that the dragons are never quite dead and might at any time be aroused, ready for another fight. But our brave act is important. It is one of the ways we stay alive, and it is the way that we convince those who live in "The Land of the Well People" that we aren't all that different from them.

As much as I rely on the talisman of the will, I know that believing in it too much can lead to another kind of deception. There has been a great deal written (mostly by psychiatrists) about why people get cancer and which personality types are most likely to get it. Susan Sontag has pointed out that this explanation of cancer parallels the explanations for tuberculosis that were popular before the discovery of the tubercle bacillus. But it is reassuring to think that people get cancer because of their personalities, because that implies that we have some control over whether we get it. (On the other hand, if people won't give up smoking to avoid cancer, I don't see how they can be expected to change their personalities on the basis of far less compelling evidence.) The trouble with this explanation of cancer is the trouble with any talisman: it is only useful when its charms are working. If I get sick, does that mean that my will to live isn't strong enough? Is being sick a moral and psychological failure? If I feel successful, as if I had slain a dragon, because I am well, should I feel guilty, as if I have failed, if I get sick?

One of the ways that all of us avoid thinking about death is by concentrating on the details of our daily lives. The work that we do everyday and the people we love—the fabric of our lives—convince us that we are alive and that we will stay alive. William Saroyan said in a recent book, "Why am I writing this book? To save my life, to keep from dying, of course. That is why we get up in the morning." Getting up in the morning seems particularly miraculous after having seriously considered the possibility that these mornings might be limited. A year after I had my lung removed, my doctors asked me what I cared about most. I was about to go to Nova Scotia, where we have a summer home, and where I had not been able to go the previous summer because I was having radiation treatments, and I told him that what was most important to me was garden peas. Not the peas themselves, of course, though they were particularly good that year. What was extraordinary to me after that year was that I could again think that peas were important, that I could concentrate on the details of when to plant them and how much mulch they would need instead of thinking about platelets and white cells. I cherished the privilege of thinking about trivia. Thinking about death can make the details of our lives seem unimportant, and so, paradoxically, they become a burden—too much trouble to think about. This is the real meaning of depression: feeling weighed down by the concrete, unable to make the effort to move objects around, overcome by ennui. It is the fear of death that causes that ennui, because the fear of death ties us too much to the physical. We think too much about our bodies, and our bodies become too concrete—machines not functioning properly.

The other difficulty with the talisman of the moment is that it is often the very preciousness of these moments that makes the thought of death so painful. As my friend got closer to death she became rather removed from those she loved the most. She seemed to have gone to some place where we couldn't reach her—to have died what doctors sometimes call a "premature death." I much preferred to think of her enjoying precious moments. I remembered the almost ritualistic way she had her hair cut and tied in satin ribbons before brain surgery, the funny, somehow joyful afternoon that we spent trying wigs on her newly shaved head. Those moments made it seem as if it wasn't so bad to have cancer. But of course it was bad. It was unspeakably bad, and toward the end she couldn't bear to speak about it or to be too close to the people she didn't want to leave. The strength of my love for my children, my husband, my life, even my garden peas has probably been more important than anything else in keeping me alive. The intensity of this love is also what makes me so terrified of dying.

For many, of course, a response to the existential paradox is religion—Kierkegaard's irrational leap toward faith. It is no coincidence that such a high number of conversions take place in cancer hospitals; there is even a group of Catholic nurses in New York who are referred to by other members of their hospital staff as "the death squad." I don't mean to belittle such conversions or any help that religion can give to anyone. I am at this point in my life simply unqualified to talk about the power of this particular talisman.

In considering some of the talismans we all use to deny death, I don't mean to suggest that these talismans should be abandoned. However, their limits must be acknowledged. Ernest Becker, in *The Denial of Death,* says that "skepticism is a more radical experience, a more manly confrontation of potential meaninglessness than mysticism." The most important thing I know now that I didn't know four years ago is that this "potential meaninglessness" can in fact be confronted. As much as I rely on my talismans—my doctors, my will, my husband, my children, and my garden peas—I know that from time to time I will have to confront what Conrad described as "the horror." I know that we can—all of us—confront that horror and not be destroyed by it, even, to some extent, be enhanced by it. To quote Becker again: "I think that taking life seriously means something such as this: that whatever man does on this planet has to be done in the lived truth of the terror of creation, of the grotesque, of the rumble of panic underneath everything. Otherwise it is false."

It astonishes me that having faced the terror, we continue to live, even to live with a great deal of joy. It is commonplace for people who have cancer—particularly those who feel as well as I do—to talk about how much richer their lives are because they have confronted death. Yes, my life is very rich. I have even begun to understand that wonderful line in *King Lear,* "Ripeness is all." I suppose that becoming ripe means finding out that none of the really important questions have answers. I wish that life had devised a less terrifying, less risky way of making me ripe. But I wasn't given any choice about this.

William Saroyan said recently, "I'm growing old! I'm falling apart! And it's VERY INTERESTING!" I'd be willing to bet that Mr. Saroyan, like me, would much rather be young and all in one piece. But somehow his longing for youth and wholeness doesn't destroy him or stop him from getting up in the morning and writing, as he says, to save his life. We will never kill the dragon. But each morning we confront him. Then we give our children breakfast, perhaps put a bit more mulch on the peas, and hope that we can convince the dragon to stay away for a while longer.

V

The Crisis of Illness
Chronic Conditions

A simple twist of fate, an abnormal gene or a sudden serious accident, may foreshadow a lifetime of coping with the limitations imposed by chronic illness or disability. Among children and adolescents, chronic illness is mainly a family affair. Families face the difficult task of nourishing a normal homelife while coping with time-consuming therapy regimens and the problems of helping the disabled child in activities of daily living, transportation, and medical emergencies (for an overview of this area, see Milunsky[7]). Given these demands, it is not surprising that families of chronically ill children are plagued by physical and emotional fatigue, strained marital relationships, social isolation, and sibling jealousy. When a family lacks adequate economic resources, such problems are much more difficult to solve.[2] Helen Featherstone[5] has written movingly of her own and other families' struggles to cope with these issues. Her book is testimony to the reservoir of adaptive capacity shown by some families when they are tapped by adversity.

Chronically ill persons and their families must come to terms with the disability and all that it entails—loss of function, dependency, stigma, and the chance of increasing infirmity over time. For some, the key to successful coping is the ability to find meaning in misfortune. For example, one 20-year-old man's remarkable adjustment to accidental blindness was due, in part, to his ability to cognitively redefine the situation in positive terms. He noted an advantage to being blind in that appearances would no longer distract him and he could appreciate people for their deeper qualities.[6] Similarly, Maurine Venters[8] found that a successful coping strategy among families of children with cystic fibrosis entailed dwelling on the positive consequences of the illness, such as increased family closeness. Some families managed to preserve an optimistic outlook by comparing their child to those with more serious problems.

In the first article, Denton C. Buchanan and his associates describe the psychological stresses and coping styles of families of children with Duchenne muscular dystrophy. This genetically transmitted sex-linked disease is particularly devastating in that it runs an uncertain course but eventually culminates in increasing disability and death. The impact of the illness touched all aspects of family life. Marital conflict was abetted by such problems as the care and discipline of the sick child, parental fatigue, and interference by extended family members. Roles within the family and career plans changed. Some of the fathers declined job transfers, and some mothers gave up their jobs in order to care for their child. Older sisters accepted maternal responsibility for their ill brothers, whereas healthy brothers often were jealous of the attention lavished on the sick child.

Parents employed a diversity of coping strategies. Denial blunted the painful impact of the diagnosis and gave parents time to adjust to the disturbing reality. This sometimes took the form of magical thinking, as when mothers felt that their child was special and would recover, or that the disease would not progress as rapidly in their child as in other children. At the same time, parents avidly sought information about the illness. Parents sought to attain some control over the unknown course of the illness by protecting their child, but in the process they sometimes isolated the child and fostered his dependence. Parents and children both tried to accept reasonable limits to independence dictated by circumstances, while sustaining the maximum development possible within such limits. Well-adjusted parents openly expressed the anger and frustration they felt. They approached problems on a day-to-day basis, took an active role in directing their child's care outside the home, and obtained some relief by setting aside time for themselves.

Studies of parents of children with neuromuscular disease

and cystic fibrosis have identified other successful coping strategies.[1,8] Some parents deal with the care demands of their child by maintaining daily schedules, delegating tasks to various family members, and encouraging the child's independence in activities of daily living. Because they cannot control the uncertain future, families make short-range plans and often adopt a take-every-day-as-it-comes philosophy. To meet the long-term demands of chronic illness, families must learn to tap outside resources to augment their own. Many families share the burden of the illness by reaching out to friends and relatives and joining support groups for parents of ill children.

Martha Cleveland's article—the second in this section—provides an in-depth view of the changes in family structure and interpersonal relationships that occur as families learn to care for a child with a spinal cord injury. Mothers shouldered the burden of physical and emotional care, while fathers tended to assume tasks traditionally associated with men, such as heavy lifting and remodeling the home to accommodate the child's wheelchair. Siblings helped with household chores, empathized with their injured brother or sister, and downplayed their own problems in order to protect their parents.

There were significant changes in the relationships between parents and the injured child. When the child requested reassurance and support, mothers tended to provide it instead of promoting the child's independence. Their constant involvement with the child left them little time or energy for their husbands, who felt angry and abandoned. Cultural norms of emotional control also made it hard for a father to share his feelings openly, especially with his son. The family power structure was altered in that injured children exerted emotional control by becoming angry or depressed when they did not get their way. But some families experienced increased closeness and reported more open communication between patients and their siblings. The author emphasizes that strengthening the father–child bond can help the family meet the demanding challenge of coping with the disabled child.

Although chronically ill children grow up with their identity intimately linked to illness, adults who become permanently disabled as a result of an accident must forge a new identity and life-style (for a memorable personal account, see Brickner[3]). The final article by Sharon Aadalen and Florence Stroebel-Kahn traces Florence's painful struggle to adjust to quadriplegia. It describes how Florence and her physician husband tried to cope with the overwhelming physical care demands, the traumatic impact of the disability on their marriage, and the gradual depletion of family resources.

Florence, a nurse, was seven months pregnant when a car accident left her a quadriplegic. In the month after the accident, she gave birth prematurely to a baby girl who died within a few days. For the first seven months after the injury Florence struggled just to survive. Her husband acted as a "buffer" between Florence and the hospital and accepted the exhausting responsibility for coordinating her care. Once at home, Florence felt angry and depressed at not being able to be self-sufficient. She attempted to gain control over her helplessness by trying to get her caretakers to run her home as she had prior to the accident. Florence also found it hard to overcome her discomfort when strange caretakers (men in particular) were responsible for her bowel, bladder, and genital care. She slowly learned to establish working relationships with caretakers and to teach them to manage her care.

Florence and her husband tried to work out some of their problems by developing videotapes on sexual adjustment for disabled persons and a procedure manual for caretakers. But the couple were not able to alter their expectations to fit the limitations of the disability. After struggling unsuccessfully to accept the changes in his marital relationship, Florence's husband obtained a divorce and remarried soon after. Florence continued to acquire skills in independent living and to deal with her disability and the breakup of her marriage. Finally, more than five years after the accident, Florence moved into her own apartment with a caretaker and resumed her active involvement in the nursing profession. In conjunction with a coordinated holistic health care program, a strong sense of self-efficacy and the flexible use of varied coping skills helped Florence regain a remarkable measure of autonomy. This process of metamorphosis, or gradual transformation of an individual's identity, foreshadows an effective adjustment to severe physical disability.[4]

References

1. Bregman, A. M. Living with progressive childhood illness: Parental management of neuromuscular disease. *Social Work in Health Care,* 1980, *5,* 387–408.
2. Breslau, N. Family care of disabled children: Effects on siblings and mothers. In L. Rubin, G. Thompson, & R. Bilenker (Eds.), *Comprehensive management of cerebral palsy.* New York: Grune & Stratton, 1983.
3. Brickner, R. *My second twenty years: An unexpected life.* New York: Basic Books, 1976.
4. DeLoach, C., & Greer, B. *Adjustment to severe physical disability: A metamorphosis.* New York: McGraw-Hill, 1981.
5. Featherstone, H. *A difference in the family.* New York: Penguin Books, 1980.
6. Hoehn-Saric, R., Frank, E., Hirst, L. W., & Seltser, C. Single case study: Coping with sudden blindness. *The Journal of Nervous and Mental Disease,* 1981, *169,* 662–665.
7. Milunsky, A. (Ed.). *Coping with crisis and handicap.* New York: Plenum Press, 1981.
8. Venters, M. Familial coping with chronic and severe childhood illness: The case of cystic fibrosis. *Social Science and Medicine,* 1981, *15A,* 289–298.

11

Reactions of Families to Children with Duchenne Muscular Dystrophy

DENTON C. BUCHANAN, CAROLYN J. LaBARBERA,
ROBERT ROELOFS, and WILLIAM OLSON

Duchenne muscular dystrophy (DMD) is a particularly insidious neuromuscular disorder combining many of the psychologic stresses observed separately in other chronic diseases of children. It is a genetic disorder, transmitted as sex-linked recessive traits by a carrier mother to recipient son. Thus, mothers have the potential for guilt reactions, similar to those in the parents of hemophilic children[1] and the reactions to impending death found in the parents of terminally ill leukemic children.[2] Duchenne muscular dystrophy has a slow and arduous course, however, causing the strain of nonfatal chronic illnesses as well as many of the physical incapacities seen in diseases such as cerebral palsy.[3]

Reprinted by permission of the publisher from *General Hospital Psychiatry*, 1979, *1*, 3, 262–269. Copyright 1979 by Elsevier Science Publishing Co., Inc.

DENTON C. BUCHANAN • Director of Psychology, Royal Ottawa Regional Rehabilitation Center, Ottawa, Ontario, Canada K1H 8M2. **CAROLYN J. LaBARBERA** • Department of Psychiatry, Vanderbilt University School of Medicine, Nashville, Tennessee 37203. **ROBERT ROELOFS** • Department of Neurology, University of Minnesota School of Medicine, Minneapolis, Minnesota 55455. **WILLIAM OLSON** • Department of Neurology, University of North Dakota, School of Medicine, Fargo, North Dakota 58102.

Several writers have commented upon various psychologic aspects of the dystrophic child, such as care and management [4,5], intellectual changes[6,7], and personality or emotional reactions.[8,9] We have noted clinically, however, that the emotional strain in the family is a major problem in the total management of DMD; yet this aspect has received little attention from other investigators. The slow progressive chronic illness of one family member places a demand upon all healthy family members to react and adapt. Although the DMD child is the identified patient, the environment in which he lives is characterized by chronic psychologic stress and prolonged grieving, influencing his acceptance of the disease and his behavioral interactions with his siblings, peers, schools, and the medical profession.

This paper presents the results of an assessment of the family's adaptation to their child's DMD. The parents DMD children were interviewed to determine the nature of psychologic distress and coping styles in the families. Based on this information, some recommendations are made to assist in managing their illness.

The Study

Twenty-five DMD families were included in the study. All were attending the dystrophy clinic for medical treatment and were not identified specifically as in need of psychologic assistance. The mothers ranged in age from 24 to 40 years (mean 32.9, median 33), and the DMD patients (all males) ranged in age from 4 to 14 years (mean 7.9, median 8). The socioeconomic level of all families was relatively high. Only 16% (four families) had a head of household with less than a high school education.

An open-ended interview was conducted with 22 mothers, one stepmother, and two fathers of the 25 families. The interview was conducted during routine hospital visits. There was no known acute stress (other than the illness) within the families that would influence their perceptions or responses. The interview of approximately 1 hour was private and confidential. Informed consent forms were signed.

Findings

Major Identified Problem

Early in each interview the parents (essentially mothers) were asked to identify what they experienced as the major problem of DMD. Nineteen of the 25 families (76%) identified some psychologic problem. Only four of the families (16%) identified physical issues such as lifting, carrying, or turning as their primary difficulty. Two of the families could not identify any specific problem.

The most prominent psychologic issue was the parent's anticipation of some future stressor; for example, the unpredictability of the disease course was of concern. How long would the child be able to be in school or be able to walk; when would he be bedridden? Although it was implied, no parent mentioned death as a major concern. They did express the dread of having to explain DMD to their sons. Other mothers identified jealousy between normal brothers and the patient as causing significant distress. The reaction of the parents' friends and relatives toward the patient was thought to be one of pity by some mothers. Two mothers identified their own guilt about the genetic aspects as their major problem. One of these said she devoted her entire existence to her son, while the other spoke of her "gift to the generations." Only one of the 25 parents identified an emotional reaction of the patient as the major problem; she described her son's loneliness and depression as the chief concern. Similarly, only one mother described marital stress as a primary difficulty.

Parents revealed other attitudes toward DMD when asked what advice they would give other potential carriers. Twenty-one of the 25 parents (84%) would recommend to these mothers that they not have children. Two of the 21 mothers made an exception in their recommendation for their own daughters; both saw their daughters as "special cases," having been tested for creatine phosphokinase levels and found to be normal.

Except for the one stepmother, all mothers were using some form of birth control, and two had had abortions. Although no family expressed regrets that they had their son, they believed the child's disorder was unfair to both the patient and his family.

Family History

Walton and Gardner-Medwin[10] estimate that one-third of DMD children have a previous family history, one-third are new mutants, and one-third are born to unwitting and often mutant carriers. Our findings agree with these figures. Sixteen of our 25 families (64%) had no known family history, and seven families (28%) had a known history. We could not determine the presence or absence of a disease history in two families where the mothers had left.

Parental Reactions to the Diagnosis

The family history was the most significant variable influencing the reaction of the parents to the diagnosis of DMD. The parents who knew of a history described their reaction to the diagnosis as "suspected," "I knew what to expect from the way he walked," "not surprised," "I was tense during the pregnancy," and "I knew the day he was born!" These parents had had the opportunity to anticipate the diagnosis and thereby reduce the psychologic impact.

The families with no prior warning of or experience with the disease described their reactions in more dramatic terms, such as "shocked," "stunned," "refused to believe it," "numb," "crushed," and "I couldn't even cry." Five of these mothers needed sedatives for the first few months, and one sought psychotherapy. One father had a coronary occlusion within 2 months of diagnosis, while another father had a brief psychiatric hospitalization. One mother attempted suicide, and two mothers abandoned the family.

The families without a history invested considerable effort in tracing their family line through grandparents, great aunts, cousins, and various offspring. All 16 families reported they could determine the absence of DMD for at least three generations. Four families had gathered information for four generations, and one had gone back six generations. This effort demonstrates the profound impact of the diagnosis upon the entire family network and the frantic search for its source.

Marital Relationships

Marital conflict reportedly has been high in the families of children with other handicaps, e.g., cerebral palsy[11], mental retardation[12], and cystic fibrosis.[13] Muscular dystrophy also seems to fall into this category. Combining the incidence of divorced and severely strained marriages, approximately 50% of our sample had marital conflict.

Of the 22 existing marriages (including three remarried), six (27%) were experiencing a strain significant enough to threaten the union. The primary difficulties in these marriages seemed to relate to DMD. Arguments focused upon caring for the child, discipline, constant fatigue from the labor involved, and interference from the extended family. One mother had experienced her own parents' divorce over her DMD brother and now had constant apprehension that her own husband would leave. To cope, she threatened to be the one to leave if he should ever give the slightest indication of anger or blame. Another couple with a strained marriage devoted their lives to their two DMD sons, yet constantly fought. They had never been away from their sons in six years.

Divorce had occurred in an additional six of the 25 families (24%). Of the six divorces, three seemed to relate primarily to the presence of DMD. One mother deserted the family upon learning the diagnosis, leaving a startled and confused father to care for the young child. A second mother left the family within a year. The third divorce occurred after some months of argument in which the husband used the genetic aspects of DMD as a weapon against his wife.

On the other hand, four of the families believed that their marriage was stronger as a result of having a DMD child. They believed that the stress united them with a common purpose and function to care for the child. The remaining 12 married couples (54%) seemed to have a reasonably stable marital relationship that had not altered markedly as the result of having a DMD child.

Even in the strongest marriages, other problems existed within the family. Interview data suggested that fathers experienced a crushing blow to their expectations of their son. They had looked forward to observing their son's development and progress in athletic events and, in general, to being a companion. These ordinarily expectable father–son activities had to be sublimated into passive activities such as playing cards or working puzzles.

Some parents changed their usual roles, with fathers taking a more active part in homemaking. At least two of the families made alterations in their career plans. The fathers jeopardized future promotions by refusing job transfers that would necessitate leaving their son's treatment center. Mothers had to quit their jobs or end their plans to reenter the work force because of the care needed by their son.

The increased daily chores, duties, and responsibilities of caring for their child produced a cumulative effect upon the families. As the DMD progressed, demands upon the parents also increased. Practical problems such as transportation, increased physical labor in lifting, the increase in medical attention, and the tremendous financial burden upon the family were all observed to some degree. The presence of a DMD child placed a perpetual restriction on the family's freedom and activities. None of these families was as socially active as one would have expected under normal circumstances.

Coping Mechanisms

The chronic stress of this progressive debilitating disease led the parents to utilize many coping mechanisms. The most common defense maneuver was some form of denial. Usually early in the adjustment process, parents refused to believe the diagnosis and sought other opinions. Several mothers demonstrated isolation of affect as a form of denial. They were unable to admit any emotional reaction whatever to DMD but could easily discuss the factual material.

Magical thinking was also encountered. Three of the mothers believed their son was different from other DMD children and did not show the same symptoms. They were convinced that his disease would not progress as quickly or that he could recover completely. Early in the adjustment process, denial was an effective way to reduce the impact and, as time progressed, the parents were better able to face the diagnosis.

Thirteen of the 25 families (52%) exhibited overprotection of the child. Their sense of guilt and total helplessness in eliminating the disease resulted in efforts to exert control over the situation in ways that seemed excessive and frequently maladaptive.

The most common form of overprotection socially isolated the child. Neighborhood children were refused permission to play with the patient because they were "too rough." Some patients were removed from the public school system and placed in private schools that would hopefully "understand" the unique problems of the child. Some parents tended to go to excessive lengths to buy items that would keep the children occupied at home. For example, one family built a swimming pool for entertainment and exercise despite financial strain.

Overprotection was also manifest in a conscious lack of discipline, with the underlying implication that the child had suffered enough. Nine families intentionally avoided any form of spanking or withdrawal of privileges.

Parents were finicky about baby-sitters, with establishment of stringent requirements and a basic distrust of the competence of anyone who had not had extensive experience with DMD. This attitude applied not only to bedridden patients but also to ambulatory patients or those with only minimal impairments. Two of the mothers slept in the same bedroom as the child to be available if needed.

Reactions of Siblings

Five of the 25 families (20%) either had no other children or the sibling was still an infant. Eight of the remaining 20 families (40%) stated they could not identify any particular emotional impact upon the well siblings. Two of these eight families, however, had not yet told the other children about the presence of DMD, although one five-year-old sister inquired about the reasons for her brother's hospitalization and asked numerous questions concerning death. The other mother stated quite candidly that she was afraid to tell her older daughter (age 9) because she anticipated a great emotional upheaval and was attempting to avoid that additional trauma in the family. It is therefore estimated, based upon mothers' opinions, that in 12 of the 20 families (60%)

(or 14 families, 70% if the two above are included), siblings experienced some degree of emotional distress.

There was a tendency for older sisters to adopt a maternal role and to overprotect their ill brother; this was observed in eight of the ten families with older sisters. One older sister, living in a poor family, quit school in order to stay home to take care of her brother. Sisters tended to spoil their brothers and to be very defensive in response to the actions and attitudes of people outside the family toward the patient but showed their own ambivalence through occasional arguments and physical fights with the patient. The patients played with their sisters more than with their brothers, perhaps encouraged by the parents to avoid the rough-and-tumble play between boys. Mothers described the patient–sister interaction in terms of quieter games and less physically strenuous activities.

Competition between brothers posed a major problem in most families with a normal son. Parents were placed in the awkward position of either restricting the activity of the well brother in order to reduce the discrepancy between him and the patient, or tolerating the frustration and anger felt by the patient in not being able to keep up with his sibling. In three families, the brothers clearly were jealous of the attention given to the patient and tended to provoke arguments and fights. One brother claimed that the patient was faking and refused to believe that the illness was real. Another older brother expressed pity for his brother to his parents but was cold and aloof with the patient. One older brother would not talk about the disease, changing the subject whenever it came up; he became a severe discipline problem in school and required the assistance of a psychiatrist. He seemed both jealous of the attention his brother received and guilty that he himself was well.

Our findings emphasize the need to attend to the well siblings' reactions to the child's illness. Parents often were so engrossed in the patient's difficulties that they missed the more subtle emotional concerns of their other children. In particular, the sisters of the patients were, by implication, identified as "deformed," resulting in a variety of emotional reactions. Parents should be made aware of this possibility. On the other hand, there is potential for misdiagnosing siblings' reactions and behaviors as attributable to an emotional reaction to DMD. For example, one of the patients had an older brother with a perceptual disability that caused learning difficulties and behavioral problems in school. Both the parents and the pediatrician assumed the difficulties were related to jealousy over the patient and failed to take proper diagnostic steps for the brother.

Patients' Responses

Parents were asked for their perception of the patient's response to his disease. Six of the 25 children (24%) had not been told they had DMD. Physicians' evaluations and other factors, however, continually drew attention to their muscular weakness. They were aware they were "different" from their peers, with a sense that the weakness was something within their control, that is, the result of their own incompetence. One 13-year-old, who had not had his disease explained, visited an uncle with DMD who was immobilized in a wheelchair. He asked his parents repeatedly about his uncle's deficit in relation to his own weakness. Three other children exhibited behavioral difficulties and discipline problems in school, presumably in response to their frustration.

The other 19 children had been told some of the details regarding their disability. The usual explanation was that they had "weak muscles." Only one child, age 14, knew he had a terminal illness and tended to be withdrawn and depressed. He tried his best to philosophize but in general was moody and irritable. He carried a cartoon of an elderly patient sitting in a wheelchair, wheeling himself with one hand and shaking a cane in front of him the other, chasing a short-skirted, attractive nurse. The caption read, "I am *not* a dirty old man, I am a sexy senior citizen." This cartoon seemed to symbolize all the psychologic distress this patient was feeling: frustration over the lack of sexual expression; impending death; lack of attractiveness; physical immobility; and the perception of a critical, negative attitude toward him.

Some parents allowed the children to believe that they would get better in the future. Most of these children exhibited sporadic behavioral problems, likely in response to the frustration of not having their hopes for improvement realized. They were generally disruptive, expressing their anger in school and at home by impulsive outbursts. One child set fire to the bathroom of his home apparently after difficulty in transferring from his wheelchair to the commode. Another child developed a conversion reaction paralysis when school was to begin in the fall, necessitating a homebound teacher. In the spring, he was able to get out of bed and go outside during the warm weather.

Support Systems

The chronic stress of living with a patient who has a progressively deteriorating disease often motivates families to seek emotional support from groups and institutions around them. Two major support systems were identified by the families in our sample.

The Extended Family.   In general, the extended family was helpful and assisted the parents in coping, but difficulties occurred primarily with parents and sisters of the patient's mother. Some relatives tended to spoil the patient and to undermine normal discipline. Out of apparent anger and anxiety toward the disease one patient's maternal grandfather told his daughter, "It's the end of the line for my family." Other grandparents denied the issue entirely, stating, "It won't happen," but heaped attention and gifts on the patient.

In at least two families the paternal grandparents were excessively intrusive. They tended to arouse considerable guilt by continually asking whether the father and mother were doing everything they could and urging them to go elsewhere for another opinion. One family had moved to another state to avoid the intrusion of the grandparents. In another family, the grandparents had not been told of the disease, although the diagnosis had been known for 6 months. This case in particular demonstrates the difficulties that the parents had in interacting with their own parents and siblings. It seemed that, early in the adjustment process, while the parents were working through their own reactions, an additional emotional upheaval in their family was too much for them to bear.

Sisters of the mothers had a unique problem in interacting because of the implication that they, too, might have the genetic disorder. One sister was pregnant at the time of diagnosis and required sedation upon hearing the news.

Schools. The school system influences both the patient and his family. Despite the ideal opportunity for this social setting to provide support, all 18 children in school were having problems obtaining a normal education as a result of their DMD. Ten of these children (56%) were in private schools or special education classes, although one private school refused to allow the patient to continue when they learned he had muscular dystrophy.

Children often were placed in special education classes to avoid obvious physical competition with normal boys and to allay parent's fear that their children were being abused in public school. Although special settings offered more individual attention, mothers complained that the curriculum was oriented toward play, not academics, and believed their son's education was deficient.

Two patients lived in rural areas offering only special classrooms for the mentally retarded and cerebral palsied and the school system believed these were inappropriate for DMD patients. Unfortunately, the use of homebound teachers for these boys contributed to their social isolation.

The eight children in public schools and regular classrooms (44%) manifested behavior and discipline problems. Mothers thought that competition with normal boys was the major difficulty. They also believed that some teachers did not understand their children and tended to spoil them, refusing to discipline them and excusing their behavior because of the illness or expecting more from them than they could physically perform.

Recommendations for Patient Management

Several observations can be made about these 25 families to assist in the management of the patient's and the family's well-being.

The most well-adjusted families seemed to have four points in common: (a) open and frank communication between the mother and father; (b) an orientation toward present activities and accomplishments; (c) an organized and routine form of recreation for the parents; and (d) some form of supportive institution outside of the nuclear family.

Anger and frustration were common to all parents, but the better adjusted parents felt free to express their feelings to one another and felt reciprocal support. Some parents said their physicians encouraged expression of feelings by explaining that these were normal emotions and not an indication of psychologic weakness. Such counsel diminished the tendency toward isolation engendered by inherent guilt feelings. Similarly, it was helpful for parents to communicate the child's capabilities and parental discipline patterns to the extended family and the school system. Families with problems seemed to avoid taking an active role in directing the child's care outside the home.

Dealing with the difficulties of muscular dystrophy on a day-to-day basis was an important strategy in the strongest couples. They avoided dwelling on past events and their child's past accomplishments. They also avoided fantasies about the future. Focusing on the past or the future typically brought about feelings of gloom, hopelessness, and helplessness that interfered with daily adjustment.

The better adjusted parents scheduled a day or an evening for themselves away from the patient, usually once a week. Some of these parents at first felt guilty and were reluctant to experience even brief separations. The encouragement of their physician helped them to seek recreation, which soon became an expected and accepted routine.

Some form of support outside of the primary family such as religion, medical staff, community agencies, extended family, or neighbors was beneficial. Parents felt they had someone close at hand upon whom they could rely if needed. It seemed that the mere knowledge of the presence of support was reassuring and anxiety reducing, unless the supportive individual or group became overly solicitous and intrusive in family affairs.

The treatment staff was not always perceived by families as supportive, although they were frequently turned to for this purpose. Yet, [there were] reported negative feelings toward the staff, ranging from outright anger and hostility to belief that the staff was disinterested and aloof. This negative reaction was particularly noted in families that had no previously known history of DMD. Presumably, during the stage of initial shock to the diagnosis, parents misinterpreted or perhaps did not hear the offer of support.

Education and information are an important form of support. A common complaint from parents was that they were inadequately educated about DMD. The time of diagnosis was a period of high stress, probably making it difficult to perceive information correctly. Some mothers complained they were told too much too soon; information overload was as frightening as no information. Parents appreciated receiving information repeatedly or the gradual presentation of partial information over periods of time. Parents also benefited from being directed to appropriate sources of information such as the local muscular dystrophy association.

The quest for knowledge was a common activity among our parents. Information seeking is a normal psychologic defense in anxious individuals and can be turned to both the parents' and treatment staff's advantage. Public libraries, home encyclopedias, and neighborhood gossip could nonetheless be sources of information as well as misinformation. Well-meaning but uninformed friends often did much harm in providing inaccurate folklore. Anxiety and fear raised by misinformation were a burdensome addition to the existing psychologic trauma.

Parents also turned to treatment staff for advice during the early school years, a time of major trauma for the DMD child. School presented more social peer contact than the child had ever had, presenting him with peer differences and self-perceived inadequacies.

The DMD children in our sample seemed to adjust better in special education classes or private schools than in public schools and normal classrooms, perhaps a function of the age of children in our sample. Nineteen of the children were in grades kindergarten through four and were mildly to moderately impaired. Older children with obvious muscular weakness may not receive the same challenge to compete, since the visual stimulus of orthopedic aids, such as braces, crutches, or wheelchairs, communicate ground rules for play to their peers. The patients in our sample were primarily without orthopedic aids, yet they were impaired enough to find the comparison and competition stressful.

Parents also requested staff assistance in telling the child about his disease. Understandably, parents were apprehensive about discussing the illness with their children. It seemed that the children with emotional and/or behavior difficulties, however, were those without information about their disease or who had partial truths. Without clear understanding of the presence of a disease, children blamed themselves for their incompetence and attempted to prove themselves physically through aggressive acts. The results of this study suggest that the patient can benefit from information about his condition and an explanation that the weakness is beyond their control.

References

1. Mattsson, A., & Gross, S. Adaptational and defensive behavior in young hemophiliacs and their parents. *American Journal of Psychiatry*, 1966, *122*, 1349–1356.
2. Friedman, S. B. Care of the family of the child with cancer. *Pediatrics*, 1967, *40*, 498–507.
3. McMichael, J. K. *Handicap: A study of physically handicapped children and their families.* Pittsburgh: University of Pittsburgh Press, 1971.
4. Green, M. Care of the child with a long-term, life-threatening illness: Some principles of management. *Pediatrics*, 1967, *39*, 441–445.
5. Taft, L. T. The care and management of the child with muscular dystrophy. *Developmental Medicine and Child Neurology*, 1973, *15*, 510–518.
6. Cohen, H. J., Molnar, G. E., & Taft, L. T. The genetic relationship of progressive muscular dystrophy (Duchenne type) and mental retardation. *Developmental Medicine and Child Neurology*, 1968, *10*, 754–765.
7. Robinow, M. Mental retardation in Duchenne muscular dystrophy: Its relation to the maternal carrier state. *Pediatrics*, 1976, *88*, 896–897.
8. Morrow, R. S., & Cohen, J. The psychosocial factors in muscular dystrophy. *Child Psychiatry*, 1954, *3*, 70–80.
9. Schoelly, M. L., & Fraser, A. W. Emotional reactions in muscular dystrophy. *American Journal of Physical Medicine*, 1955, *34*, 119–123.
10. Walton, J. N., & Gardner-Medwin, D. Progressive muscular dystrophy and the myotonic disorders. In J. N. Walton (Ed.), *Disorders of voluntary muscles.* London: Churchill-Livingstone, 1974.
11. Boles, G. Personality factors in mothers of cerebral palsied children. *Genetic Psychological Monographs*, 1959, *59*, 159–218.
12. Farber, B. Effects of a severely mentally retarded child on family integration. *Monographs of the Society for Research in Child Development*, 1959, *24*(2).
13. Patterson, P. R. Psychosocial aspects of cystic fibrosis. In P. R. Patterson, C. R. Denning, & A. H. Kutscher (Eds.), *Psychosocial aspects of cystic fibrosis.* New York: Columbia University Press, 1973.

12

Family Adaptation to Traumatic Spinal Cord Injury
Response to Crisis

MARTHA CLEVELAND

An important effect of the application of systems theory to families is the increasing interest of both family academicians and practitioners in the response of the family unit to crisis situations. To date, family stress and adaptation literature seems to have been focused on families' response to traumatic natural and/or social disaster such as economic depression or war.[1] Families suffering from these kinds of stressors share their trauma with many other families, their circumstance is socially common rather than socially isolated, and they receive much social support. Other than Farber's[2] work on families of retarded children, little systematic research attention has been directed toward families suffering from traumatic events which occur randomly to individual families. These families are socially isolated and receive little social support. The research described in this article focuses on a so-

MARTHA CLEVELAND • Licensed Consulting Psychologist, 6185 Apple Road, Excelsior, Minnesota 55331.

cially isolated crisis, that is, the traumatic physical disablement of a family member.

In terms of family reaction to a stressor event, traumatic spinal cord injury to a son or daughter can be considered to produce a severe crisis. It meets Hill's definition of crisis as a "sharp or decisive change for which old, or ongoing, roles are inadequate" as well as Burr's "situation in which a change has brought about disruption in the family system".[3] By Hill's criteria this stressor yields a high potential for family vulnerability: All families define the event as producing an extreme crisis; it is very difficult to externalize blame for the stressor; the family has not time to anticipate the change; there are no norms allowing for anticipatory socialization; the crisis producing stressor is permanent; and there are, in general, no collective support groups with which the family may identify or become involved.[4] In addition to fulfilling the criteria for a high degree of family vulnerability to crisis, traumatic spinal cord injury families fit the classification which Hill reports to be most difficult of crisis resolution: dismemberment ("death" of the uninjured family member as s/he normally was) plus accession ("birth" of the injured family member as a disabled person) plus demoralization (the culture's strong negative view of disabled persons). Finally, there are no clear normative guidelines or expectations for a family in which a person becomes traumatically paralyzed; these families must find their way out of the crisis alone. Traumatic spinal cord injury to a family member is an extreme stressor, which strikes isolated families and, as such, may provide a prototype for the examination of family adaptation to crisis.

It is becoming increasingly clear that stress is a very complex factor, made up of physiological, emotional, and behavioral components. Studies of family stress need to consider the impact of the stressor on an incredibly enmeshed system of individual and family processes. As we attempt to describe and explain family stress we need to examine how the stressor affects many different aspects of the family system. The following study attempts to analyze the impact of traumatic spinal cord injury first on family structures and second, on specific interpersonal relationships of family members.

Method

Sample

The sample consisted of families of traumatically spinal cord injured young people who were unmarried and for whom their family of orientation took primary responsibility. All families were intact at the time of the injury, husband, wife, and children residing together. The group contained families of the entire population of patients who met the criteria and were treated at the most extensive rehabilitation facilities serving Minnesota and North and South Dakota.* Data were gathered from April of 1975 through November of 1976. Seventeen of 19 injured were male and 17 of 19 families had more than three children. Consequently, family adaptation to the injury of a son could not be compared with that of injury to a daughter, nor could adaptation patterns of large families be compared with those of families with less than four children. Statistical breakdown of the sample in terms of residence, socioeconomic status, and age at injury showed no significant differences between adaptation patterns of rural and urban families, families with high or low socioeconomic status, or families in which the young person was injured before or after graduation from high school. . . .

Data Collection

Data were collected in two phases, Phase I, at the beginning of rehabilitation treatment, and Phase II, six months following the injured's release from the rehab institution. The Phase I contact was carried out at the hospital or the rehabilitation facility; the Phase II contact in the family home. The length of time between Phase I and Phase II was between nine and twelve months. This range, which was based on variations in length of rehabilitation treatment, did not appear to affect the findings. At the time of each contact, conjoint family and individual interviews were

*University of Minnesota Hospitals, Minneapolis Sister Kenny Institute, Minneapolis.

held, based on structured interview schedules. In addition, fathers, mothers, the injured, and siblings completed lengthy ques-
tionnaries. All instruments were developed by the author for the
study. Comparison of data from the families of quadriplegics with
data from families of paraplegics indicated no significant differences. Therefore, the results and discussion . . . include data
from both groups.

Results

Impact on Family Structure

Task Organization.   Following the injury mothers spent most
of their time at the hospital, which significantly disrupted family
task organization. Families coped with this problem in one of two
ways. Fourteen families reallocated household tasks within the
residential nuclear unit, five brought in an outside female relative
to take on the role of mother substitute. In general, fathers were
not incorporated into the reallocation of household tasks; rather,
they acted as general overseer while siblings carried out mothers'
duties.

Following the injured child's return home from rehabilitation
there was almost no change in the distribution of preinjury tasks.
However, there were major increases in the overall task repetoire
of each family member. The new tasks which resulted from the
condition of the injured were allocated within the previously existing conceptual framework of appropriate mother, father, and
sibling roles. Mothers were physical/emotional caretakers of the
injured, fathers helped with heavy lifting and did remodeling
tasks to make the house more accessible to the wheelchair. Most
siblings carried on household tasks and also carried out newly
derived tasks oriented toward helping the injured.

In looking at the effect of postinjury task organization on the
family, an important question concerns whether this organizational adaptation results in any family members experiencing
what Goode[5] defines as "role strain," a felt difficulty in fulfilling
role obligations. Across time fathers and siblings reported a rela-

tive lack of role strain; however, mothers experienced such strain as continual and increasing. Maternal involvement with the injured resulted in reported wife/mother role strain for all women. In addition they suffered severe role strain within the maternal role cluster itself. The nurturant maternal role prescription to care for their dependent offspring conflicted with the cultural maternal role prescription to help their child toward independence. Role strain was also reported by the injured son or daughter, most of whom felt they had lost all of their preinjury roles and expressed feelings of helplessness and powerlessness.

Affection Structure.   Traumatic spinal cord injury to a child had a significant impact on family affection structure, and a clear adaptation pattern emerged. Following the injury there was an immediate upsurge in feelings of intrafamily closeness. Fifty % or more of all respondents reported themselves as feeling closer to each of the other members of their family. In addition, over 50% perceived other family members as having closer relationships since the injury. Gradually, across time, the affection structure became more complex and discriminate in terms of developing specific "close" dyadic relationships. Individual family members tended to feel "close to" those for whom they held specific responsibility or on whom they felt particularly dependent. Mothers and fathers reported feeling closer to the injured, sibs to mother and father, and injured to the entire family.

A discrepancy in postinjury adaptation of the affection structure was that although family members reported increased feelings of closeness following the stressor, they reported no change in the affectional behavior of the family. There was no report of postinjury increase in physical or verbal affection, nor did family members perceive themselves as "getting along better" with each other.

Communication Structure.   Following the stressor, communication became centered on the injured, and mother took on the role of interpreter between injured and the family. When the injured returned home this interpreter role was generally taken over by an older sib. Both injured and noninjured sibs reported more postinjury openness among themselves. For example, they said they discussed the crisis situation with each other rather than with their parents. Several siblings spontaneously mentioned that these were such hard times for mother and dad that they, the sibs, had an obligation not to upset their parents with the sibs' own difficulties. Intrasib openness seemed to be the only significant change in the family communication structure.

Analysis of communication data made it possible to examine husbands', wives', and disabled childrens' empathy concerning levels of adjustment to the injureds' condition. . . . Across time mothers' empathy remained relatively stable, showing moderate empathy for the injured and very low empathy for father. From Phase I to Phase II fathers' empathy for the injureds' feelings of adjustment dropped radically, as their empathy for mothers' rose dramatically. The injureds' empathy for their parents' adjustment rose over time. Phase II empathy may be an indicator of conflicted relationships among husband, wife, and injured child. Mother and injured share a fair amount of reciprocal empathy for each others' feelings of adjustment; Father and injured report lower reciprocal empathy; fathers' empathy for mothers is moderate, mothers' for fathers is very low.

Power Structure.   At the Phase I contact no respondent reported the injured to hold excessive power in the family system; all reported father and/or mother to be the most powerful family figures. By Phase II there was a change in the family power structure; a clear conflict had developed between father and injured. Although the father continued to be perceived by family members as having the "most power," the injured was reported to be struggling with him for this position. With only two exceptions (both female), the injured reported themselves as holding the most power within the family.

Study results indicated that across time injured sons and daughters came to hold an extraordinary amount of control within the family unit. Perhaps the most critical was the emotional power which they developed over noninjured family members. Most of the injured had the ability to cause emotional suffering in their parents and siblings and to ease that suffering whenever they wished. They did this by selectively activating and deactivating parental or sibling guilt. As Phase II interviews and family contacts were conducted it became clear that the major mechanism used by the injured to activate parental guilt was manipulation of his or her own mood. If parents, brothers, or sisters didn't respond to the wishes of the injured s/he would become angry, or more often depressed, which had the effect of making parent or sibling feel guilty. When questioned about their guilt, noninjured family members expressed the feeling that they must do everything in their power to help the injured and "keep him happy."

Family Unity. Data gathered at the first contact indicated that although families perceived the situation brought about by the child's disablement to be a serious crisis, they also saw themselves as integrated units able to deal with the problem. By the time of the Phase II contact, the realities of living with a physically disabled person were reflected in a lowered feeling of family unity. Two-thirds of the fathers and sibs and one-half of the mothers reported that this kind of situation caused significant problems in terms of "holding the family together." They also reported a sharp decrease in the "closeness" of the family as a whole. Behavioral data from family members reflected the decrease of family closeness. At Phase I most respondents felt unable to maintain social contacts outside the home. They reported anxiety, and even fear, at exposing themselves to the community and turned to each other for support. Nine months later this pattern had changed, and siblings (but not husbands and wives) reported turning outward to peers for relief from the pressures and tensions at home.

There is some literature to suggest that in this type of situation family unity might be maintained by scapegoating the injured.[6] It was the author's judgment that this process did not occur to any significant degree; families did not mask other relationship problems by focusing on the injured's condition. Respondents recognized "noninjury"-related family problems but indicated that those problems must be dealt with in the context of a reality which demanded excessive physical and emotional involvement with the injured at this point in the family's career.

Impact on Specific Interpersonal Relationships

An important question concerning postinjury adaptation patterns concerns the effect of the injured's condition on specific interpersonal relationships within the family. The situation did not seem to have a significant impact on relationships between parents and noninjured sibs, and, in fact, sibs indicated more open communication among themselves following the injury. The most significant changes in interpersonal relationships occurred between the injured and each parent and in the husband/wife relationship.

Father/Injured. Most fathers and sons reported that the injury had led to a closer relationship between them. Sons said their fathers were more nurturant than in the past, and that they, the sons, enjoyed this nurturance. Data also indicated two significant problem areas for fathers and their injured sons.

The first problem area concerned our cultural definition of "male." Fathers in the sample were reared within the traditional value structure of the 1930s, believing that their job as fathers was to teach their sons to "become men." To become men meant to learn to hunt, to fish, to participate in sports, to date girls, and to be stoic in the face of hurt. Following the injury most of these values were incompatible with the injureds' physical condition. Consequently, fathers reported being confused and frightened about their sons' overall sexual identity. Injured sons faced the same dilemma, yet "male" values for stoicism and repression of feelings stood between father/son discussion of their mutual fears and confusions.

A second problem area for fathers and sons centered around mother. All fathers reported that mother's involvement with the injured interfered with her role as wife. They believed that their sons deliberately intensified this problem by making excessive demands which took mothers' time and emotional energy. This often resulted in fathers feeling serious resentment toward the needs of their injured sons.

Mother/Injured. The relationship between mothers and injured seemed to be the critical focus of the postinjury family system. It was around this dyad that the family organized itself. Mother and injured were forced into a close relationship, both physically and emotionally. Mothers were physical caretakers for the injured, and as culturally designated "guardians of affective needs," they took on primary responsibility for the injured's emotional adjustment.

Given this situation, it is not surprising that although over 70% of mothers and sons reported a closer postinjury relationship, major mother/injured problems arose in the area of mother's overprotectiveness. Data indicated that mothers did not underestimate the physical capabilities of the injured but were unable to allow them to function to their maximum potential. The injured added to this problem by frequently asking for help or support and then criticizing mothers for giving it. On the other hand, if mothers refused to help, the injured would become angry or depressed. Mothers responded to the anger/depression by soliciting or cajoling which, in turn, gave positive reinforcement to the injured's use of his own mood as a mechanism of control.

Husband/Wife. Data showed the postinjury marital relationship to be significantly affected by mothers' involvement with the injured. Her physical involvement decreased the time she had to spend with her husband, and her emotional involvement resulted in a decreased ability to make an active investment in her marriage. As a result of this situation, husbands became angry with wives, and wives reciprocated that anger for husbands' "lack of understanding."

Husbands and wives also reported ongoing tension between them in terms of mothers' protectiveness toward the injured. Typically, fathers reported that mothers' overprotectiveness impeded both the physical and emotional adjustment of their injured sons.

In general, both husbands and wives reported that marriage had been neither improved nor harmed by the injury and expressed a deep regret that due to their child's condition they would never feel free from parenthood. Many reported feeling that plans for themselves as a couple would always be contingent on the injured's life situation.

Discussion

In adapting to the stressor, family tasks and organization were not renegotiated in a load-equalizing way. Consequently, mothers in the sample experienced continuing and increasing role strain across time. This tended to decrease her effectiveness as a mother to noninjured children, as wife to husband, and as individual to self. Changes in family affection structure which occurred on a feeling level were not reflected in behavior. This seemed to result in confusion and discomfort in affective relationships. Also, the differentiating of "close" dyads on the basis of dependency/responsibility seemed to isolate some family members from each other. Changes in communication structures tended to separate parents from children, rigidifying boundaries between generations. In terms of power, the father/injured struggle for dominance apparently resulted in ambiguity and confusion. In addition, the power of the injured to control through the manipulation of his own mood can be described as destructive. It was destructive for the entire family because the power structure was not an equitable one; the injured held excessive control in many areas of family life.

Marris[7] claims that people can adjust to life change only when they are able to find meaning in, to make sense of, the change. During the course of this study each respondent in the sample came to rationalize the situation in terms of his or her previous life philosophy; none reported any basic change in attitudes toward God, fate, or the meaning of life. Under the severe stress of traumatic spinal cord injury to a family member, the great majority of respondents in this sample maintained their previous coping behaviors as well as the philosophies and attitudes underlying these behaviors.

Implications for Intervention

As a practitioner, the author has determined several goals which she has found useful when working with families of spinal cord injured young people.

Minimize Involvement between Mother and Injured

In a family facing this situation, it is crucial to their long-term postinjury adjustment that the physical and emotional enmeshment between mother and injured be untangled. The author has found it helpful to explore with the mother and her injured son or daughter the symbiotic nature of their relationship and the part each plays in maintaining it. Once the pattern of interaction is recognized, the enmeshment can be broken down. When the mother/child system begins to change, the mother may feel guilty and useless, as though she is somehow not fulfilling the duties expected of her. The practitioner plays an important role in supporting the mother toward a realistic appraisal of the situation and of the part she can play in her injured child's life.

One of the things that can be most helpful in working with mothers through this process is their own recognition that fathers may be as important to the injured's adjustment as are mothers. Mothers almost invariably recognize that their son or daughter responds more maturely, more at their age level, with their father. Practitioners can utilize this understanding on the part of mothers to help deintensify the mother/injured relationship while encouraging increasing father/injured involvement.

Maximize Involvement between Father and Injured

The relationship between father and injured is often a potentially strong element in the postinjury family system. They feel closer to each other and tend to "get along better." A major obstacle to the development of their relationship is their problem in communicating, particularly about affective or relationship issues. The practitioner can serve a valuable function by facilitating communication between them concerning their fears about sexuality, their conflict over mother, and specific expectations each has for the future independence of the injured. Each of these topics is important in the development of a mature relationship between father and son, and each, if ignored, has the potential to be destructive to their relationship. Skillful facilitation can bring the issues into clear focus and set the pattern for an ongoing rational dialogue between father and son.

Maximize the Relationship between Husband and Wife

A way to help mothers break out of enmeshed relationships with their injured child is to work with them toward an improved marital relationship and increasing marital involvement. Satir[8] calls parents the "architects of the family" and claims that as the marriage goes, so goes the family system. Focusing on the marital relationship in a family with a cord-injured child seems to have three important results. First, husbands and wives come to see their marriage as an avenue of emotional support and personal development and as a viable alternative to a stultifying overinvolved parental relationship. Second, when a couple consciously focuses on their relationship as husband and wife they are not apt to displace their interpersonal problems onto the condition of their injured son or daughter. Finally, the couple's involvement with each other allows the injured the psychological room he or she needs to face the situation of physical disability, to grow into that situation, and to reach his or her potential of physical and emotional independence.

Through contact with families of traumatically disabled young people it has become clear to the author that without clinical intervention the great majority of these families do not move toward goals which have been suggested as important to posttrauma functioning. Typically, grief is dealt with intrapersonally, fear of depression becomes a powerful factor in family relationships, mothers remain enmeshed with disabled children, and husbands and wives remain conflicted in areas concerning the injured.

Conclusion

The ... discussion of families which experience traumatic spinal cord injury to a son or daughter is necessarily brief. However, the results of the study clearly show that following this particular stressor event families are in crisis, and that family systems adapt to the crisis by making structural change. A fascinating, and unanswered, question growing out of this study relates to the rigid application of pre-injury family principles to postinjury adaptation. Is postinjury family dysfunction due to the reliance on previous coping strategies? Beyond this: Do families experiencing other severe stressors typically respond in this way? Are less severe stressors, or those which are "socially common," more apt to be dealt with creatively? Is it the nature of the stressor event or the type of prestressor family structure which most influences poststressor adaptation patterns? Many such questions exist. Unfortunately, the present study can only lead to speculation, perhaps further research may lead to answers.

References

1. McCubbin, H. I. Integrating coping behavior in family stress theory. *Journal of Marriage and the Family*, 1979, *41*, 237–244.
2. Farber, B. Effects of a severely mentally retarded child on family integration. *Monograph of the Society for Research in Child Development*, 1959, *71* 24(2).
3. Burr, W. *Theory construction and the sociology of the family*. New York: Wiley, 1973.
4. Hill, R. Social stresses on the family. *Social Casework*, 1958, *39*, 139–150.
5. Goode, W. A. A theory of role strain. *American Sociological Review*, 1960, *25*, 488–496.
6. Vogel, E., & Bell, N. The emotionally distrubed child as the family scapegoat. In E. Vogel & N. Bell (Eds.), *A modern introduction to the family*. New York: Free Press, 1960.
7. Marris, P. *Loss and change*. New York: Pantheon, 1974.
8. Satir, V. *Peoplemaking*. Palo Alto, Calif.: Science and Behavior Books, 1972.

13

Coping with Quadriplegia

SHARON PRICE AADALEN and
FLORENCE STROEBEL-KAHN

The accident, which left me a C5-6 quadriplegic, occurred June 8, 1973. Stopped at a red light, I was hit from behind by a moving car. Because I was seven months pregnant I did not have the seat belt fastened. The car seat came loose, my head hit the top of the car, and the sudden anterior neck flexion caused collapse and total fragmentation of the centrum of C-5. Complete motor paralysis and incomplete sensory interruption was the result.

I lost consciousness and awoke as the neurosurgeon was placing Crutchfield tongs in my head. I remember thinking, "There goes my life," but otherwise I have little memory of that initial period.

Within two weeks of the accident I had surgery to stabilize my neck fracture. Postoperatively, I developed shock lung. It is terribly frightening when you can't breathe. The insertion and continued presence of the endotracheal tube is extremely painful.

I remember thinking about the baby, the poor baby, trying to get oxygen. I was crying and whining in pain. Following an emergency tracheostomy I was put on a respirator. I fought the respirator, so they snowed me with morphine. I don't remember much that happened for the next two to three

SHARON PRICE AADALEN • Continuing Education Consultant, Educator, and Researcher, Edina, Minnesota. **FLORENCE STROEBEL-KAHN** • Independent Consultant, Speaker, and Educator, Minneapolis, Minnesota.

months. Any awareness I had was of my body. All my energy was focused on physical survival. My family was there all the time, but I wasn't aware of them.

The adaptive mechanisms Florence used in the first three months postinjury are *regression* and *denial*. These mechanisms served to screen out her inner feelings and her external reality, so that only awareness of her body remained. It is not unusual for the patient and family to have some degree of amnesia for this period.

The following incident occurred during the first month postinjury, when Florence's survival was very much in doubt. It shows how patients can be helped to cope even under extremely difficult circumstances. Florence had delivered a premature baby girl who died of pulmonary and gastrointestinal complications a few days after delivery.

No one knew if I would be able to hear or respond to the reality of my baby's death. But my husband, my parents, and our baby's pediatrician approached me as if I could. They played a tape of me singing "Lord Have Mercy on Me" while they told me about the baby. Momentarily I was able to respond and tell them my wishes about the baby, funeral, and burial. The news of my baby's death provided an opportunity for me to "split up the grief" into manageable segments.

Listening to the tape of herself singing helped Florence to regain, at least momentarily, an adult developmental level of functioning; she was able to move beyond body awareness, receive the message that her baby had died, expend emotional energy in grieving, and make decisions about the funeral.

Another example of Florence's coping concerned the difficult task of weaning her from the respirator.

By August, when it was time for weaning, I felt that there was no way I could breathe on my own. My diaphragm was floppy, and the idea of one day off the respirator seemed like an eternity. My doctor broke the process of breathing down into manageable, teachable, endurable components; and with the support of the nursing staff, I became willing to relearn breathing.

For most of the first seven to eight months postinjury, Flo's condition was so life threatening that defense and fragmentation processes predominated.

I was fighting for my life. I couldn't imagine dying. Often I would say or think, "I wish I were dead," but that is not the same thing as wanting to die or losing the will to live.

When the shock lung condition improved, I became increasingly aware of my surroundings. The intensive care unit was like an open operating room with five or six beds. It was frightening. There were times that I felt I was floating around and was incapable of getting back to my bed. I don't know whether this was a protective mechanism or related to the morphine, but I literally left that place and went across the street.

When her fear, pain, discomfort, and total dependence on caretakers and complex equipment were totally overwhelming, Flo unconsciously managed her feelings by the fragmentation processes of depersonalization, perceptual distortion, and delusions.

During a difficult night when I thought the flowers on the overbed table were flowers on an altar at a funeral, I was lucky to be cared for by a nurse who responded to my distorted perception of reality. She moved my bed as I asked her to and, also at my request, called my mother into the hospital at 2:00 A.M. As soon as I saw Mom, I calmed down. With her at my bedside, the unbearable became bearable. Her presence provided me with a secure boundary, and I drifted into sleep.

This is a period when the family, too, need support as they struggle to always be there for a loved one who is in grave danger. Flo received much "stroking" from her family members, who were experiencing terrible pain and emotional suffering themselves.

Because of the trach I could only mouth words. People couldn't understand me, and I would get exhausted trying to communicate. I would clam up in anger and frustration. At this time, the silent presence of a loved one was tremendously important. My husband and I shared our sadness. He is a physician and was, therefore, able to be a buffer between me and the "zoo"—the hospital. He was also a buffer between the rest of my family and the hospital "zoo." Then he would go home and cry and scream alone at night.

The Postacute Phase

I had a rich and fulfilling life before my accident. I had lived on my own, advanced in my profession, attended graduate school, traveled, pursued such interests as singing, knitting, sculpting, sewing, gardening, and cooking. I married in my early thirties and had a beautiful relationship with my husband. I knew what it felt like to be important without being focused on.

Since the accident I've tried to deal with so many losses (my marriage as it existed before the accident, our baby, my hands, my legs and feet, my singing voice) that most of my energy has gone into holding myself together. Working with other people had always filled me up. Now, my attention and energy were focused on me and my body functions—activities that I used to take for granted.

I just kind of floated along, letting other people plan my rehabilitation program, which was being structured by occupational therapy, physical therapy, my husband, a couple of nurses, a male attendant. . . . I was so exhausted at the end of the evening I could hardly hold up my head. I did not, could not, assert myself to be involved in planning my rehabilitation. But if I had been asked, invited to be involved . . . .

The immediate postacute phase was profoundly fatiguing for Florence and her family. She had little to no reserve energy. Physiologically, she was demonstrating the stress response that Hans Selye has called the general adaptation syndrome.[1] Prolonged stress eventually overcomes the body's intrinsic homeostatic mechanisms, and exhaustion ensues. Florence did not develop a stress ulcer (a classic example of adaptive exhaustion) nor skin breakdown, but she did develop shock lung and a tracheoesophageal fistula. By October, five months postinjury, her hair had begun to fall out.

The focus of the care givers was on Flo's life-threatening condition—on saving her life, so that the exhaustion being experienced by Flo's family was not noticed. After five months of assuming the role of coordinator of the various services involved in his wife's care, Flo's husband recognized his own exhaustion and asked another physician to assume this role. The needs of spouse and other family members were not assessed, nor was any ongoing contact established by social service personnel.

When the tracheoesophageal fistula was diagnosed, surgery

to close it was discussed but ruled out because of Flo's condition. She was fed by gastrostomy tube, but her nutritional state was deteriorating. During this time, Flo's mother was away for two weeks. On her return, she was so appalled at Flo's deterioration that she went to the surgeons and insisted that they repair the fistula.

Surgery was done, but the repair broke down. Flo and her husband cried as they tried to cope with one more setback. With time, the fistula did heal, but the scar tissue left an hourglass-shaped stricture in Flo's trachea, making closure of the tracheostomy impossible.

During this period, Flo received hand splints and began getting up in a wheelchair. She did not, however, find pleasure in these assistive devices; rather, she became depressed. The fact that she needed these devices underlined the permanence of her disability. She was starting to mourn the loss of her able body.

> *When I stood, I stood tall. I look crummy in a wheelchair . . . long torso, short arms . . . it is really hard to hold up my head and shoulders.*

Flo was transferred to the Rehabilitation Service in January 1974. She still had the tracheostomy, but a Montgomery T-tube allowed her to talk.

> *It was while I was on this service that I attended a conference on my rehab progress. No one at the conference ever addressed me directly, not once. "How is Flo doing in OT?" was addressed to the occupational therapist. I was disappointed and utterly devastated. I had a lot of confidence in the physician present, but I was treated like a piece of wood by everyone, including him. Back in my room I cried. Finally, I was able to tell a male nursing assistant how hurt and angry I was; he subsequently communicated this to the physician. It is hard to know how much one's total physical dependence affects one's ability to express anger. I do know that all my life I have tended to manage anger by turning it inward to some degree, and its blocked expression comes out as crying, as sadness.*

Gradually, Florence began to take pleasure in the world again. She delighted in sights, sounds, and smells when she went on outings with her husband.

Her coping during the postacute phase of hospitalization was supported by personalized care (shampooing her hair and hand massages) given by nurses and friends. These acts of caring supported Florence's sense of herself as a whole and worthy person.

Her coping was inhibited by the tendency of well-meaning care givers to unload some of their problems on her. With the tracheostomy, talking was difficult. Flo's eyes expressed empathy, and the staff responded with self-disclosure. While this form of communication bolstered Flo's feeling of worthiness, it also allowed her to hide from some of the issues she needed to begin dealing with before going home.

She was mortified at being dependent on others for her bowel, bladder, and genital care. She was afraid of the possible negative effect on her sexual relationship with her husband were he to be involved with her bowel program, catheter care, or menses care. She sensed that her husband did not want to be involved in these aspects of her care, and she didn't want him to be. Their mutual avoidance of discussion of this aspect of their relationship was not recognized by hospital personnel. Perhaps their avoidance of the subject was reinforced by the societal attitude that it is appropriate for a woman to nurse her sick husband but not for a man to nurse a sick wife. For whatever reason, they were not adequately prepared for the next step—going home.

Going Home

Following three months on the rehab floor, we began to make plans for me to go home. I still had the tracheostomy and the Montgomery T-tube. Therefore, arrangements had to be made for round-the-clock attendants who could handle both the tracheostomy and quadriplegic care.

My doctor said it would be "tough," but urged me not to be scared. My response was disbelief . . . "I'm not scared. Why, I can hardly wait to go home!" He urged me to give myself time and said it would take me at least five to six years to cope with all that had happened to me. He knew that I was facing one of the biggest adjustments I would face in the long struggle to climb back up my mountain. If he had been more direct in his communication it might have helped, but I don't know if I was ready to hear what he was saying. I do feel, however, that he could have helped my family to understand and anticipate how difficult the days would be. Written materials would have been very helpful as a resource for the day-to-day problems that arose. But perhaps the family couldn't have heard either. After 10 long months, in terms of coping, they were drowning. If I had let myself, I could have had three nervous breakdowns by the time I went home because of what my family was going through.

I could not have been prepared for what it would be like to experience myself as a quadriplegic within my own home—the home I had cared for, the gardens I had tended, the arrangements I had made of our furniture and knickknacks. I resented my caretaker's ability to "do."

My feelings were raw. I tried to regain some control over my sense of utter helplessness by giving directions to caretakers and my husband. I'd bite out at the people closest to me. . . . I was angry I couldn't do it myself, I was willing to sit home, immobile, rather than ask caretakers to do things for me and help me get out. In the first three months, we had three or four caretakers. I was driving them nuts.

After I had been home four months, my husband confronted me: "Flo, you can't expect others to do all the things you've done the way you've done them. You can't expect caretakers to garden for your pleasure."

The true meaning of the loss doesn't really hit until you are home for the first time. I was experiencing the most profound depression yet in the year-long struggle for survival. Jumping the gun on caretakers was one of the ways I was still denying my reality. But my energy level for the emotional work I had to do continued to be very low, because of complex physiological problems. Having the tracheostomy was exhausting because of the tracheopulmonary secretions and the effort it took to communicate. Furthermore, I had autonomic dysreflexia.

Autonomic dysreflexia is an exaggerated response of the autonomic nervous system, and it is most likely to occur in patients with cervical or high thoracic cord lesions. The symptoms include extreme blood pressure elevation, diaphoresis, severe headache, bradycardia, and nasal stuffiness.[2] Florence was completely unprepared for this problem. She does not recall any teaching for her or her family about this syndrome. Not only should the patient and family know about autonomic dysreflexia, but they should be well enough informed so that they can educate caretakers.

By July 1974, I was having so much trouble with autonomic dysreflexia that we needed to seek assistance. (In restrospect I realize that I experienced the syndrome in the intensive care unit. I would wake up dripping wet and the nurses would put cornstarch on me to absorb the perspiration.) My husband could no longer cope with the idea of multiple teams at the hospital, so we went to a smaller, local rehabilitation institute.

Our physician there reached out to my husband; it was the first time anyone had. This physician said, "When you get tired, come see us." By August, my husband and I were both tired, and so I spent several weeks at the institute. We experimented with drugs, trying to find some relief from the dysreflexia, but relief for one problem was usually accompanied by side effects in another system. For me respiratory side effects were the most difficult. My husband continued trying to solve the problem of my trach, hoping to find some way to improve my ability to communicate.

When I returned home in September we were better prepared to work out our problems with our home life. We had been involved in developing some videotapes on sexual relationships for spinal-cord injured persons and their spouses, something we were working on in our own lives. We also developed a procedure manual for caretakers. I think it would have been helpful if I had been involved in the preparation of such a manual while hospitalized that first year.

We established contact with a fine social worker at the institute who assumed responsibility for coordinating our ongoing care.

On my return home we began a new schedule. An LPN was with me during the day; a college student took the evening responsibility. We found that advertising in the newspaper worked best for recruiting help. I slept in our king-size bed with an air mattress. We wanted it that way, even though the lowness of the bed and lack of siderails made transfers difficult.

We had learned a lot at the institute, and we had a good autumn. I probably didn't realize it at the time, but I had begun to learn the difference between effective home and self-management and acting out my anger at my losses.

While my motor paralysis is complete, my sensory deficit is incomplete and changing all the time. Many people think quads have no feeling, and, therefore, don't check with the person about what sensations he or she had. Attendants often do not realize that tripping over a catheter tubing or bumping into or applying pressure to parts of the body can cause the person extreme discomfort. I have sensory differences between the two sides of my body, and I have a kind of buzzing in my whole body. Few people realize that quads often have to learn to live with a significant amount of constant discomfort. There are strange autonomic hookups.

During the first year at home, the impact of the loss of the use of my hands (I call it the loss of my hands) confronted me at every turn. I was a "touching person." For me the inability to use my hands expressively, to reach out, to comfort, to caress, was profound. My inability to actively hold my husband, to actively love him, deeply affected my perception of our sexual relationship. My husband and I shared our feelings, trying to get them out on the table. As I look back now, I see that my husband encouraged and supported me in getting my feelings out, but he was careful not to lay his sad feelings on me. I compared our life before the accident to what it was now. There were so many holes. I was physically drained, low on energy, and unable to respond to spur-of-the-moment suggestions or impulses. My husband was using so much energy in day-to-day coping that his sex drive decreased.

I had not been able to establish appropriate criteria of worthiness for myself as a quadriplegic. Our society values productivity and ascribes a lesser value to, or devalues, pure being. We tried to work out our losses intellectually, but we seemed to get stuck in comparisons of our life before and our life since the accident. Warm, touching, caring, physical closeness is something I miss so much. Being in a chair is so distancing. I realized this recently when I saw two able-bodied persons stand and hug each other, body to body, arms entwined. I just burst into tears.

The Next Step

    In the winter of 1975 I was scheduled for surgery to close the tracheostomy. I had waited so long for this, but the day of surgery I was scared to death. Fortunately, I had such a long trachea that the surgeon was able to remove 2.5 cm of scarred trachea and anastomose a healthy, patent, tubal trachea. The surgery was a success, the intensive respiratory care was superb, and we were able to return home in three weeks. Thus, two-and-a-half years after the accident, I was free of intensive trach care for the first time. We were in awe of the added time, the increased energy, and the improvement in communication that closure of the trach afforded. It was a very Merry Christmas!

    In April of 1976, I went to a major rehabilitation center. I was so glad to get there. I can't say enough about the center. I discovered that I had developed increased risk-taking skills. When you've been really hurt, you develop accommodating skills. You're not taking in everything, just one thing at a time. Learning this, you see that you can tackle most anything by breaking it down into bits and pieces of challenge. At the center you work on overall, absolute independence, whatever your limitations. And you are given permission to be, and expected to be, an autonomous individual. Oh, how I worked—on weakened muscles, on activities of daily living, such as leg bag emptying, on learning all about my care, and my responsibility for intelligent management of it.

    I had particularly hoped to meet another female quad who might serve as a role model for me. I wanted and needed to be able to develop relationships with other women struggling with quadriplegia. I did meet female quads, but I had to learn that a similar disability does not translate into similar adaptation.

My husband was hoping for a miracle—that I would be walking, that I would be the "old Flo" when I came home. Psychologically, he could not handle the reality of the five- to six-year rehabilitation period or my total disability.

I was so happy to be back home again after my experience at the center. My self-pity had decreased. I was not sure I had been able to assimilate all that I had learned, but I returned armed with an excellent manual for reference. I had begun dealing with the hurts and losses in relationship to my husband, but once I got home, depression reared its ugly head again because I had yet to work on, work out, and let go of my losses.

My husband was finding the living situation at home, with attendants ever present, increasingly difficult. When he traveled, he wanted companionship, and although I went along sometimes, it wasn't enough. My fear of dysreflexia and my diminished energy affected my perspective on going anywhere.

In December, 1976, my husband consulted a psychiatrist for an assessment of our situation. My husband had had it trying to deal with Flo in the chair. But he still wasn't able to talk about his depression and exhaustion. He was denying the reality and totality of the loss. Denial is one of the ways we get through hell. And yet, ultimately, the whole family has to come to terms with the loss, the permanent change.

The visit was disturbing because the psychiatrist failed to look at our whole family system and to realize that both my husband and I were depressed. The visit did, however, make us aware of some things. My husband was hurting terribly; his coping resources were depleted. And I was in a rut again. My husband had seen me functioning in a supportive role at the center and urged me to get out and do some volunteer work with families of disabled children, but I didn't.

Near our home there was a new residence for severely disabled young adults. My husband suggested that it might provide the setting for me to get remobilized professionally. At first, I wasn't interested in or willing to enter the facility, but an unexpected opening in March 1977 led to my moving to the residence.

My husband was wiped out from carrying so much responsibility. He loves to make decisions and get things going, but, at that point, he was in a great empty space, and he couldn't cope with it. He loves, needs, and misses me, but a couple of months after I moved to the residence, he initiated divorce proceedings.

Residential Living

The implications of leaving home were not clear to me at first, although when my husband came to visit each day, I felt strange, separated. He was anticipating a job at a geographical distance, so, with planned finality, I packed things at the house, held a garage sale, yet, I thought that after two years (my anticipated stay at the residence) we would live together again. This was an odd type of denial because I dreaded coming to the residence. It was the beginning of saying good-bye; on an unconscious level I knew it.

"Busy-ness" characterized the flurry of activity in which Flo immersed herself as she relocated at the residence. It was a useful mechanism for hiding her fears, her anger, and her anxiety, especially from herself.

It was yet another devastating personal loss that helped Florence get in touch with her feelings.

The news that my sister-in-law, someone very close to me, had committed suicide released the floodgate. Somehow this tragic and shattering news helped me to cope with my feelings. It is most significant that my parents communicated directly with me. I do not know what I would have done if a stranger had been the bearer of such news. I had to begin to get in touch with my sadness and my resistance to developing an identity as a permanently disabled person.

When I emerged from the body-focused fog of near-death, I comprehended, at some level, that I was totally dependent on others for my care; that was one level of awareness. But it was not the emotional level of awareness of how dependent I am for my very life on the safe and competent care of others. It was not the emotional awareness of being totally dependent on others for all personal care (bowel, bladder, and perineal care). That emotional realization of dependency was yet to come.

The physical dependence of quadriplegia demands ongoing interaction with caretakers, and this makes it necessary for the spinal-cord injured person to develop management skills.

The residence was the first setting in which I began to confront the adaptive task of my own self-management vis-à-vis caretakers. In the privacy of my own home I was in control of whom we hired as caretakers, and we chose females. But at the residence I had no say in the caretakers (resident assistants) assigned to me. When a policy was established that female quads would have to adjust to having their perineal care and bowel program done my male assistants, I had to accept the policy. At the residence I learned that my energy level correlates with the degree of skill my caretaker has, and with how well I know and whether I trust that person. Caretaker ineptness increases my sense of dependency, decreases my trust level, arouses my perceptual sensitivity, and is emotionally exhausting.

Certainly one of the ironies of life as a quad is having to constantly meet, interact with, and orient strangers to one's most intimate physical care. During a period when, in the beginning of most relationships, a very cautious kind of distanced checking-out is going on, the physically disabled person has to instantly open her or his most private physical parts to the strange caretaker's view and handling.

I don't know if I will ever adjust to the time and energy required to plan anything, undertake any activity, go anywhere. It freaks me out—it is such a putdown! "Would you mind opening the door?" "Would you please get me my bag?" "Would you mind . . . would you please . . . ?" I had to realize how much I can do by myself. I had to relearn to carry out activities of daily living. In the end, I learned that I have to decide how much of my limited energy I will expend on independent functioning, and how much I will conserve by asking for assistance.

During the summer of 1977 divorce proceedings were initiated.

From then on, nursing and counseling personnel at the residence made assumptions about how I should be feeling and judgments about what I was or was not feeling or expressing. I am aware that I put things on hold, such as dealing or not dealing with feelings, and I do need a kick in the butt to get going at times, but I want to be respected as an adult who is competent and who can make choices about me and for my own life.

Florence's first year at the residence included several major areas of adaptive demand: physical care, emotional status (she began participation in a transactional analysis group), the divorce, and the issue of a subsequent relationship with her husband, accepting male caretakers, maintaining relationships with old friends, developing new friendships at the residence, involvement in self-governance at the residence, preliminary thinking about professional remobilization, decision making about priorities for energy expenditure, and speculation about long-term living arrangements.

I went to my parents' home for Christmas in 1977. Until that time my parents' response to the divorce was "Well, you can live with us after your stay at the residence." It was a good Christmas and an important period of reality testing. With the help of visiting nurses, Mom was able to care for me, and she loved doing it. But when I returned to the residence, we knew that it would never work on a long-term basis.

No adaptive demand was greater, more stressful, or more wrenching for Florence than the divorce.

We finally could discuss our future—divorce—yet clung to the hope for a special relationship. Since then, with time and more crises, I've learned you can understand something intellectually, but when the time comes, the gut kicks out with all the feelings involved. When my husband first brought up the subject of divorce he couched it in terms of financial drain. But by midwinter 1977–78, he finally was able to acknowledge that there was no way he could live with me and have his needs met. It had taken a long time for him to be able to face this, and it had been important to him to know that I had enough internal strength to be able to accept it. We both feel rotten about getting a divorce. Each feels very alone. But, I am developing a whole network of meaningful people and relationships in my life. I am alone but not lonely. My husband, on the other hand, has close ties with very few people.

To me the divorce is a manifestation of our inability to change and grow together to meet the facts, facets, and crises of our lives.

Moving On

As I began the second year, I wanted to withdraw the energy investment I had in the transactional analysis group and begin planning to move back to the community. Psychological goals took priority the first year. The TA group was very important. I did a lot of grief work, I learned a lot about myself, and I am amazed at how desensitized I became. Perhaps that is a matter of taking charge of me and my needs and behaviors, instead of allowing someone or something out there to do it for me. I am learning to take responsibility for experiencing and expressing my emotions.

A counselor at the residence told me that my feelings about my losses are like a switchboard with many blinking red lights, representing feelings that are put on "hold." That is a fairly accurate description of a pattern I have had all my life and that I will probably continue to have. My involvement in the governance of the residence, my interest in planning and participating in fun times for myself, and my responsiveness to analysis of my own coping and that of my family since the accident might be interpreted by some as putting feelings on hold and not dealing with them. But for me this "holding pattern" has enabled me to reconstruct my life. I have had to let go of my losses and say good-bye to my standing self. Until I was thirty I lived as a single, fulfilled, self-sufficient woman. I see my rehabilitation as a spiraling process with each succeeding loop more expansive than the last, as I have gradually assimilated the full meaning of my disability. With skills of self-management, I will continue my life plan.

In this period of Florence's rehabilitation, her husband's defensive processes impoverished and exhausted him, and he was finally able to acknowledge that fact. Did health professionals assume that because he is a physician he could care for himself and needed no outside assistance? Was he unable to seek or ask for help? He has had to cope with guilt about choosing to divorce Flo in order to meet his own needs for physical care, security, and love; to be free to remarry. For a long time he couldn't admit these needs to himself, much less to Flo.

One month after the divorce was final, he remarried. Flo was devastated, but each of them now acknowledge responsibility for meeting their own needs. This is direct coping, for each is facing reality with empathy, compassion, and no small amount of pain.

Permanently Disabled, Yes, but . . .

Prior to the accident, Florence had completed the developmental tasks of young adulthood, but many of these tasks had to be reworked as she struggled to come to terms with her new identity—permanently disabled, yes, but capable of aspiring to a full, healthy, productive life.

Maximizing her physical potential (to be able to empty her own leg bag, feed herself, flush the toilet, propel her wheelchair, apply her own makeup, use a typewriter, and write longhand) was an ongoing challenge. The experience at the center had provided the opportunity for such achievement. She also had to learn to manage herself and others, to accomplish tasks requiring joint effort. She was confronted with the need to do this when she first went home from the hospital. Developing the kind of expertise in self-other management, which a spinal-cord injured person needs in order to supervise caretakers, is very difficult for an adult who has already achieved significant maturity. Managing emotions is a tremendous challenge for the person with an acquired disability. The physical outlets for aggression that were once available are no longer options. Counseling provides the opportunity to assimilate this loss. All the emotions of the grief reaction need to be fully experienced. The support to do this work and the encouragement to develop new means of getting positive emotional input are very important for the spinal-cord injured person.

Florence had to deal with the loss of physical independence, while trying to develop strength and assertiveness as a person-in-a-chair—a person who not only has the right to, but can and does have, something to say about her own life.

Identity reestablishment also means developing new support systems and new fulfilling human relationships. During the first year at the residence, Florence worked extremely hard on assimilating the realities of her losses and adjusting to her future. During the second year she focused her energies on the goal of independent living. Discharge planning, attempting to get her driver's license, finding an apartment, locating furniture, hiring attendants, and working on developing vocational options were uppermost in her mind.

> *Vocationally, I didn't do as many things as I thought I would, but I did work on a primary nursing conference, and that involved commitment and followthrough. My colleagues told me I changed and grew greatly while working on the project. Visualizing and planning for the future, in terms of professional involvement and self-actualization are ongoing processes. Regarding discharge, it really takes planning, help, and luck. I had a great pair of friends who made it possible.*

In January 1979, Florence moved to her own apartment with a live-in caretaker. The crises are not over, but as a result of experience and with some professional help, Florence and her family have developed coping skills that have enabled them to move beyond a survival existence to a self-actualized one.

Following the move to her apartment, Florence developed

some physical problems. The first one began with an exacerbation of bladder spasms and mucus production that led to blockage of her catheter. This triggered a serious episode of autonomic dysreflexia, and Flo had to talk her weekend caretaker through a catheter change. Shortly after that, she developed an upper respiratory infection that progressed to bronchitis.

Another issue she has had to deal with is interviewing, hiring, and training caretakers and developing workable and mutually satisfying relationships with them. She knows how important dealing with this challenge is if she is to be able to continue to sustain and develop the autonomy she has struggled to achieve.

In the past, her husband was a buffer between her and the various medical and rehabilitation services. Flo has now assumed much of this responsibility for herself, and she has a few close friends who maintain almost daily contact with her and who also act as buffers.

We have shared a perspective on the rehabilitation of the spinal-cord injured individual in which the person injured is viewed within the context of a family system. We believe that the ability of the client and family to cope with the prolonged stress of spinal cord injury is based on intrinsic biopsychological processes, ego strength, family structure, and extrinsic environmental supports. We believe that intrinsic biopsychological coping processes are supported by superb and coordinated interdisciplinary care. We believe that individual and family system processes of coping and defense can be positively affected by the interdisciplinary design and implementation of supportive educational programs that reach out to victims and families at every stage of rehabilitation. And finally, we believe that external environmental support systems and resources can be mobilized in an optimally effective way by nursing care delivery systems that affirm preventive health care and health promotion philosophies.

References

1. Selye, Hans. *The stress of life* (2nd ed.). New York: McGraw-Hill, 1978.
2. Taylor, A. G. Autonomic dysreflexia in spinal cord injury. *Nursing Clinics of North America*, 1974, *9*, 717–725.

VI

The Crisis of Treatment
Hospital Environments

Although hospitals are designed to deliver specialized medical care and promote healing, they can be intimidating and de-humanizing places. Because of the unfamiliar equipment and procedures, many patients are as upset and frightened by their hospital experience as they are reassured by the medical resources made available to them. Patients are separated from their families, examined by a series of seemingly aloof strangers; they are exposed to unfamiliar technical equipment such as scanners and lasers; and they are subjected to painful treatment. Anxiety about diagnostic and therapeutic procedures may be heightened by mandatory consent forms that graphically outline the risks associated with exposure to invasive tests such as cardiac catheterization, surgery, and powerful chemicals (for example, see Chapter 17).

Intensive care units are well known for the stress they elicit in patients, their families, and staff. Coronary care units (CCU) have received special attention because of the unexpected delerium some patients report in these specialized settings. Patients who have experienced a heart attack are frightened when they are left alone; when they witness a fellow patient suffer a cardiac arrest; and (not surprisingly), when a priest comes to administer last rites. Unlike other critically ill patients, those who have just had a heart attack are often alert and aware of their surroundings. Their stay in the CCU gives them time to think about the prospect of greater dependence and other changes in their life-style, the damage to their heart, and the reality of death. Although many find the array of monitoring equipment reassuring, it is also evidence of the imminent danger their lives are in.[4]

The stressors involved in hospitalization led Norman Cousins[1] to conclude that "a hospital is no place for a person who is seriously ill." He cited such problems as lack of respect for basic sanitation, the high risk of exposure to infectious agents, and the overly extensive use of x-ray and other technical equipment. Cousins[1] noted a circular paradox to intensive care units in which patients are provided with "better electronic aids than ever before for dealing with emergencies that are often intensified because they communicate a sense of imminent disaster" (p. 133). Although most patients cannot cope with the hospital environment by abandoning it, Cousins dealt with these issues by moving into a hotel room that afforded peace and quiet and cost only about one-third as much as his hospital room. (For an overview of this area, see references 5 and 6.)

In the discussion of adult cancer (Part IV), we saw how some patients handled their illness and treatment by using action-oriented coping strategies. Because children do not have as many coping options available to them as do adults, hospitalization poses unique problems for them. In the first article, Donald Brunnquell and Marian D. Hall highlight some of the issues that have evolved as medical technology prolongs the lives of children with cancer. The authors identify specific stressful aspects of the hospital setting and of treatment, and they note how they trigger the underlying issues of separation and loss and the maintenance of control and competence. For instance, the restriction in activity and mobility and the lack of stimulation that come with being confined to a hospital bed or an isolation room are special threats to an active child's sense of competence. Children also feel powerless in the face of multiple invasive tests and the frightening side effects of treatment. Staff who enable children to regain some control by involving them in their own care are often rewarded with increased cooperation. (For ideas about how children can maintain control during diagnostic uroradiologic procedures, see Fischman.)[3]

When previously healthy persons are suddenly struck with a life-threatening health crisis, family members are likely to be overwhelmed by the stress of hospitalization and the intensity of treatment. If they obtain only scant information from staff, as is often the case, their fears and misconceptions may be intensified. In the second article, Peter Rothstein examines patients' reactions when a child suddenly becomes seriously ill and is hospitalized in a pediatric intensive care unit (ICU). The initial shock and help-lessness parents experience may last for several days, especially if the child's condition does not improve or complicated treatment is required. The parents' shock is intensified when they see their child covered with bandages or connected to monitors, tubes, or urinary catheters. During this phase, parents may cope by deny-ing reality, glossing over information provided by staff, or becom-ing angry when bad news is imparted.

These parental reactions are moderated during the phase of anticipatory waiting, which begins once the child's condition im-proves. But parents whose children remain unconscious face a special dilemma in that they cannot comfort or reassure their child. Parent–staff conflicts may arise when staff withdraw from the family, which sometimes happens when a child is dying (see Chapter 5) or when staff believe parents share responsibility for the child's illness. Such communication breakdowns contribute to the vulnerability of parents who have a child in an ICU. Unlike parents of leukemic children who can assist in their child's care, such parents typically feel like helpless bystanders because the complex equipment and knowledge required make it difficult for them to participate actively in their child's care.

Hospital environments create an atmosphere that can con-tribute to the use of certain coping mechanisms by patients and their families. The physical setting of the ICU, the sophisticated equipment, the flurry of health care professionals who quickly respond when a patient is in serious danger, all serve to instill hope among distraught families that their loved ones can be saved. When expected miracles fail to occur and family members are told that there is little or no chance for recovery, the informa-tion may be met with disbelief and denial.

In the third article, David Waller and his associates examine the conflicts that arise when staff use a coping mechanism called "hanging of crepe" (that is, communicating a hopeless prognosis) and parents respond by behaving as though their child will recover. In essence, this "Cassandra prophecy" phenomenon places physicians in a position analogous to Cassandra—the Greek prophetess of doom—whose portent of dreaded events was disregarded. Physicians interpret parents' failure to accept the prognosis as a rejection of their professional expertise. Nurses feel resentful toward parents who accuse them of not doing everything possible for their child.

Coping mechanisms such as the "hanging of crepe" and parental denial are a function of the environmental, illness-related, and interpersonal context. Aspects of the illness and of the overall setting both contribute to parental denial. Because the children described by Waller and his associates did not have cancer, parents were not as likely to associate their child's condition with death. Moreover, the technical equipment and intensive treatment of children in an ICU testifies to the fact that staff try to and can save lives. For the distraught parents, therefore, the hopeless prognosis is not congruent with the underlying purpose of the intensive care setting. Moreover, in their communication with social workers, parents showed their awareness of the gravity of their child's situation. Parents were concerned that an "understanding" of the poor prognosis might be interpreted as acquiescence and would permit physicians and nurses to give up aggressive treatment of their child. As the authors point out, *denial* can be a social act intended to influence other people's behavior.

The prediction of a grave outcome also has interpersonal overtones because it may free the physician from the responsibility of waging a losing battle. In a more complex manner, the two coping strategies can amplify each other: Parental "certainty" of a child's recovery may stimulate a grave prognosis, whereas such a prognosis may intensify parental denial. In order to allay parents' fears that their child will be abandoned, staff can couple honest information about the prognosis with a promise that everything possible will be done to help the child. Also, by sharing parental perceptions of the situation with each other, staff members can identify different levels and purposes of parental denial.

Much can be done to humanize hospitals. Some of the problems associated with the physical environment of intensive care settings may be alleviated by placing patients in individual cubicles that offer some privacy, turning down the lights at night, scheduling procedures so patients have some free time, keeping monitors out of patient rooms, and providing a more cheerful environment by using color on walls and in linens and curtains. Moreover, hospital designers can meet the unique goals of specific groups of patients, such as maintaining a sense of identity among young adults. This goal can be promoted by placing each bed next to a window and in a corner of the room, surrounding the bed with screens or dividers, leaving sufficient space for medical equipment and personal effects, and clearly defining a place in which each patient can keep possessions and personalize the environment.

Patients forfeit control over most of the tasks they customarily perform when they enter a hospital. Because the lack of control creates reactions of depression and helplessness that can hinder the treatment and recovery process, staff are trying to establish more viable roles for hospitalized patients and their family members.[7] For instance, patient participation in rehabilitation can be promoted by increased staff–patient interaction, explicit staff expectations for patients, ongoing opportunities for information exchange among staff and family members, and shared staff decision making.[2] Patients who are actively involved in the treatment process and who see illness management as a collaborative endeavor are more motivated and effective in keeping their illness under control. More generally, attention to both physical and social design can improve hospital settings and their beneficial impact.

References

1. Cousins, N. *Anatomy of an illness as perceived by the patient.* New York: Norton, 1979.
2. Davis, M. Z. The organizational, interactional, and care-oriented conditions for patient participation in continuity of care: A framework for staff intervention. *Social Science and Medicine,* 1980, *14A,* 39–47.
3. Fischman, S. Cooperation. In G. W. Friedland & associates (Eds.), *Uroradiology: An integrated approach* New York: Churchill Livingstone, 1983.
4. Kimball, C. P. Reactions to illness, the acute phase: The interplay of environmental factors in intensive care units. *Psychiatric Clinics of North America,* 1979, *2,* 307–319.
5. Kornfeld, D., & Politser, P. The hospital environment: Understanding and modifying its impact on the patient. In R. H. Price & P. E. Politser (Eds.), *Evaluation and action in the social environment.* New York: Academic Press, 1980.

6. Shumaker, S., & Reizenstein, J. Environmental factors affecting inpatient stress in acute care hospitals. In G. Evans (Ed.), *Environmental stress.* New York: Cambridge University Press, 1982.
7. Taylor, S. Hospital patient behavior: Reactance, helplessness, or control? *Journal of Social Issues,* 1979, *35,* 156–184.

14

Issues in the Psychological Care of Pediatric Oncology Patients

DONALD BRUNNQUELL and MARIAN D. HALL

As a result of the enormous changes in mode and efficacy of treatment, a new population with distinct psychological needs is rapidly developing: the pediatric cancer survivor. The rigors of the medical treatment, pattern of hospitalizations, remissions, and relapses, and the ever-present fear of death all require enormous psychological adjustment on the part of patients and their families. Although each case presents a unique picture of strengths and difficulties, certain similarities in problems exhibited by these children are beginning to be seen.

Geist[1] referred to a "developmental lag" between provision of medical and psychological services, with medical technology advancing so rapidly that the adjustments required of the human systems are very difficult. His review of the area of psychological care of chronically ill patients provides an important basis for

Adapted from the *American Journal of Orthopsychiatry,* 1982, *52,* 32–44. Copyright 1982 the American Orthopsychiatric Association, Inc. Reproduced by permission.

DONALD BRUNNQUELL and MARIAN D. HALL • Staff Members, the Children's Health Center, Minneapolis, Minnesota 55404.

understanding both the patients' and caregivers' reactions. But due precisely to the stress on *all* involved, provision of optimal care is difficult. The aggression, regression, and depression of patients as well as the feelings of guilt, helplessness, anger, and depression of the family and the staff must all be taken into account in dealing with pediatric oncology patients.

Specific Concerns

Mobility, Activity, and Isolation

A frequent problem in many hospital situations is impairment of mobility and activity. This is often so with oncology patients because of testing procedures and intravenous administration of medication, blood, fluids, or nutrients. This is, of course, in addition to any pre- or postsurgical restrictions, bodily weakness, pain, or nausea that can cause disturbance of mobility and activity. Additionally, one must consider self-imposed "psychological" restrictions.

Motor activity is an important form of self-expression for all children and helps them develop competent relations with the world. Murphy[4] noted that "the time–space dimensions of freedom" contribute not only to the child's bodily development but "to his inner image of the world" and his place in that world. The effects of hospitalization and interventions in this realm must therefore be carefully weighed. To older children, being in bed constantly, especially in a bed with side rails, which is associated with babies, has clear regressive implications. In such cases, some means should be provided to help motivate greater and more age-appropriate activity. Simply allowing the child to wear his own clothes or to decorate the hospital room, for example, can serve this purpose.

Jim, a very ill 11-year-old hospitalized briefly for a transfusion and medication, was not only physically weak but could, for the day, use only one arm. He was very irritable and angry through the day, finally insisting that he be brought something to do. He worked intensely on simple snap-together models of cars. While these were below his usual competence level, he accepted them and proved to himself, his parents, and nurses that he was still able to do things that boys of his age "should be able to do." After completing the models, he was able to relax considerably and cooperate more fully with the treatment.

At times, restriction of activity combines with realistic pain, the child's fears, and the parents' reactions to the child's condition to hinder recovery.

Karl, a six-year-old with Hodgkins disease, was very resistant to any activity following surgery. He simply lay in bed in a darkened room, with his mother constantly present and meeting all his needs. Before any progress with Karl could be made, his mother's fears of leaving him alone had to be dealt with; finally, when she was out of the room with the psychologist, the nurses were able to engage Karl to sit up, and eventually stand up to go to the bathroom. He did at first experience pain from his incision and was fearful of separation from his mother, but within two days was acting as an independent, curious, though somewhat stiff, six-year-old.

The restriction of contact and activity entered into by this boy and his mother gave clear messages of a more severe situation than existed. If not interrupted by a return to more normal activity, a much more disturbed, symbiotic situation could easily have developed.

Periods of isolation constitute a special problem for many oncology patients. This is due not only to the enforced separation from one's family and peers but to the restriction of mobility over a long period of time. A small, private hospital room is not a stimulating environment for a child and in time can contribute significantly to depression and fears. The restlessness that grows as children stay in such a room contributes greatly to irritability and noncooperation. Even brief excursions, if they can be safely arranged, can help alleviate "cabin fever." Since peer relations are so important to latency-age children, isolation has serious effects on their self-esteem as well. This increases the fear of never again having friends or relating competently to other aspects of the environment.

Bill, an 11-year-old boy with leukemia, was in isolation for about a week, with steady decrease in his mood and ease of relationship with staff and parents. When he was finally free to leave his room and to go outside, he said he didn't want to. This refusal continued for a time, and he was finally able to confide his fears that the air pollution would make him sick again. He held to this fear in spite of reassurance that it was unfounded, clearly indicating the broader effect on his own sense of control and competence and fears stirred up by his isolation.

Accommodations to such psychological repercussions of isolation can come in various forms, such as living-in parents or visiting sibs and friends. Two private rooms in our facility, built for isolation and often used for oncology patients, were recently slightly changed by installing a window and intercom phone. In the past, patients in these rooms have often spoken on the phone or exchanged notes and pictures. The change is intended to allow more direct contact and interaction, thereby relieving the effects of isolation to some extent.

Sequelae of Treatment and Issues of Self-Control

Because of the aggressive therapy regiments now in widespread use, side effects of therapy present adjustment problems as great as the illness itself, and consultation is often sought to deal with the adjustment problems. Perhaps most prominent is difficulty with nausea. This is a frequent side effect of cancer therapies, but its severity varies greatly from child to child, in part because of psychological factors. A very great difficulty in dealing with nausea is separating out the physiological and psychological aspects. Children very quickly learn that vomiting elicits immediate concern, sympathy, and attention from parents and staff. Such responses are appropriate but quite often come to be manipulated by patients. As a psychological symptom, nausea is very closely tied to issues of self-control, regulation of relations with others, and one's sense of competence.

Michael, a 15-year-old with an abdominal tumor, had developed a habit pattern that involved vomiting as a major vehicle for relating to other people. He would lay in his bed curled around an emesis basin. When a nurse or visitor said they were going to leave, he would begin to wretch violently. Similarly, when emotionally difficult topics were raised, he would immediately complain of nausea and begin to throw up, requiring that nurses clean him up. He had a great need for affective physical contact and used his nausea as a means of achieving that contact. He once told a nurse to come back to talk to him in 20 minutes, because he knew he would throw up then if she didn't come back.

This boy, having lost the more positive, age-appropriate means of relating to other people, used his nausea, in part a real physical side effect, to manipulate others. This tied in to other regressive aspects of his case (lack of activity, no ongoing peer relations, and no eating), and presented a major problem to the staff. It was handled, after determining no medical cause for frequent vomiting, by removing "rewards" of attention and physical contact, and restoring self-control by requiring the boy to clean himself. The emesis basin was removed (he was allowed to have towels, but had to dispose of them himself, leading to more activity), and staff and family did not stay with him during his vomiting, but returned afterward to engage him in positive interaction.

Eating is frequently an issue, as a result of nausea or of surgical requirements or protocol. It should be noted that eating is the quintessential instance or example of nurturance and self-control, and any change of eating patterns can be expected to raise psychological issues. For children up to age seven or eight, feeding one's self is an issue of considerable importance simply because it is a relatively new learned skill; as children grow up, the complexity of their feeding themselves increases, and they are frequently told to "eat like a big boy (or girl)." When they are suddenly told not to eat and are fed passively through a tube, a great blow to their self-esteem has been struck. When they can again eat, children sometimes are eager and cooperative; at other times, because of specific fears or a more general regression, eating becomes an activity laden with many affective and control issues (they can make me take the medicine, but they can't make me eat!).

Peter, an eight-year-old who had been transferred from two previous hospitals, was now many miles from his home. He had become increasingly withdrawn and irritable after many procedures and considerable difficulty with IV [intravenous] sites. The last straw came when he was placed on a no-food regimen. After this he became extremely uncooperative and almost totally uncommunicative. He eventually was set to be transferred to yet another, more specialized hospital. He said he did not want to go, but raised little fuss until the morning of his transfer, when he wrapped his legs around the bed and refused to let go until he had something to eat. He said even one bite would be enough. His doctor talked with him and agreed to let him have one pancake; he ate only half and was afterward very cooperative.

This illustrates the importance both of eating and of small accommodations when they are medically feasible. Unusual requests often are made around food, and can have a positive as well as negative meaning.

Bill, mentioned above, had had no food for almost a week. When asked what he would like to eat, he refused the standard fare for a few days. Eventually, on his own time, he said he was ready to eat something and chose a very salty fish dish that was traditional holiday fare for his family. He surprised his family and staff by not only eating and keeping it down but by asking for seconds. While some difficulties continued, this signaled his desire to move back to more normal patterns of eating, self-control, and relating to his family.

It should be mentioned here that intake of fluids is also a frequent problem, and has much of the same significance as intake of solid foods. Often issues of food or beverage intake become confrontations with staff or parents, in which the child takes a stand based on not eating as an assertion of self-control. Helping the child reformulate his concern around eating, so that the activity implying greater self-control is the act of eating, is a useful strategy in dealing with this problem.

The issue of "cares and procedures" also relates clearly to the treatment and to the child's sense of competence and control. Oncology patients are constantly bombarded by cares and procedures that invade their body—IVs, [intravenous punctures], dressing changes, bone marrows, spinal taps, biopsies, NG tubes, and *-oscopies, -ostomies,* and *-ectopies* of various sorts. It is little wonder that the issue of bodily control is a major one. Certainly, fears play a major role in the child's reaction, ranging from fear of disfigurement to fear of all their blood running out, to fear of bursting like an overfilled balloon. These must be dealt with, but are in general much more obvious than the insidious loss of control and of self-esteem occasioned by constantly "having things done" to them. This can be among the strongest forces pushing children towards aggression, dependence, and depression. In every case it is important to enlist the child's involvement as much as possible. This is especially important in light of the feeling of loss of control over the body occasioned by any disease, but especially by cancer. Even small acts of cooperation can help the child maintain such feelings of control and thus a cooperative and helpful attitude toward the treatments.

> *Peter, mentioned above, had been on the receiving end of so many procedures and changes, at three different hospitals, that he had no sense of having any role at all in his care, and would complain about and make more difficult the regular nursing tasks. Before long, the nurses here discovered that by explaining what had to be done and letting him do as much as possible, the cares could be accomplished with little struggle. While the cares took longer overall for the nurses to perform, enlisting his help made the cares easier and began to engage Peter in an active way in fighting his disease. He thus helped with changing tape, dressings, and even, under close supervision, IV changes. When his help was engaged, the cares went smoothly; when done "to him," he made them extremely difficult.*

Related to the issue of control in the face of numerous procedures are issues of control in the face of sedative or antinausea drugs, with side effects of drowsiness, loss of awareness, or dyscoordination. These can be very frightening to a child, and are highly overdetermined fears since they reflect in great detail fears of separation, loss, and death. Children's fantasies about the loss of control involved in death often include effects similar to the loss of awareness or control that are side effects of tranquilizers.

> *Cindy, an eight-year-old receiving extremely high chemotherapeutic doses, was very fearful of, and resistant to, receiving doses of Thorazine to help reduce nausea and promote relaxation. At other times she had described her feelings while receiving these as "talking to angels" and "thinking she'd gone up to Heaven." She did not want to "have to" go to sleep unless she wanted to, and was extremely resistant to receiving the medication. Rational explanations, while important to give, were not sufficient to allay her fears, which clearly reflected her larger fear of death.*

While this girl was able to receive the medication with some working through, the panic that the specter of loss of control raised is important to note. In her case, where other issues of control were not major problems, she was able, with support, to handle her fears.

Interpersonal Issues

As in all areas of functioning, a child's social relations are often greatly altered by disease, hospitalization, and treatment. Issues of a balance of dependence and independence are extremely difficult, not only for the children but for family and staff. Yet a balance of those forces appropriate to the child's developmental level must be reached if the child is to maintain self-control and feel competent in the world.

Michael, mentioned above, who had developed a manipulatory pattern with vomiting, had been very adept at using the sympathy of staff to maintain such patterns. At another hospital, the staff and family, feeling great sympathy for a young man with a terminal illness, had begun to take care of his every need. In an attempt to remove "burdensome cares" from him, they removed his active role in caring for himself, giving him an indication of their own hopelessness. He responded by insisting on more and more cares carried out by staff, until he was very regressed. His need for physical affective contact recalled that of a toddler. By yielding to and encouraging natural regressive tendencies (in a situation in which he must in part be dependent) rather than encouraging his independence or maintenance of the developmental milestones he had achieved, his regression was massive and required great effort to overcome. As he became more regressed, he became more fearful of his state and more depressed, leading to still further regression.

That cycle of dependence, regression, being frightened by the regression, and becoming more regressed and dependent is present in some way in almost every case, and must continually be prevented by careful staff monitoring of their own and family behavior.

One frequent issue in a complex case is the sheer number of professionals involved. Effective team relations is an important issue,[2,3] complicated by growing numbers of disciplines concerned in total care management. A young child's natural fears of separation from parents can easily be compounded by many professionals trooping in and out, no matter how caring those people are. They can heighten fears of being left at the hospital or taken away from parents. Frequent disturbance can also prevent a child from forming the close relationship he needs with a select few staff members in whom he might confide. Every person who interacts with the child places further emotional demands on him; demands as simple as polite conversation can prevent a child from working through the more significant issues at his own time or speed. Simple numbers also increase general confusion and stress level for patients and their families.

Of special importance is consistency in nursing care. The trust that develops between a long-term patient and a nurse can be a major source of strength for the child in times of particular stress. The assignment of the same nurse to a child regularly in the course of a hospital stay and on return visits is extremely valuable. It is, of course, also more taxing on the nurse, since it leads to a closer relationship to the child and family. This can at times be a treatment issue, and therefore must be watched closely by the nurse and her peers; provision of support for nurses dealing frequently with chronically or terminally ill patients must be made.

Another frequent issue in this area is open discussion of the patient's condition. Discussions among staff or between staff and parents often take place in a child's room. While it is important for the child to see doctors and parents communicating and to have a chance to be informed, a number of complications can arise. Children frequently misinterpret technical or jargon terms and invent very frightening explanations for routine events. Due to their not fully developed sense of time, misunderstandings can occur. Events that are in fact difficult, but which with proper verbal preparation can be adequately handled, are raised before the preparation can occur. Parents' reactions to new information can be anxiety provoking to the children in an unnecessary way. Finally, the child's sense of exclusion from control can be emphasized by a discussion in which the child feels more like an object than a person. All of these issues frequently arise.

Claude, present during discussion of a minor surgical procedure on his leg between surgeon and mother, interpreted the talk to mean that his leg would be cut off. While not reporting this fear to parents or nurses, he raised considerable fuss whenever any procedure was done, even long after the event that was originally misinterpreted, continuing to fear that his leg would be removed. Eventually he did, in panic, express his fear, and the misunderstanding was dealt with.

This incident points out not only the danger of discussion in front of children, but the need for careful and frequent work with them to help understand what will be done. Fantasy can always be, and often is, worse than the fact. It is therefore of great importance to help children deal with the facts without providing further grist for fantasy. A routine of the doctor talking alone to the patient and alone to the parent, and sharing information appropriately with each can be useful.

It is furthermore important to mention that discussions in the presence of "sleeping" children are a real problem, precisely because both staff and parents feel more free when the child "can't hear." Leaving aside the issue of incorporation of environmental events into sleep and dreams, children waking up or feigning sleep is a frequent occurrence when such discussions are taking place. Parents have reported numerous times that the child "could not have known, since he was asleep when it was discussed." Once again, care and consideration are constantly important in this regard. We do not advocate hiding information from children. One must, however, be aware that giving even "correct" information in confusing ways, or at times when it will be misinterpreted or not open to discussion, is tantamount to giving incorrect information. There is, of course, a need to answer questions that arise, based on the child's cues of his or her readiness for the information. This must be done honestly, to maintain trust and open communication, but in such a way that hope is maintained and adaptation facilitated. Flexibility and attentiveness to the child's need to know are the basic principles.

Interaction with other oncology patients is a frequent issue. While such contact can be extremely valuable, it must be approached and handled with extreme sensitivity. The affected children can offer each other a type of support that no one else can offer, and as friendships develop, patterns of dealing with the disease and treatments are exchanged, including coping strategies, fears, anxieties, and possible misconceptions. It is not a priori bad for children to discuss their fears with one another, and, in fact, it is often helpful. But all of the factors affecting relationships of children in more usual circumstances are at play here, including rivalry, comparison of condition, and selfish motivation as well as sharing, exploring, and growing. Of course, the physical condition of a child influences his feelings, and a child who is very weak, withdrawn, and depressed may not want to be with other children, or may frighten other children. Difficulty also arises in informing children of the relapse or death of a friend. It is unfair to expect any child to relate always in a positive, uplifting manner; adults must be careful not to expect one child simply to minister to or support another. Their relationship will, of necessity, be more complex. None of these difficulties is reason for discouraging friendship among oncology patients; in fact, the difficulties can become growth experiences. Parents and staff should, however, remember that such difficulties may arise and be prepared to deal with them.

Time, Change, and Adjustment

Because of the severity of the disease and the necessity of immediate intensive treatment, many of these children are exposed, especially in a first hospitalization, to many major changes with great rapidity. Some of these have been noted above—isolation, mobility restriction, medical procedures, complications with eating, chemotherapy, disfigurement, large numbers of strangers, a new environment, and the life-threatening nature of the disease itself. Adjustment to each of these factors takes time. For some children almost all of these occur simultaneously, with many additional difficulties such as surgery and anesthesia complicating the picture. The greater the number of changes instituted at a given time, the more difficult the adjustment period generally is. Modulating the pace of such adjustment, when possible, can be extremely important to the child. For example, a child confused and bewildered because of isolation, bone marrow and other procedures, and an exploratory surgery has many adjustments to make; beginning chemotherapy immediately can affect the entire course of treatment in major ways. If adjustment problems are evident, consideration should be given to a brief delay in adjusting to what has happened. This may permit a more mature reaction to the therapy, which can significantly affect long-term adjustment.

Amos, a 3-year-old with a lymphoma, underwent exploratory surgery shortly after initial hospitalization. Two days after that, a second surgery was performed to make a vein available for IV work. His return to normal mood and activity after the second surgery took much longer, and was in fact not complete before a third surgery, for the same reason as the second, was undertaken. After this third surgery, the boy was extremely depressed, showing almost no activity, withdrawal, general dysphoria, refusal of food, and very little verbalization outside of whining. Long after the physiological effects of the third surgery had disappeared, his depression remained as the only adjustment he could make to the rapid and continued major changes to which he was subject. Such massive disruption so overwhelmed this usually talkative, expressive boy that no adaptive adjustment was possible; instead, he withdrew from any interaction with external events or persons.

In every case, one must keep the pace of change and adjustment in mind; the more changes, the greater the adjustments that are necessary, the longer they will generally take. This cumulative impact must be taken into account in the total care picture of the patient. The child's sense of control and competence is affected by the quantity of change as well as the specifics of each individual adjustment.

The Whole Child

While it is convenient to discuss specific psychosocial issues separately, it is essential to recognize how these issues interact with each other. All of these concerns have impact on two broad areas with which each patient struggles: competence and loss. The disease, by its threat of death, is inherently a threat to all attachments and relationships. Loss and separation therefore become an issue in every interaction that the child has. Even minor events such as a parent's leaving a room for lunch can take on added importance based not on the real event but on its connection to the threat of loss. Similarly, the disease and treatment are a constant threat to competence and a positive self-image, and seemingly minor tasks or activities can have costs or rewards far beyond their typical meaning. Every interaction with the child is influenced by and influences these areas of loss and competence.

References

1. Geist, R. Onset of chronic illness in children and adolescents: Psychotherapeutic and consultative intervention. *American Journal of Orthopsychiatry, 49,* 1979, 4–23.
2. Koocher, G., Sourkes, B., & Keane, W. Pediatric oncology consultations: A generalizable model for medical settings. *Professional Psychology, 10,* 1979, 467–474.
3. Lansky, S. B., Lowman, J. T., Gyulay, J., & Briscoe, K. A team approach to coping with cancer. In J. Cullen, B. Fox, & R. Isom (Eds.), *Cancer: The behavioral dimensions.* New York: Raven Press, 1976.
4. Murphy, L. *Personality in young children* (Vol. 1). New York: Basic Books, 1956.

15

Psychological Stress in Families of Children in a Pediatric Intensive Care Unit

PETER ROTHSTEIN

In recent years tremendous growth and development of pediatric intensive care units has occurred. New units have been established, and new forms of therapy have been introduced for the critically ill child. Children who in the past were too sick to move are being transported to referral centers sometimes hundreds of miles away. Children who would have died from respiratory failure are being saved with modern techniques of ventilation; children with intracranial disease are being monitored and treated to prevent intracranial hypertension; dialysis is readily available for children with renal failure.

While our understanding of the pathophysiology of critical illness has increased, our knowledge of the psychological impact of critical illness on the child and his family is still quite rudimentary. Because illness severe enough to warrant hospitalization in

Reprinted in abridged form from *Pediatric Clinics of North America,* August 1980, *27,* 613–620.

PETER ROTHSTEIN • Department of Anesthesiology and Pediatrics, Yale University School of Medicine and Director, Pediatric Intensive Care Unit, Yale New Haven Hospital, New Haven, Connecticut 06504.

an intensive care unit (ICU) is so far removed from the everyday experience of most people, even stable families need help in coping with the psychological and emotional distress associated with the hospitalization of a child.

As progress is made in the practice of intensive care medicine, attention must be also given to the families of patients. Major investments in time must be made by the ICU staff to help parents cope with the period of acute hospitalization; for parents of children who die, this support must continue after the child's death. Hospitalization of a child is a stress-producing situation for a family. When the illness is severe, when there has been little or no preparation for hospitalization, when the etiology is not always clear, and when the outcome is often uncertain, stress will be increased. Awareness of how families deal with the stress of the ICU allows us to help them deal with that stress and provide support to the family at this critical time.

Patterns of Parental Reactions

The family of the previously healthy child who is admitted with severe life-threatening disease will be stressed most severely by hospitalization in the ICU and is most prone to be disrupted.[4] Studies in the Pediatric ICU at Yale-New Haven Hospital have shown that initially all parents go through a period of overwhelming shock and disbelief accompanied by a feeling of helplessness. Information given to parents during this time often has to be repeated several hours later and over the course of the succeeding several days. This phase of parental shock lasts as long as the child is unstable and may be intensified by sleep deprivation. For most parents, the initial stage of overwhelming shock passes during the first day. However, when the child is in an unstable condition without signs of improvement and when more complex modalities of therapy are introduced to support organ systems, the initial stage of shock may last many days. The shock and disbelief experienced by the parents may be intensified by the physical appearance of the child as a result of trauma, dermatologic manifestations of the disease, bandages, endotracheal tubes, chest tubes, monitoring lines, and urinary catheters.

During the hours following admission of the child to the ICU, parents grope for explanations and causes for the illness. It is incomprehensible to them that their previously healthy child is now so sick. For children in whom the diagnosis and etiology are clear cut, parents will search for the reason that their particular child became ill. When the precise etiology is not known, parents seem to be more anxious. Not only is their child critically ill, but the physicians are not sure of the cause.

Because of the inability to explain why the child is so ill, all parents experience a period of self-blame. Had they disregarded earlier signs of illness? Did the child become ill because of an appointment missed at the well child clinic? If they had been able to stop the child's vomiting, would the child still have developed Reye syndrome? Many parents choose to explain the child's illness as a manifestation of either God's will or God's punishment of the parents through the child.

Once the child has stabilized in the ICU and survival seems likely, the phase of parental shock merges into one of anticipatory waiting. Parents become concerned over the long-term effects of the disease on the brain, lungs, and other organs. Will the child be brain damaged? Will there be a need for amputation or reconstructive surgery? It is during this time that the parents watch the monitor at the child's bedside and eagerly look for signs of change. The parents focus on insignificant changes in heart rate, blood pressure, or intracranial pressure, hoping to see immediate improvement. During this waiting time parents are more demanding of the staff, and anger may be expressed toward the staff when progress is slow. The guilt and helplessness that parents experience during the early stages of the child's illness are carried over into the period of waiting. These feelings do not begin to subside until the child starts to show marked improvement.

A small number of parents find themselves unable to be with their child. The sight of the child may be too overwhelming. In some instances, parents are afraid of losing control of emotions and of crying in the presence of spouses or staff.

EXAMPLE. *A 12-year-old boy was admitted in status epilepticus caused by California encephalitis. The child required mechanical ventilation and despite very high doses of anticonvulsants, the seizures were difficult to control. On the day following admission, the boy's father was hesitant about visiting his son. Overwhelmed by the tragedy, it was only with great difficulty that he was able to express grief or sadness. Following discussions with the staff, he was able to talk more about what he was feeling and was then able to be with his son.*

Most parents initially understand little about the pathophysiology of the disease affecting their child. During the period of anticipatory waiting, the questions the parents ask of staff reflect a range of understanding of illness from primitive to the sophisticated.

After anticipatory waiting, the next parental reaction is elation or mourning. As the time approaches when the child will be discharged from the ICU to a general care floor, the parents see the discharge as a tremendous step forward, even though recovery might be months away. This excitement is at times short-lived when it is followed by a long and arduous recovery on the ward. Separation from the ICU and its familiar faces and surroundings creates parental anxiety in the days immediately following discharge from the ICU. While the child is in the ICU, he or she is constantly surrounded by many physicians, and one or two nurses are with the child around the clock. Meetings with physicians occur several times during the day. When the child goes to the ward, he or she becomes one of many children and the level of attention is not as great.

A special problem faced by families of children in the ICU arises when a child is unconscious on admission and dies without regaining consciousness. Not being able to talk to the child and have the child answer the parents prevents the parents from feeling that they can comfort and protect their child. They are concerned about whether their child can hear them and if the child is in pain. Parents of children who have died may continue to blame themselves for the child's death for many months following the death.

When the child's stay in the ICU is a long one and when the child remains in a nonresponsive state, parents find themselves experiencing ambivalent and frightening feelings. Parents are faced with what appears to be a hopeless situation, yet they often resist thoughts that would suggest that their child will never regain his or her previous state of health. Acknowledgment of this fact is necessary for parents to accept a decision not to reinstitute mechanical ventilation should respiratory failure ensue in a nonresponsive child. Parents may resent the fact that their child, who is incapable of any form of interaction, may be draining precious family financial resources, yet feel extremely guilty about wishing that their child will die.

> *EXAMPLE. The previously described child with California encephalitis was in electrical status for four weeks. The parents felt tremendous anguish over the situation. If the parents prayed for the ordeal of their child to be over, they felt they were asking that the life of their child be taken. On the other hand, if they prayed for the child to continue to survive in a vegatative state, they felt that they were causing their child to continue to suffer.*

When a previously healthy child dies in the ICU, mourning is often preceded by and later accompanied by anger. Faced with the "meaningless" death of their child, some parents react with rage. This rage may be directed toward referring physicians for what is perceived to be poor care prior to referral to the ICU or toward the staff in the ICU for saying that nothing more could be done for the child. The period of mourning may last for many months and is an extremely difficult time for parents. Parental depression during the months following the death of the child may be more intense at times of special meaning to families such as birthdays, holidays, and vacation time.

Understanding Parental Reactions

To help understand how a family will deal with the stress of the situation, a comprehensive family history should be obtained. It is important to have information concerning family structure, previous patterns of coping with situations of stress, family experience with illness and hospitals, and religious affiliations and beliefs to help understand the coping mechanisms that the family will use during this crisis.

The period of acute illness requires that a family utilize and be offered every possible means of support that is appropriate.

One must pay attention to support systems within the family that predate the present crisis. It is important to know if one parent blames the other for the child's illness. One should observe whether parents provide physical and emotional support for each other while visiting their child or during conferences with staff or whether they are distant from each other.

Previously established patterns of coping with stress will be brought to bear on the current situation. Parents will have various coping mechanism such as denial, projection, intellectualization, and anger.

> EXAMPLE. *A 14-year-old girl was admitted to the ICU with severe meningococcal sepsis. At the time of admission she was encephalopathic, hypotensive, and had lost circulation in her lower extremities because of thrombosis. Her father was an ambulance attendant. During the initial hours of hospitalization, any information given to the father was dutifully written down in his ambulance log book, as if he were recording information at the scene of the accident. The child's mother implored the doctors to tell her good news at a time when there was very little good news. During the first several days in the ICU, the family relied heavily on a minister for comfort. It was only after their daughter's condition stabilized, when she was awake and no longer required mechanical ventilation, that the father put his notebook away and the mother was able to talk about her child's illness.*

Families that have had previous contacts with hospitals tend to be less overwhelmed by the large number of people involved with their child and with hospital routines. Just knowing where cafeterias and bathrooms are and knowing faces around the hospital helps parents to adapt. Providing places to sleep and making provision for bathrooms and showers for parents helps to allow them to deal with the sudden disruption of their lives. Equally important is the need of the family for privacy during discussions with staff or at a time when they need to be alone.

A major concept that is central to our discussion is that the illness is a sudden unexplained event. Although the disease may be described in exquisite technical terms, it is most difficult to explain it in *human* terms. Why was *their* child afflicted? Many families turn to religious explanations. They see the illness as a part of a greater plan.

> EXAMPLE. *A six-month-old boy was admitted with meningitis caused*

by Hemophilus influenzae. *The child required mechanical ventilation during the first 24 hours in the ICU. In the hours following admission, the child's mother was convinced that the child would die. She would not believe information that the child was stable and that he was slowly improving. Two days later, during discussions with the ICU attending physician, she said that her initial convictions about her son's fate were due to "guilt—overwhelming guilt." She felt she was being punished by God for having had an abortion three months earlier, and that now God was going to take her son for her transgression.*

Many families will want to have their minister, rabbi, or religious counselor with them during discussions with the ICU staff, particularly when critical decisions are to be made concerning their child's care or when the staff must discuss a worsening in the condition of the child. . . .

Reactions of Siblings

Up to this point the discussion has concerned the reactions of parents. It must be recognized that siblings also need care. They need to be told about their brother or sister in language and concepts that are appropriate for their age. They have fears that they too may become ill or might have played some role in the illness of their brother or sister. They are also worried about whether their brother or sister is going to die. Siblings may be asked what they think is wrong with their brother or sister; if they have difficulty with verbal expression, they may wish to share this information through drawings.

> EXAMPLE. *An 11-year-old boy was admitted with Reye syndrome. He had a prolonged course with severe intracranial hypertension. During his three weeks in the ICU, his 10-year-old syster visited several times and made several drawings of her brother. In the drawings, equipment is faithfully reproduced and monitors and hyperalimentation fluids well drawn. Captions were included such as "He recognized me!" and "He is stronger than I thought." However, prior to his discharge from the unit, her drawings of her brother were reduced dramatically in size compared to herself, who she also included in the drawings. On the day of discharge from the ICU, her drawing of her brother suddenly increased in size to a true representation of*

*his size as compared to hers. As he was restored to health and her anxieties
about him decreased, she was able to restore him to normal size.*

We allow brothers and sisters to visit in the ICU when they
express the desire to do so. Before visiting, a member of the staff
will sit down with them and explain what is going on. After the
visit, we again sit down with them to talk about what they have
seen. We have found children to be very astute observers of what
is occurring in the ICU. It is essential for the children and parents
to know that we are available to talk about what the child has seen
and experienced at any time after the visit. Following discharge
from the ICU, the parents should know that the ICU staff is still
available to them for counseling.

Death

For the child who is beyond hope and who is dying, the
burden on the parents is immense. This is the time that support is
needed more than ever. If brain death is ascertained and a decision is made to withdraw support, this decision must be presented
to parents as a staff decision. The family must not feel that they
are being asked to make the decision. We have sometimes found
ourselves in situations in which parents could not acknowledge
the death of their child because there was still a heartbeat or blood
pressure. This situation sometimes takes hours to days of pa-
tiently working with the family to allow them to acknowledge that
their child had died.

Conflicts between Parents and Staff Members

There are a number of situations that create conflicts between staff members and parents. Denial is a defense that all
parents use to a greater or lesser extent. In its extreme form,
parents do not hear what the staff has to say. This happens when
the child is most ill, has the poorest prognosis, or is dying[6] (see
Chapter 16). Because parents deny the fact that the child is dying
or seems to be severely damaged, they may become quite angry

with the staff for giving them the information that they do not want to hear. In dealing with impending death, anger may be directed toward staff, themselves, a spouse, or God. When there is a problem with transmission of information resulting from either language or general level of understanding, there is great potential for misunderstandings.

Staff conflicts over treatment of a child inevitably spill over to the family. This usually occurs when two services are both caring for a patient and have different approaches to a problem. Such differences should be settled during rounds or on the telephone—not by open disagreements in the middle of the ICU, or by trying to engage the parents to take sides. Parents are confused by different options and generally do not have the knowledge to choose between different courses of action.

Withdrawal on the part of the staff produces tremendous anxiety and defensiveness in the parents. This usually happens when an attending physician does not take active control of the care of the child and avoids the family, when the ICU staff sees the parents as having contributed to the child's condition through neglect or abuse, or when the parents do not meet staff expectations in terms of visiting or conduct (such as the use of alcohol or drugs). Withdrawal of the staff sometimes is felt by parents when a child is dying. This makes parents feel isolated, defensive, and angry. The ICU staff as well as the parents must be supported when a child is dying, and they must be able to express their grief and frustration. If they cannot or are not allowed to do this, the final result is a chasm between parents and staff when the need for closeness is paramount.

Differences between the Intensive Care Unit and Other Pediatric Care Situations

Hospitalization in a pediatric ICU has many characteristics that differentiate it from other stress-producing situations in the hospital. A study of stress in families of children with leukemia has shown a period of great stress following hospitalization.[1,3] Many of those parents, however, knew or strongly suspected the diagnosis of leukemia prior to hospitalization and knew they were facing a chronic illness that might last for years. Despite this fore-knowledge, these parents also go through a period of shock and denial following the confirmation of the diagnosis. In most cases the diagnosis is rapidly established, and the parents are able to assist with their child's care in the hospital. They are also able to freely communicate with their child. Because of the rapid changes in the child's condition that may occur in the ICU, phases of parental reactions are not as well defined as in the parents of leukemic children. Denial, a defense mechanism that appears im-mediately following admission, becomes less important once sta-bilization and recovery start. Helplessness on the part of the par-ents of children in the ICU is to some extent augmented by the fact that they are excluded from taking an active role in the care of their child. Unlike the situation with the leukemic child, the parents of children in the ICU are not able to help feed their child, nor are they often able to comfort their child. For the child in a coma or the child on a respirator who is heavily sedated or receiving muscle relaxants, communication is not possible. The lack of feedback from the child and the inability of the child to acknowledge the presence of the parents is frustrating for the parents and adds to their feeling of helplessness.

In the case of the child born with congenital malformations, the parents had been expecting a normal child and a normal delivery, but the definitive bonds with the child had not yet been formed.[2] Postponing of bond formation is a defense parents may use in facing the burden of the deformed child. Children hospi-talized in the pediatric ICU have already established bonds with their parents, and these bonds have taken on special significance depending on the child's age.

References

1. Binger, C. M., Ablin, A. R., Feverstein, R. C., Kushner, J. H., & Zoger, S. Childhood leukemia—Emotional impact on patient and family. *New England Journal of Medicine*, 1969, *280*, 414–418.
2. Drotar, D., Baskiewicz, A., Irvin, N., Kennell, J., & Klaus, M. The adaptation of parents to the birth of an infant with a congenital malformation: A hypothetical model. *Pedi-atrics*, 1975, *56*, 710–717.
3. Friedman, S. B., Chodoff, P., Mason, J. W. & Hamburg, D. A., Behavioral observations on parents anticipating the death of a child. *Pediatrics*, 1963, *32*, 610–625.

4. Rothstein, P. Family reaction to acute overwhelming illness in children. *Critical Care Medicine,* 1979, *7,* 130.

5. Siegler, M. Pascal's wager and the handing of the crepe. *New England Journal of Medicine,* 1975, *293,* 853–857.

6. Waller, D. A., Todres, I. D., Cassem, N. H., & Anderten, A. Coping with poor prognosis in the pediatric intensive care unit. *American Journal of Diseases of Children,* 1979, *133,* 1121–1125.

16

Coping with Poor Prognosis in the Pediatric Intensive Care Unit
The Cassandra Prophecy

DAVID A. WALLER, I. DAVID TODRES, NED H. CASSEM, and ANDE ANDERTEN

When the pediatrician in a hospital intensive care unit (ICU) predicts to parents that a poor outcome is likely, he may sometimes encounter disbelief and even animosity. "We've told the parents their child's chances for a healthy recovery are extremely poor, but they don't appear to understand—they seem to be totally unrealistic" was a comment not infrequently made by pediatric medical staff and nursing staff in our pediatric intensive care unit. The physician may compare his plight to that of Cassandra—the mythical Greek prophetess of doom, who was cursed to see into

Reprinted from the *American Journal of Diseases of Children,* 1979, *133,* 1121–1125. Copyright 1979, American Medical Association.

DAVID A. WALLER • Director, Child and Adolescent Psychiatry, Department of Psychiatry, University of Texas Health Science Center, Dallas, Texas 75235. I. DAVID TODRES • Joseph S. Barr Pediatric Intensive Care Unit, Children's Service, Massachusetts General Hospital, Boston, Massachusetts 02114. NED H. CASSEM • Department of Psychiatry, Massachusetts General Hospital, Boston, Massachusetts 02114. ANDE ANDERTEN • Department of Social Services, Massachusetts General Hospital, Boston, Massachusetts 02114.

the future and not be believed. The purpose of this report is to describe the Cassandra prophecy phenomenon and to present our hypotheses about its meaning and how it might be dealt with effectively.

Report of Cases

To illustrate the context in which the Cassandra prophecy was made, four cases will be briefly cited; and examples will be given of physician–parent and nurse–parent interchanges that followed this prediction.

> CASE 1. *An 8-month-old male infant with telecanthus-hypospadias syndrome and multiple midline defects had increasing respiratory distress, eventually resulting in complete dependence on mechanical ventilation. Although the specific etiology of respiratory failure was never proved, severe small-airway disease related to a congenital defect seemed the most likely cause. As his condition deteriorated and all attempts at weaning him from the respirator failed, his mother was noted to be increasing her conviction that some type of medical intervention could result in a "cure." The multitude of daily medical procedures bore little relationship to overall prognosis, yet she focused on each as though it might be the long-awaited "solution," only to experience frustration as her child's condition worsened. She stated that initially, she and her husband "had experienced some disappointment at their child's problems," but now they had "accepted" the situation and were determined to help him "conquer it," a goal viewed as totally unrealistic by the medical and nursing staff.*
>
> CASE 2. *A 3-month-old male infant with biliary atresia and severe congenital heart disease, both inoperable, had increasing liver failure. Despite the hopeless prognosis, his parents remained convinced that he would ultimately recover. As he lay moribund, they filled his crib with new toys and blankets, a poignant testimony to their conviction. One day, when the futility of medical intervention seemed inescapable, his mother suddenly announced that her child was "possessed by the devil" and that he would be cured by an exorcist in two weeks.*
>
> CASE 3. *A 10-year-old boy accidentally touched a high voltage wire while playing, resulting in cardiac arrest and a period of cerebral anoxia of between five and ten minutes before resuscitation was begun. After a month in the ICU, he was still breathing spontaneously but was decerebrate. Nevertheless, his parents brought him daily reports of inquiries from friends and*

family, talking with him as they would with a fully alert person. His mother asked one of the nurses whether she thought her son might have to repeat a year of school after he recovered. The nurses and physicians involved with this case were upset by the parents' apparent inability to acknowledge the reality of poor prognosis.

  CASE *4. A newborn infant weighing 2.4 kg was admitted to the ICU on the first day of life, with multiple congenital anomalies and severe respiratory distress requiring mechanical respiratory support. The anomalies included severe defects of the heart and genitourinary tract. In addition, the child showed evidence of diffuse brain damage. Physicians informed the parents that their infant's multiple problems were not amenable to any therapy that would lead to survival beyond a period of months. This reality seemed not to be shared by the parents, who persistently clung to the belief that somehow all the heroic measures applied would result in the recovery of their infant. The endotrachael tube and respiratory connections coming from the infant's critical condition, were practically dismissed by the mother. When asked by the doctor what she perceived, she replied, "It's just like a pacifier."*

Results: Physician–Parent Interactions

  In each of these cases, when physicians gave parents an honest appraisal of poor prognosis, they were met with what seemed to the physicians to be a hostile denial of the realities of the situation. It was in the context of the doctor–parent relationship that parental denial seemed most extreme and the consequences most severe. Parents viewed physicians with frustration and suspicion since they were seen as possessing the ability to effect a cure if they really wanted to. One father said, "I want to believe that you're doing all that you can, but I just can't."

  In an apparent attempt to sustain their denial, parents often posed leading questions to the physician: for example, "Is his temperature down today? That's better than yesterday, isn't it? We're glad to hear that he's getting better"—in a case in which fever was not relevant to overall prognosis. If the physician, on the other hand, presented an honest opinion about the prognosis, the parent sometimes responded with a personal rejection. Said one, "If that's what you're going to say, I don't want to talk with you anymore." Out of an apparent need to see at least a confused picture rather than accept the hopeless one, parents would "play off" one physician's comments against the others' and would make accusations that they were getting "conflicting information" when, in fact, they were distorting fairly consistent messages. Parents found it all the more difficult to accept bad news from house staff who they knew were relatively inexperienced: "Wasn't there possibly some chance for recovery that the young doctor didn't know about?" Indeed, any physician can be wrong—fallibility is part of every medical judgment.

If the physician said that there was "always a one in a million chance," it seemed to constitute "playing a statistical game" in a situation where the outlook was really hopeless. But the parent would often seize on "that one chance" and assume that with work and enthusiasm, a competent pediatric ICU could turn that one chance into reality—why should not their child be the "one in a million" to recover?

Physicians had the uneasy sense that medical care was being dictated by parental attitudes they viewed as "pathological" but could not change. Medical staff seemed genuinely concerned that "nothing positive" could come from the parents' position. They feared that other children in the family were being neglected; that the parents' marital relationship was suffering from their exclusive focus on their sick child; and that the parents were being "selfish in not appreciating their child's suffering."

Furthermore, they were angry that these parents' reactions frustrated mutual understanding of the inadvisability of extraordinary heroic measures. They regarded parents who did not accept their view of the prognosis as "noncooperative." One said, "Why don't they get on with the grieving process—that's where they should be." Physicians felt "not allied" with the parents and regretted "having to fight with them." It was painful "to be the bearer of bad news and to be made to feel that the parent was on the child's side, and I wasn't." One doctor reported he felt like telling the parents, "Wake up! What you're believing isn't true."

Physicians developed personal stakes in the parents' acceptance of their opinions concerning prognoses. When they did not, it was taken as a personal affront: "They were disregarding the physician's expertise." Physicians felt more inclined to tell parents information, and they were uncomfortable having to be receptive to "where the parents were," especially if the parents' views contradicted the physicians'. Sensing this atmosphere of disagreement, physicians were less inclined to attend to the child in the parents' presence, thus giving the impression to the parents that the child was being neglected although the physicians would dutifully attend to the child once the parents left the room.

Interactions between Parents and Nurses

Relationships between nurses and parents were sometimes as strained as those involving parents and physicians. As part of their denial of their child's poor prognosis, parents viewed nurses with suspicion for "not doing enough." They accused the nurses of outright neglect in one instance. Nurses felt resentful toward the parents, and they missed the positive parental support that is usually given nurses even in tragic cases with a poor outlook. One nurse said that she began to doubt her own competence when parental support was lacking. The parents in these cases tended to "see past" the various equipment being used in treating their child. This equipment was testimony to the severity of the illness, but after a time, the parents in these cases no longer saw their children as critically ill. They became totally immersed in the details of day-to-day medical and nursing procedures as though each held the key to realizing the possibility of recovery. In a sense, then, parents were often isolated psychologically from the medical and nursing staff since staff members could not share their belief in the real possibility of recovery. In view of the relatively unrewarding medical, and nonsupportive psychological, aspects of these cases, nurses sometimes found themselves hoping not to be assigned to the care of that child and yet felt guilty about that hope.

Outcome of Cases

The children in cases 1, 2, and 4 unfortunately followed the courses their physicians had predicted for them and eventually died despite valiant attempts to reverse the courses of their illnesses. But to the amazement of all but his parents, the child in case 3 made a miraculous recovery. Every clinical and laboratory indicator (length of coma; decerebrate behavior; persistent, "diffuse, slow-wave, low voltage" EEG, brain scan evidence of cortical atrophy) pointed to a prognosis at best of severe handicap, with a significant chance of surviving in a nearly vegetative state. Three months later, he was playing outside with friends; learning to ride his bicycle again; and being tutored at home because of some learning difficulties, with an especially pronounced defect in short-term memory. The parents described his personality as quieter and "more pleasant" than before his accident. His speech at the time of follow-up examination seemed less spontaneous. Many of the staff found the reality of his overall recovery as difficult to believe as the reality of poor prognosis had been for the parents.

Comment

In an attempt to generate hypotheses concerning the meaning of the Cassandra prophecy phenomenon, a series of team meetings was held involving members of the unit's medical staff, social service staff, and consulting psychiatrists. One way of understanding the observations in this report is that in coping with the tragedy of poor prognosis on the pediatric ICU, parents and staff may have used conflicting coping mechanisms.

Coping with Poor Prognosis: Parental Denial

In 1955, Richmond and Waisman[1] described how parents facing the impending loss of their child from malignant disease experienced painful feelings of sadness, emptiness, and guilt. Some of the reasons parents in the present report felt guilty were for passing on a genetic condition, for having a child at age 35 when risks were greater, and for not starting adequate resuscitation in time. Denial can be defined as the conscious or unconscious repudiation of part or all of the meaning of an event to allay fear, anxiety, or other unpleasant feelings.[2] Friedman et al.[3]

noted that parental denial of the seriousness of illness and prognosis was generally present in greater or lesser degree and served, along with other defense patterns and coping mechanisms, to buffer the parent in a helpful way from the impact of having a child with a fatal disease. Illustrative of the maladaptive aspect of the absence of denial was the instance of a father who wanted to be with his son, but who found it intolerable to do so because he was so preoccupied with thoughts of the boy ultimately dying.

One explanation for apparent extreme denial in the situations described in this report is that for some parents, painful feelings were unbearable, to the point where they had to convince themselves that the events causing the intolerable pain were not really happening. "Partializing," or focusing on one small aspect of the child's condition or treatment, is a related coping mechanism. For example, the concept of fluctuation in body temperature as an indicator of advancing or resolving illness is a familiar one, making it more understandable that a parent in this situation might focus on a downward turn in fever as a hopeful sign, even to the point of disregarding what might be more relevant data. Similarly, laboratory tests, mechanical life supports, and other means of diagnosis and treatment are the concrete representations of attempts to help, and parents may become immersed in the minute details of one or more of these matters, seemingly excluding from awareness other, more general data that are more important, but that are also intolerably painful in implication.

The nature of the children's medical problems and of the pediatric ICU setting may have combined to foster the extreme parental denial in these cases. The patients in this report followed a long course characterized by neither recovering nor dying, for a long period of time. Usually, on the ICU, time resolved the direction of patients' courses much more rapidly. Whereas the outlooks for all of these children were grim, their situations differed from that of the child who is dying from a fatal form of cancer, in that the parents did not as readily associate these conditions with the possibility of death. The situations were more analogous to the common outpatient one involving a seriously retarded child, whose parents cling to the hope that if only appropriate help can be obtained, their child will recover completely and avoid lifelong handicap.

Indeed, it is the goal of the pediatric ICU to provide intensive care to children until they recover sufficiently to be transferred to other facilities. For the child with an essentially hopeless prognosis to be treated in the ICU is a contradiction in terms, and this gives the parents a double message: "We are providing intensive care, doing everything we can, and will continue to; but there is no hope." Whereas a chronic care facility might have as a goal that of making a child more comfortable, the orientation of a pediatric ICU is that of saving the child's life. Moreover, the fact that it is a *pediatric* ICU gives special meaning to the aggressive efforts to save the child. They imply feelings of hope, often absent when serious illness interrupts the life of an adult. Few can bear denying a child the chance for a life to be lived.

Coping with Poor Prognosis: The "Hanging of Crepe"

Just as denial is an important defense mechanism enabling some parents to cope with the painful reality of their child's poor prognosis, so is predicting a grave outcome a means by which the physician copes with the painful reality of having as his patient a child he may not be able to cure. The defensive aspects of predicting outcome can easily be obscured by the fact that it is part of the physician's job to inform parents of the outlook for their child; and in all of the cases reported here, the content of the prediction was logical and rational. We must ask, however, what feelings might prompt a physician to give parents a particular prediction at a particular time and to continue confronting parents with that information when it seems they are having difficulty hearing it.

In a recent description of "the doctor's job," Oken[4] noted that an important psychological theme common to the profession is the denial and undoing of anxiety about death. For the physician who sees his job as conquering death and illness, each instance of disease progression "is not merely a task failure, but strikes to this core feature of his personality."[4] Siegler[5] coined the phrase "hanging of crepe" to describe the strategy used by physicians who in communicating prognosis to families, offer the bleakest, most pessimistic prediction of the patient's outcome.

Aside from its ostensible purpose of lessening the family's suffering if the patient dies of his illness, Siegler noted that this strategy could function as a psychologic defense for the physician: Since death is seen as inevitable, the physician is freed from the responsibility of a losing battle; if death occurs, he is exonerated from what he might otherwise see as a professional failure.

In the cases reported here, the parents, having not reached in the course of their grieving the point of being able to accept a poor prognosis, clung to the reality that the future was unpredictable and denied the gravity of the situation at hand. The medical staff was more in touch with the reality of the likelihood of poor outcome, but they tended to deny any other possibility. Unlike Cassandra, no physician has the gift of divine prophecy. Though he or she may at times make grave predictions and be met with disbelief, nevertheless, the physician cannot see with certainty into the future as the outcome in case 3 demonstrates. Some physicians ordinarily careful not to overestimate their powers of prediction felt that they had done so in case 3 as a response to the parents' unrealistic certainty that their child would recover.

Moreover, as human beings concerned for the welfare of children, physicians are, like parents, subject to the full range of human emotion and motivation. One physician recalled that when the child in case 3 had been critically ill, each of his encounters with the parents heightened a sense of guilt he felt about not being able to make the outcome they wished for a reality. Repeated confrontations with parents about prognoses may be motivated by more than our well-intended desire that they come to grips with "reality" for the sake of themselves and their children. The situation may once again be analogous to that involving the retarded child, for whom Solnit and Stark[6] recommended a "conservative attitude toward prognosticating," based on (1) the expectation that parents will need time and help to deal with their reactions to having a defective child, and (2) "the awareness of the physician's own feeling of helplessness and resentment that his work has failed to produce a normal child."

Conflicting Coping Mechanisms: Denial as a Social Act

The conflict seemingly brought about by the physicians' insistent dire predictions on the one hand and parental denials of prognoses on the other did not occur between parents and social workers, bringing into focus the extent to which parental denial may have been in part a product of the confrontation between medical staff and parents. For among the most surprising and important information to emerge from the team meetings was evidence that in the cases reported here, the poor prognosis of the child was denied by the parents to *varying* degrees. When conversing with the parents, the physicians received no clue that the parents recognized how hopeless their child's chances were. The doctor's efforts to convince the parents of this were met only by increasingly unrealistic statements that the child would actually recover. As one house officer said, "The faith-healer—the belief in it—that's the ultimate extension of denial."

But the social workers, in each case, had been given some glimpse that the parents recognized how close to death the child actually was. For example, in case 3, whereas the father never indicated to the doctors that he considered the prognosis poor, he said to the social workers, "We will take care of our son even if he is a vegetable." Thus, the social service staff felt that the parents knew that the chances for meaningful improvement seemed negligible; why then did the parents not communicate this to the physician?

Subsequent staff team discussions suggested that the decision to prophesy to parents that the outlook was hopeless, arising in part perhaps from feelings described previously, meant that medical and nursing staff had reached an opinion not only about outcome, but also about the nature of medical and nursing care that should now be given—usually a kind of "pulling back." Physicians and nurses hoped that by sharing their prediction of grave outcome with parents, the parents would then accede to this shift in approach to care. But the parents in the cases reported here, viewed from the social service perspective, resented the medical and nursing staff's pressure to agree to a kind of "giving up." A mother said, "This child was too wanted to let go." One family feared the staff would "play God." The father said, "When God is ready, He will take my child." One parent said that if she did not maintain a hopeful attitude in the presence of the physician, she was sure he would "give up," and she did not want him to; whereas in conversations with the social worker, she discussed the poor prognosis realistically.

Weisman and Hackett[7] have pointed out that denial is a social act. A person's use of it will fluctuate according to his psychic needs. In these cases, it seemed the parents could not disclose to the doctors their awareness of how hopeless their children's illnesses seemed to be because they feared the physicians (and sometimes the nurses), learning this, would give up trying. But they felt more free to speak with a social worker, who was not giving immediate care to the child. Indeed, the social worker may have been more tolerant of parental attitudes because of feeling less burdened personally and professionally by the continuing poor medical condition of the child.

Management

What constitutes a rational approach to treatment in these circumstances? Physicians and parents in these cases reached differing opinions based on differences in the way they perceived the same situation. An event the staff viewed as evidence of hopelessness and failure was not necessarily seen in the same way by parents. The father in case 3 was pleased to report one day while his son was still nearly comatose that "it almost looked as though he was watching TV." A physician saw the same situation as a previously healthy 10-year-old boy whose "brain was now gone." Each interpretation carries a different implication for aggressiveness of treatment.

The boy's eventual recovery makes one wonder if the parent was able to see something in the situation that the physician could not, and it raises the question of whether the kind of care administered should take into account the prognosis. One physician postulated that the physician–parent conflicts described here might be avoided if the medical staff automatically did everything for every child, including starting extremely heroic measures and continuing them, without regard for prognosis—hoping for the best. Some parents, however, may want from physicians an appraisal of probable outcome and may believe that the kind of care administered should take into account predictions that a poor quality of life is likely to follow heroic efforts. Since the children in this report were treated, the Massachusetts Supreme Judicial Court[8] ruled that:

> the question of whether potentially life-prolonging treatment should be withheld from a person incapable of making his own decision . . . [is] our responsibility and that of the lower court, and is not to be entrusted to any group purporting to represent the "morality and conscience" of our society no matter how highly motivated or impressively constituted.

The following guidelines may be useful in the prevention and/or early recognition and management of the Cassandra prophecy phenomenon:

1. Information concerning prognosis is probably best given to parents, and best heard by them, at those times they request it, with appropriate attention to our inability to see with certainty into the future.

2. If parents are not asking for the information the medical staff believe they should have, it should be presented tactfully to them, with careful sensitivity to their degree of acceptance of it. Honesty is essential, but it should be combined with a promise of therapeutic commitment and continued communication; for example, "Recovery from biliary atresia may not be possible, but we'll examine absolutely every possibility and discuss it with you." When parents ask for miracles, the doctor might reply, "I wish I could promise you a cure; I do promise you we'll do everything we can to help your child."

3. When parents subsequently want further information, they should be asked first to describe what others have already told them. In this way, it is possible in answering their questions to build on their prior basis of understanding and to better recognize when a parent is having to resort to extreme denial.

4. When parents seem to be denying the prognosis, recourse to the other members of the ICU team (nurses, social workers, consulting psychiatrists) can provide insights withheld from the physician by the parents for protective reasons. A team approach may provide the best chance of achieving a clear perspective of the various aspects of reality in these complicated cases and of correcting for individual distortions.

5. Parents can be given additional emotional support so that

they are better able to endure the situation rather than having to resort to denial. Caplan[9] has outlined how physicians can help individuals who are having difficulty with grieving, as were the parents in this report: Engaging parents in a discussion of some subject other than their child's prognosis and talking with them about what their child had been like before the illness or about what have been their plans and hopes for their newborn seem to be helpful ways of reaching out to these parents.

6. We must ask to what extent our impatience with parents who do not accept their child's poor prognosis reflects our own need for relief from the pain of being confronted with our professional limitations. Are parental "unrealistic hopes" and anger at the lot that has befallen them intensifying our own feelings of frustration? Frequent staff meetings may provide the safe and supportive setting needed to address this important question and thereby enable medical and nursing staff to be more tolerant of parents who must bear the anguish of having a child who is gravely ill.

7. Situations may arise in which staff and parent positions are so polarized as to preclude resolution with the interventions. An example might be the child being maintained on a respirator who is determined by physicians to be dead, but whose parents will not permit discontinuation of life-support systems. It may be impossible for some parents ever to see the familiar physical form of their child, with some physiologic function maintained, as "lifeless." A court ruling may become necessary, but one would hope that with empathic understanding, with identification of staff attitudes that may be perpetuating confrontation, and with the passage of time, communication between staff and parents could be restored, and eventually, a mutually acceptable decision could be reached.

In the case of a child with a poor prognosis, relationships between doctor and family, and among the members of the pediatric ICU team, seem to be extremely important, and these relationships may influence medical decisions. Careful attention to these interpersonal relationships from the outset may result in the kind of working alliance and the sharing of concerns that can provide strength and possibly a degree of satisfaction in situations which tax the coping skills of everyone.

ACKNOWLEDGMENTS

The nursing personnel of the Massachusetts General Hospital Pediatric Intensive Care Unit, Boston, contributed to the preparation of this article.

References

1. Richmond, J. B., & Waisman, H. A. Psychologic aspects of management of children with malignant diseases. *American Journal of Diseases of Children*, 1955, *89,* 42–47.
2. Weisman, A. D., & Hackett, T. P. Predilection to death: Death and dying as a psychiatric problem. *Psychosomatic Medicine*, 1961, *23,* 232–256.
3. Friedman, S. B., Chodoff, P., Mason, J. W., & Hamburg, D. A. Behavioral observations on parents anticipating the death of a child. *Pediatrics*, 1963, *32,* 610–625.
4. Oken, D. The doctor's job: An update. *Psychosomatic Medicine*, 1978, *40,* 449–461.
5. Siegler, M. Pascal's wager and the hanging of crepe. *New England Journal of Medicine*, 1975, *293,* 853–857.
6. Solnit, A. J., & Stark, M. H. Mourning and the birth of a defective child. *Psychoanalytic Study of the Child*, 1961, *16,* 523–537.
7. Weisman, A. D., & Hackett, T. P. Denial as a social act. In S. Levin & R. Kahana (Eds.), *Geriatric psychiatry: Creativity, reminiscing and dying.* New York: International University Press, 1966.
8. *Superintendent of Belchertown State School* vs. *Saikewicz,*—Mass—, 370 NE 2d 417, 1977.
9. Caplan, G. Practical steps for the family physician in the prevention of emotional disorder. *JAMA*, 1959, *170,* 1497–1506.

VII

The Crisis of Treatment
Bone Marrow Transplantation

Radical experimental treatment sometimes is the only option remaining to a patient. One such treatment, bone marrow transplantation, provides a final, slim hope for patients who otherwise are destined to die of leukemia, immunodeficiency, or severe aplastic anemia (an acquired disease in which the bone marrow fails to produce normal blood cells). In this procedure, the patient's own malignant or deficient bone marrow is destroyed by total body irradiation or chemotherapy and is replaced by bone marrow from a healthy, immunologically compatible donor, usually a sibling (for an overview of the issues involved in bone marrow transplantation, see Thomas[6]). Although the transplant offers a chance for cure, it is a life-threatening procedure that may lead to a more painful and troubled death than would the disease itself. At a time when their life hangs in the balance, patients face extreme discomfort and isolation in an alien treatment setting—a germ-free room in which they are not allowed to have direct physical contact with other people.

Coping with the painful treatment and the isolation of a protected environment is a formidable challenge for patients and their families.[2] Children feel especially helpless in the face of multiple painful procedures and may try to reduce their tension by venting anger at the nursing staff or their parents. Some children deny symptoms in order to avoid further tests, whereas others try to gain control over their situation by refusing to eat or hesitating to take medications (see Chapter 14). Some children seek to meet their need for physical contact by asking to be kissed and hugged through the barrier curtains. Lack of privacy is also a problem, as patients suffer from the "fishbowl" effect while in isolation. One man coped by keeping the curtains of his room closed for prolonged periods of time.[5] Although patients want privacy, they also rely on contacts with other patients to assimilate the transplant experience. Patients identify with each other and judge their progress by what happens to their peers (see Chapter 9 for the use of similar coping mechanisms by leukemia patients in remission). Shared experiences enable patients to reassure each other, but when one patient dies, the survivors suffer emotional turmoil and grief as well as the fear that they will also die.[3]

Bone marrow transplantation is especially trying for parents because they may regret the decision to subject their child to the pain and risk of treatment. Parents who watch their child become progressively weaker during total body irradiation see the procedure as an "execution." In general, parents cope with the emotional strain of the transplant experience by hovering over their ill child and seeking information and support from staff and parents of other transplant patients.[1,4] Friends and relatives may be less salient sources of emotional aid at this time because it is hard for them to comprehend the acute stress elicited by the child's rapidly changing condition.

In the first article, Herbert N. Brown and Martin J. Kelly outline eight stages of the bone marrow transplantation process and patients' typical psychological responses to them. Patients seek information in the process of deciding whether or not to accept a transplant, though they also try to control their emotions and deny their fear in the service of maintaining hope for a cure. As expected, the type and prior history of the illness shapes patients' initial reactions. Leukemia patients who have experienced repeated relapses see the transplant as a last chance and eagerly accept it, whereas aplastic anemia patients are more cautious and hesitant because they often are asymptomatic and less thoroughly convinced that they have a fatal disease. Once the decision is made to proceed, the patient's immune system is suppressed in preparation for the transplant. Immunosuppression marks "the point of no return" because the patient is left without adequate defense against infection if the transplant fails. Not surprisingly, increased concern about death surfaces at this time, although there may also be a period of relative calm and acceptance.

After the transplant occurs, there is an agonizing one-to-five-week wait to see if it will take. However, even the hopeful signs of bone marrow engraftment prompt an added worry about the chance of graft-versus-host disease (a potentially life-threatening immune reaction of the marrow graft against the patient's tissue). One patient coped with the tension aroused by his precarious physical status by carefully monitoring his blood counts and various procedures—a quite understandable response given their life and death significance. By encouraging his involvement in self-care activities, staff supported the patient's coping strategy and enabled him to control his fear.[5]

Anticipation and joy arise as patients prepare for discharge. Having successfully weathered the acute medical crisis, adults may think about returning to work, whereas adolescents plan to resume their friendships and school activities. Nevertheless, most patients have mixed feelings about leaving the protected hospital environment and exposing themselves to the risk of infection. Because an implanted immune system may take a year to mature fully, patients and their family members must learn to maintain a clean environment, prepare special meals, and carefully control their exposure to nonfamily members. Once at home, patients also must come to grips with contrasting feelings of being indebted to donors and others, while believing that they are entitled to special status as survivors of an experimental treatment.

The second article by Margarita Kutsanellou-Meyer and Grace Hyslop Christ explores the process of coping with the bone marrow transplant and reverse isolation unit among adolescents with aplastic anemia. Some adolescents sought information about their disease and its treatment in an effort to promote their sense of mastery. Some coped with hair loss and other physical changes associated with chemotherapy by avoiding mirrors to temporarily block out distressing bodily changes. Other adolescents tried to offset the lack of privacy by turning out the light in their room so they could not be seen by staff or visitors. One way to maintain personal contact entailed asking staff and family members to stand just outside the glass partition to the room so that their faces could be seen without masks. Peer contact proved to be an important way of coping with illness and isolation; telephoning friends and other adolescent patients was a popular activity.

Family reactions to the illness had a significant impact on the adolescents' coping style.[5] One boy reacted to his mother's excessive involvement and concern by becoming very independent. Conversely, a girl whose parents visited infrequently and expected her to function on her own coped by forming close relationships with the nursing staff. In addition, when parents are especially distraught, children may try to protect them by avoiding an open display of pain or fear of death (see Chapter 7).

Kutsanellou-Meyer and Christ also studied the families of infants with severe combined immunodeficiency disease (SCID). The knowledge that SCID was transmitted genetically was an added strain for some parents, especially those with another child or relative who had died from the disease. These parents had to cope with the fact that they knowingly conceived a child at risk of SCID. Mothers tended to be the primary caregivers. Those who functioned best had the support of their spouse and had come to terms with their grief over the death of other family members from SCID. The mothers' coping strategies emphasized information seeking and cognitive mastery. The depth of knowledge they obtained about SCID promoted their self-esteem. Another positive outcome from this health crisis was that the mothers set new goals for themselves such as obtaining more education and better jobs.

Because bone marrow transplant patients and their families are somewhat isolated from their usual sources of support, health care staff play an especially valuable role in promoting the coping process. Staff can help patients by preparing them for stressful events, such as the side effects of powerful drugs and total body irradiation. Moreover, patients and their families appreciate a thorough orientation and an opportunity to visit the isolation room. Staff also need to recognize that their own reactions may be incongruent or "out of phase" with those of patients. Patients may be depressed about the pain and nausea of treatment just as staff start to feel optimistic in response to positive lab results. In such a situation, staff members can be most helpful by acknowledging and empathizing with patients' concerns rather than by trying to counteract them.

References

1. Gardner, G. G., August, C. S., & Githens, J. Psychological issues in bone marrow transplantation. *Pediatrics,* 1977, *60,* 625–631.
2. Holland, J., Plumb, M., Yates, J., Harris, S., Tuttolomondo, A., Holmes, J., & Holland, J. F. Psychological response of patients with acute leukemia to germ-free environments. *Cancer,* 1977, *40,* 871–879.
3. Patenaude, A. F., & Rappeport, J. M. Surviving bone marrow transplantation: The patient in the other bed. *Annals of Internal Medicine,* 1982, *97,* 915–918.
4. Patenaude, A. F., Szymanski, L., & Rappeport, J. Psychological costs of bone marrow transplantation in children. *American Journal of Orthopsychiatry,* 1979, *49,* 409–422.
5. Popkin, M. K., Moldow, C. F., Hall, R. C. W., Branda, R. F., & Yarchoan, R. Psychiatric aspects of allogenic bone marrow transplantation for aplastic anemia. *Diseases of the Nervous System,* 1977, *38,* 925–927.
6. Thomas, E. D. Bone marrow transplantation: A lifesaving applied art. *Journal of the American Medical Association,* 1983, *249,* 2528–2536.

17

Stages of Bone Marrow Transplantation
A Psychiatric Perspective

HERBERT N. BROWN and MARTIN J. KELLY

Introduction

Human bone marrow grafting procedures were first attempted in the late 1950's, and since then they have been increasing in frequency and success. As progress continues in histocompatibility typing, immunosuppressive techniques, and intensive care procedures, even greater numbers of these transplants can be expected to be undertaken for selected patients with severe aplastic anemia, leukemia, or certain other conditions.[1,2] Concurrently, there has been an expanded interest in the social and psychological factors that may influence the course and experience of disease,[3,4] specifically including increased attention to the psychological aspects of organ transplantation.

The following report summarizes the experience of a psychi-

Reprinted by permission of the publisher from *Psychosomatic Medicine, 38*, 6, 439–446. Copyright 1976 by the American Psychosomatic Society, Inc.

HERBERT N. BROWN • Director, Adult Psychiatric Resident Training Program, Cambridge Hospital, Cambridge, Massachusetts 02139. MARTIN J. KELLY • Associate Director, Psychiatry Division, Peter Bent Bringham Hospital, Boston, Massachusetts 02115.

atric service that functions as part of a multidisciplinary team caring for patients admitted for bone marrow transplantation. The observations were made during intensive work with six adolescent and adult patients (three with leukemia and three with aplastic anemia); however, they also stem from experience with 28 other patients who have received transplants here in the Children's Hospital Medical Center and the Peter Bent Brigham Hospital.

Stages of the Bone Marrow Transplantation Process and Associated Psychiatric Aspects

The entire bone marrow transplantation process has been divided into eight stages. While we by no means wish to imply adherence to a rigid outline and, in fact, would emphasize that greatest attention be devoted to understanding the coping reactions and needs of each individual patient, we do believe that it is possible to anticipate specific psychological stresses at various points in the treatment course and to plan appropriate management.

Stage 1: The Decision to Accept Treatment—"Anticipation"

The decision about whether or not to undergo transplantation has almost always been made some distance from the treatment center. Because of this, patients are often unaware of specific procedures (especially the more distressing ones) and are faced with the task of dealing with tremendous stress while away from their usual social setting. Therefore, an evaluation of expectations and available social supports is made immediately for each new patient.

Like all transplantation procedures, bone marrow transplantation raises the hope of cure. The initial decision about treatment is often perceived differently, however, depending on whether the patient has aplastic anemia or leukemia. Patients with aplastic anemia have a less familiar disease and generally are not as frightened as the leukemic patients, who are confronted with the well-known specter of cancer and death associated with their illness. In addition, patients with aplastic anemia tend to be relatively asymptomatic and, therefore, have a sense of disbelief that their illness is severe enough to warrant an "experimental" treatment that is life-threatening in itself. Since there is a possibility of spontaneous remission and that the treatment will require many weeks or months in relative isolation from friends and families, they are understandably hesitant acceptors. Also, they usually feel that there is too little time to make a decision about the transplant—a feeling of pressure intensified by the recommendation, for certain patients, that the earlier the transplant is done the greater the chance of success. On the other hand, patients with leukemia have typically been through stressful chemotherapeutic and irradiation therapies that have failed to bring about prolonged remission. As a result, they are more likely to accept eagerly, often stating that they are at the point of "trying anything," while simultaneously fearing that "this is the end of the road."

Due to the experimental nature of this treatment, after several preliminary sessions to explain the procedure and answer questions, each patient must read and sign a frighteningly explicit consent form that outlines the entire bone marrow transplantation process in detail. The following example is included to describe more explicitly the treatment procedures as well as to convey some of the psychological impact of such a document and decision.

It is my understanding that I have advanced leukemia, for which I have received many chemotherapeutic agents as well as X-ray therapy. The chances of my responding to any further conventional therapy for any prolonged period are extremely remote and, when I no longer respond, my chances for survival become virtually nil. There is a chance of responding with a prolonged remission if I receive a bone marrow transplant using my brother, who is immunologically compatible, as a source of marrow.

I will be isolated in a germ-free environment, and will undergo treatment with extremely high doses of cyclophosphamide, total body irradiation (TBI), procarbazine, and anti-thymocyte serum (ATS). This preparatory treatment is necessary both to destroy the leukemia cells and to suppress my immune system so as to enable me to accept the donated marrow. When this initial preparation is completed, bone marrow obtained from my brother will be given as an intravenous infusion. It is hoped that this infusion of bone marrow will reconstitute my marrow.

The risks of this procedure to me are extreme. The preparatory therapy is probably lethal unless the transplant succeeds, since any remaining normal marrow which I have will have been destroyed. There is also a chance that the leukemia will recur. Even if a successful graft does occur, there is a significant risk of the graft reacting against me despite careful matching of me and my brother. This is called graft-versus-host disease (GVHD). This disease may vary in intensity from minimal to severe, but, if severe, it may be lethal. Another medication, methotrexate, will be given posttransplant in an attempt to mitigate this problem. Methotrexate can cause lung, liver, and intestinal damage. ATS may also be of help in treating established graft-versus-host disease.

Even if all goes well, my immune system will not function fully for 6–12 months. During this time, I will have to be watched carefully for the development of infection.

The long range effects of TBI include probable sterility, almost certain cataracts (vision is adequate using contact lenses after surgical removal), and an increased risk of developing tumors. Cyclophosphamide may cause temporary hair loss and gastrointestinal upset as well as bladder bleeding which rarely leads to permanent bladder damage. Cyclophosphamide will also contribute to the problem of sterility. Other long-term effects of high dose cyclophosphamide are largely unknown. Procarbazine may cause gastrointestinal upset as well as drowsiness, muscle pains, and joint pains. ATS is produced in rabbits and can cause rapidly fatal allergic reactions, nephritis, and serum sickness.

Using this procedure both in Seattle and in Boston, there is an approximately 30% chance of success. On the other hand, the alternative is conventional chemotherapy with virtually no chance for long-term survival. This bone marrow transplantation represents an attempt to achieve a long-standing remission. All of the doctors involved agree that a transplantation attempt should be made, despite the grave risks involved.

Accordingly, I consent to the procedure to the extent that I am legally competent to do so.

One must wonder whether such permission can ever be fully "informed," for most patients protect themselves psychologically from the helplessness and anxiety posed by this massive threat with defense mechanisms, such as denial or displacement, which maintain some sense of being less vulnerable.[6] For example, usually patients simply sign the consent form and avoid confronting the issues of death or sterility—focusing instead on relatively less threatening issues, such as hair loss or technical aspects of the procedure.

We do not know the total number of patients who refuse bone marrow transplantation, but of the 34 patients admitted for the procedure, only one patient with aplastic anemia and one patient with leukemia have declined treatment here.

Stage 2: Initial Admission Evaluation and Care Planning— "Preparation"

While the extraordinarily complex medical preparations for transplantation are being made, psychiatric assessment is simultaneously begun. We believe, as described elsewhere,[3] that a patient's way of coping with illness stems from the particular meaning the illness and treatment has for that individual. This meaning can usually be understood by evaluating the blend of three factors: (a) the nature of the specific disease process and treatment itself, (b) the patient's personality structure and past history, and (c) the patient's immediate social and psychological realities.[3] It is particularly useful to assess in detail the patient's behavior during any previous illness. When combined, these evaluations aid in anticipating characteristic reactions and, thus, yield guidelines for effective patient management.[7]

In addition to developing this kind of understanding of the patient as a person, the consulting psychiatrist also looks for evidence of current major psychiatric illness, such as severe depression or psychosis, which might affect transplantation plans. Psychometric testing may also be helpful as well as evaluating the patient for possible hypnotic or relaxation techniques to deal with pain, nausea, tension, or other problems later in the course of treatment. An initial care-planning meeting is held by the team at the conclusion of all admission evaluations in order to coordinate the medical and psychological approach to each patient (as well as to members of the patient's family, who also often need an explicit plan, such as a daily schedule).

Subsequently a team meeting is held weekly to review psychiatric or social issues in the patient's care. The psychiatrist meets individually with the patient about once weekly, but this schedule can vary greatly depending on the patient's condition and needs. The medical, nursing, and social service staff have regular meetings with the family, with the psychiatrist attending frequently, and whenever specific problems arise.

Stage 3: Immunosuppression and Entry into Isolation—"The Point of No Return" (Approximately days minus 6 to 0)

Shortly following or even during the preparatory immunosuppression with TBI or chemotherapy, patients tend to consider themselves exposed and defenseless—not only immunologically but also psychologically. This is viewed as the "point of no return," when the transplant procedure, with all its uncertainties and risks, becomes significantly harder to minimize or avoid. Unlike kidney transplantation, there is no equivalent to dialysis on which to fall back once the procedure has begun.

In our experience, this period is marked by a more pronounced concern, either directly or subtly, with death and dying. Patients talk more about the possibilities of their own death or speak in displaced ways about the deaths of friends or relatives. Often, however, a period of calmness is reached just prior to TBI.

For several of our patients with aplastic anemia, the unpleasant side effects of immunosuppression became the first time they were distressingly symptomatic and led them to wonder why they agreed to the procedure in the first place. One patient complained, "I felt good until you did this to me." It is helpful to stress repeatedly the predictable physical symptoms in advance to patients who have been relatively asymptomatic.

To avoid infecting the immunologically defenseless patient, our program routinely employs rigid isolation in a sterile room. This prompts concern on the part of both patients and family members about barriers to touching and closeness, and patients tend to feel more alone during this period. Teaching patients and families to deal comfortably with sterile precautions and helping to gauge how actively family members should participate in patient care are important nursing skills in this setting.

With the combined stresses of isolation and being unable to turn back, patients' personality features usually intensify. Obsessive patients generally require even more detailed explanations about and greater control of their care than usual, whereas more dependent patients may escalate their demands for attention to the point at which limits must often be set. In a specific and extreme case, one very inhibited patient became progressively withdrawn during this period, with a buildup of tension, fear, and somatic complaints that finally culminated in a psychotic reaction, during which the patient refused her critically important anti-thymocyte serum (ATS). She expressed the fear that somehow a clot from her hematuria was going to her brain and would kill her. This transient reaction turned out to be an expression of the patient's desperate fear that the high temperature that she developed during the ATS administration was going to destroy her graft, but she had not been able to express this concern in words.

Despite the intense psychological pressure than can develop, it has been striking that no patient in our experience has ever walked out of the isolation room, although threats to do so are not uncommon.

At this stage we are watchful of the medications that can directly produce psychiatric symptoms, particularly the corticosteroids and procarbazine. Also, the immunosuppressive effects of both cytotoxic agents and corticosteroids increase the likelihood of neurological infectious processes, which can then secondarily result in mental status changes. The possible psychiatric (and neurological) effects of central nervous system irradiation do not appear to be marked,[8–10], while the question of the possible interaction between psychological factors and the immune system remains speculative.[11] We keep the use of psychotropic medications to a minimum, so as not to complicate evaluation further. Relaxation techniques appear to be quite applicable for helping with anxiety or fear.

Stage 4: The Transplant Itself (day 0)

This central event is a paradoxically brief, uncomplicated, and relatively undramatic intravenous infusion. There is almost never any physical reaction or sensation. Patients may ask whether or not they should "feel any different now," or may express affection or concern for the donor. Nonetheless, the implications of such a profound giving and taking are not usually expressed during this brief stage.

Stage 5: Graft Rejection or Take—"Waiting" (Approximately days 6 to 35)

Unless there are problems with infection or hemorrhage, patients are generally well during this period. Some want company, others do not, but none want to feel abandoned as they await the verdict of whether or not the graft their life will depend on has taken. As one patient put it, "I don't think about the days that have gone by, I just think about how long it will be before I know about the graft taking. They told me I'd know in 6 to 35 days. I want to know in 5." Taking "one day at a time" is a good approach during this period, while also paying attention to each patient's calendar of expectations. If a particular event has not occurred when the patient expects it, this leads to unnecessary anxiety if the staff is not aware of the expectation and cannot clarify it. Dreams and sometimes nightmares about the procedure are frequent during this phase.

As the days in isolation mount, the challenge of making the room as tolerable as possible for the patient increases. It is helpful to have planned the gradual introduction of a few surprises as well-suited to the patient's particular interests as possible (e.g., visit by a sports figure, flower box outside window, etc.). In general, however, relatively passive or intellectually oriented patients tend to tolerate the isolation room better, whereas active types tend to be more disturbed by the restrictions of the room. An exercise bicycle is sometimes helpful for activity-oriented patients.

During this difficult period of waiting, efforts by the staff to be psychologically helpful or understanding sometimes result in what is perceived by the patient as prying or badgering. Trying to force patients to "open up" or "ventilate" is usually counterproductive. Being observant and available to listen tends to be the best stance.

Stage 6: Graft-versus-Host Disease (Approximately days 6 to 100)

The very success of the marrow transplant sometimes brings with it a paradoxically cruel threat to the patient's life in the form of graft-versus-host-disease (GVHD). Such a turning of the transplant against the recipient is unique to bone marrow transplantation, and usually results in anger and depression in the patient who feels unfairly trapped by this situation. One patient was so angry about this turn of events that he stopped keeping a diary because he "didn't want people to remember me as being as angry as I was." The depression at this stage is often deepened by the prolonged isolation as well as by the need for further immunosuppression (this time to control GVHD) with a recurrence of unpleasant side effects. One well-adjusted patient used humor to help deal with GVHD, commenting to his donor sibling about his rash, "Now you're really getting under my skin!"

Family members, who have usually made special efforts and sacrifices through the initial stages, often feel almost equally disappointed and overwhelmed by the seemingly endless series of life-threatening situations. The donor, who is often concerned that his marrow is hurting or failing his sibling for some special reason (one of our donors worried that this might be due to past marijuana use), may particularly need clarification and reassurance.

Stage 7: Preparation for Discharge

When the transplanted marrow is functioning adequately, the long-awaited preparation for discharge is signaled by the capsules of lactobacilli that begin a controlled "contamination." The education program for self-care out of the hospital is begun at this time, and it is always striking to watch how patients begin to venture nearer to the double doors of the isolation room that they had, up to this point, assiduously avoided.

Most patients now show a heightened concern with the issues of living, which had largely been held in abeyance. They, in effect, begin attemtping to pick up their lives where they left off prior to the onset of illness. Typically, adolescent patients become more concerned about their bodies and begin wondering about whether they will be able to keep up with friends of the same sex and be attractive to members of the opposite sex. Adults tend to begin thinking about their jobs and whether and how they can be parents or spouses again. As a return to more normal activities is anticipated, there is always an admixture of joy at the anticipated discharge and fear of leaving the security of the hospital. Repeatedly going over specific follow-up plans and lines of support is crucial to most patients.

Stage 8: Adaptation Out of the Hospital

Least is known about the psychological aspects of this stage of the process, partially because only about one-third of the already small number of patients make it this far and partially because of the logistical difficulties in following patients once they leave the center. However, one issue that has emerged repeatedly concerns the balance that must be struck between the patient's feelings of entitlement, being the survivor of such a challenging process, and feelings of persistent indebtedness, having needed so much help from the donor and others. In the case of one patient who had a successful transplant, the donor shortly thereafter died in an automobile accident. This resulted in major difficulty for the recipient in working through whether she then should try to be more like her sibling, out of a combination of guilt, gratitude, and identification.

Another predictable issue is the concern, both on the part of the patient and the family, about whether the patient has been permanently altered by the original illness or the transplantation process. One family called the patient an "aplastic anemia person" largely out of this feeling that she had been permanently altered. It takes quite concrete guidance from the staff to help patients and relatives separate the important, but relatively temporary, special precautions that must be taken when the patient first leaves the hospital from the fact that the patient remains essentially the person he or she was before entering into the transplantation process.

We noted that several (especially younger) patients who had become very involved with the staff during their hospitalization were quite concerned about being replaced by the next patient admitted following their discharge. It was important to emphasize to these patients that they were not forgotten. A psychological follow-up of adaptation out of the hospital (best done in conjunction with medical follow-up) appears to help the process of adjustment, particularly in the first few months following discharge.

If the Patient Dies

In bone marrow transplantation, the relevance of the topic of death and dying is all too apparent: Most patients are relatively young and, at present, more die during the procedure than survive. Failure is often heralded by several weeks of decreasing hope by both patient and family, usually in the face of accelerating complications.

We believe a special meeting should be held with the donor and the family about 1 to 4 weeks after the patient's death, so as to address unresolved questions and to screen for any emerging problems. The very complexity of the bone marrow transplantation process makes fertile soil in which painful misconceptions can grow. One donor expressed the concern that he might somehow have acquired leukemia himself through having attempted to donate his marrow to his leukemic brother—a misconception that represented his guilt and fear about being the only surviving sibling who had not yet gotten leukemia. Family members are often desperately confused about "what went wrong" and need to discuss this. Despite the harsh explanations of the odds against survivial, virtually no one ever expects the transplant to fail. Staff members also need a chance to review and discuss their feelings about a patient's death.

Although it is still the general rule that a referring physician first suggests the possibility of bone marrow transplantation, with the increased attention the popular press has devoted to this form of treatment,[12] it is important to inquire whether any family member (or friend) feels that he first thought of or suggested the transplant. Such an individual may feel or be held responsible for the patient's death.

Acknowledgments

The authors would like to acknowledge the special assistance of Dr. Joel M. Rappeport, and also to thank Betty Palmer, R.N., Rosemary Galvin, R.N., and Mary Ann Hogan, R.N., and the rest of the nursing staff on the Clinical Center of the Peter Bent Brigham Hospital. This unit is supported by the National Institutes of Health Grant 5 MO1 RR00888.

References

1. Thomas, E. D., Storb, R., Clift, R. A., Fefer, A., Johnson, F. L., Neiman, P. E., Lerner, K. G., Glucksberg, H., & Buckner, C. D. Bone-marrow transplantation. *New England Journal of Medicine*, 1975, *292*, 832–843.
2. Buckner, C. D., Clift, R. A., Fefer, A., Neiman, P., Storb, R., & Thomas, E. D. Human marrow transplantation—Current status. *Progress in Hemotology*, 1973, *8*, 299–324.
3. Lipowski, Z. J. Physical illness, the individual and the coping process. *International Journal of Psychiatry in Medicine*, 1970, *1*, 91–102.
4. Lipowski, Z. J. Consultation-liaison psychiatry: An overview. *American Journal of Psychiatry*, 1974, *131*, 625–626.
5. Castelnuovo-Tedesco, P. (Ed.). Psychiatric aspects of organ transplantation. In *Seminars in Psychiatry*, February 1971, *3*, pp. 1, 5.
6. Weiss, R. J., & Payson, H. E. Gross stress reaction. In A. M. Fredman & H. I. Kaplan (Eds.), *Comprehensive textbook of psychiatry*. Baltimore: Williams and Wilkins, 1967.
7. Bibring, G. L., & Kahana, R. J. Personality types in medical management. In N. Zinberg (Ed.), *Psychiatry and Medical Practice in the General Hospital*. New York: International Universities Press, 1964.
8. Soni, S. S., Marten, G. W., Pitner, S. E., Duenas, D. A., & Powazek, M. Effects of central-nervous-system irradiation on neuropsychologic functioning of children with acute lymphocytic leukemia. *New England Journal of Medicine*, 1975, *293*, 113–118.
9. Gottschalk, L. A., Kunkel, R., Wohl, T. H., Saenger, E. L., & Winget, C. N. Total and half body irradiation: Effect on cognitive and emotional processes. *Archives of General Psychiatry*, 1969, *21*, 574–580.
10. Payne, R. B. Effects of ionizing radiation on human psychomotor skills. *U.S. Armed Forces Medical Journal*, 1959, *10*, 1009–1021.
11. Amkraut, A., & Solomon, G. F. From the symbolic stimulus to the pathophysiological response: Immune mechanisms. *International Journal of Psychiatric Medicine*, 1974, *5*, 541–563.
12. Honicker, L., & Honicker, D. Linda's extraordinary triumph and rebirth. *The Reader's Digest*, February 1975, pp. 77–82.

18

Factors Affecting Coping of Adolescents and Infants on a Reverse Isolation Unit

MARGARITA KUTSANELLOU-MEYER and
GRACE HYSLOP CHRIST

The treatment of such life-threatening diseases as leukemia, aplastic anemia, and severe combined immunodeficiency disease has greatly increased at least the short-term survival of many patients. The medical treatments used, however, are replete with extraordinary stress to patients, their families, and the medical and nursing staff. Bone marrow transplantation performed within the milieu of a reverse isolation unit is a treatment of this dimension.

Bone marrow transplant in the last decade has become the curative treatment of choice for aplastic anemia and severe combined immunodeficiency disease and has resulted in disease-free remissions in up to 18% of patients with chemotherapeutic resistant leukemia.[1,2,3]

Reprinted in abridged form from *Social Work in Health Care*, Winter 1978, *4*, 125–137.

MARGARITA KUTSANELLOU-MEYER • Staff Social Worker, Memorial Sloan-Kettering Cancer Center, New York, New York 10021. GRACE HYSLOP CHRIST • Assistant Director, Department of Social Work, Memorial Sloan-Kettering Cancer Center, New York, New York 10021.

253

Protected environments such as our reverse isolation unit have been increasingly used to decrease the incidence and severity of certain microbial infections particularly lethal to marrow transplant recipients immediately after radiation or chemotherapy. These radical medical treatments constitute an overt confrontation between a patient and his disease with an absolute recognition that his disease is lethal. Marrow transplantation is an extraordinarily aggressive approach that offers the potential of cure, but also a high likelihood of failure and death. Early failure and death complicate 30 to 50% of transplants in cases of aplastic anemia and leukemia. Recurrent leukemia may appear late in the transplant period of 20 to 30% of cases. A summary of the extraordinary stresses would include the reality of a lethal illness; immunosuppression, including in some instances chemotherapy and the prospect of total body irradiation in leukemia; isolation from normal body contact with others; and numerous uncomfortable and painful medical procedures. The enhancement of the survivor's coping capacities presents a new challenge to the mental health professional.

Reverse Isolation Unit

The reverse isolation unit at Memorial Sloan-Kettering Cancer Center was, prior to expansion, an intensive care facility equipped with four laminar flow isolation rooms designed to maintain a patient in a relatively germ-free environment. The rooms had no windows and were separated from the central nursing station by a large glass partition that contained an intercom system allowing verbal access between patient, family, and staff. A small corridor between rooms was utilized by staff or family to put on mask, hat, and boots before walking to the scrub area. Direct contact with the patient was possible only after a 10-minute scrub and the completion of sterile dressing, which consisted of two sets of gloves and a sterile gown. The procedure was obviously time consuming and limited the number of people entering the room. Although the diagnoses treated in a reverse isolation unit vary, as do the ages of the patients, what is common is the added stress of the isolation with its concomitant drastic reduction in normal emotional supports.

Population

There are three different diagnostic groups admitted to this unit. The first consists of children born with severe combined immunodeficiency disease, hereafter called SCID. These are genetically transmitted defects. The second group are patients diagnosed with aplastic anemia, an acquired disease in which there is a failure of production of normal blood cells by the bone marrow. These are primarily adolescents and young adults. Leukemia is the diagnosis of the third group. At the time of this report, only three patients with the diagnosis of leukemia had been treated on the unit during the period covered. Leukemics treated with bone marrow transplants have been discussed elsehwere.[4,5,6]

Pertinent Literature

The available literature on psychosocial aspects of bone marrow transplantation and reverse isolation is sparse and derived from experiences with a small number of child and adolescent patients. Pffeferbaum et al.[6] studied bone marrow transplantation in 19 children and adolescents. They correlated psychosocial factors of parent–child interaction with survival rates. No statistically significant correlation was made. The weakness of this study is that it focused on only one aspect of coping, namely, parent–child interaction, and related it to survival. We have been impressed that coping is affected by at least three groups of interacting variables: (a) stresses of different diagnoses, treatment, and disease course; (b) coping strategies as they are available to the patient at each developmental level and enhanced by his or her support system (i.e., family and nonfamily members); and (c) psychosocial interventions provided by medical and nonmedical staff. Because of the interaction of variables, statistically correlating an aspect of any one of these to survival rate could lead to insignificant findings.

Brown and Kelly[4] described the psychosocial implications of the process in six adolescents and adults (see Chapter 17). Adaptive measures were employed by patients at various stages of bone marrow transplantation procedures. In general, our patient population differed in that all the 19 patients were either children or adolescents. The importance of the developmental level of the child in determining the impact of the stress and selection of coping strategies proved particularly important.

Stresses on Patients with Aplastic Anemia

Eleven patients, aged 2 to 22, were diagnosed with aplastic anemia (see Table 1). Their mean length of stay on the reverse isolation unit was 3.6 months. All but two patients had one bone marrow transplant, one had two, and another had three. Seven patients have been discharged and are doing well; two are still on the unit. The two 22-year-old patients, whose disease had a much longer history before treatment, died 8 months and 3 months after the bone marrow transplant.

The most severe psychosocial stress for these patients is the stark isolation, particularly from normal body contact, at the very time experimental treatment for their life-threatening illness is being undertaken. Holland et al. [5] have emphasized that the lack of direct physical contact is the most distressing aspect of reverse isolation, producing a sense of loneliness and distance from others.

Children and adolescents find their initial entrance into the

Table 1. Patients on a Reverse Isolation Unit

	Age					
Diagnosis	0–2	5–8	14–16	22	23–40	Mean length of stay
SCID	8	—	—	—	—	19.7 months
Aplastic anemia	1	2	6	2	—	3.6 months
Leukemia	—	—	—	—	3	3 months

isolation rooms frightening in a way different from adults. Children are more distressed by the separation from people, objects, and activities important to them than by the possibility of death. One 13-year-old patient refused entrance into the room for several hours until he could be reassured that he was not being abandoned by his family. Families also have misconceptions and anxieties about the degree of isolation. Even though they learn that they will be able to enter the room, they are extremely apprehensive about the possibility of contaminating the patient.

We have observed a fairly typical sequence in the way a patient with aplastic anemia and the family react to bone marrow transplantation and isolation. A phase of optimism and hope, excitement, even euphoria, follows the family's hearing about the treatment. A cure has been found. As the time for admission draws close, the patient's and family's denial is broken down by repeated descriptions of the following facts and procedures. Immunosuppression to insure engraftment involves high dose chemotherapy which results in nausea, vomiting, loss of hair, and increased susceptibility to infection. This emphasizes the severity of the undertaking. In addition, patients are made aware of the possibility of graft versus host disease, that is, an immune reaction by the marrow graft against the patient's tissue resulting in severe skin reactions, hepatitis, diarrhea, and occasionally death. The high possibility of developing lethal pneumonia as a complication of the immunodeficiency induced and the graft versus host disease process is also explained. Children, adolescents, and their families continue to express misconceptions about the transplant procedure itself, although it has been carefully described to them by the physician and nursing staff prior to admission and during the initial period of treatment. For example, most express the belief that the treatment involves a surgical procedure removing a bone from the donor and transplanting it in the patient.

Heightened feelings of aloneness occur when the adult or adolescent patients enter the sterile room. They express awareness of the "no return" aspect of the procedure.

We have been impressed by one further stress that is developmentally specific to the adolescent. The loss of hair and other physical changes resulting from chemotherapy and medical procedures cause painful feelings of alteration in body image. This could be further complicated by the limitation in movement which is part of hospitalization. Several patients stated they felt that they looked quite different from their previous appearance and refused to look into mirrors.

Special Stresses to Other Family Members

The psychological relationship of the donor to the patient may be another area of stress for patient, donor, and family. It has been observed that the adult donor has few strong psychological reactions to this procedure, especially when compared to the reactions of donors of organ transplants.[7] However, we have found that the child and adolescent donors often experience a variety of misconceptions and distressing emotional reactions. Careful attention to communication, such as giving concrete information on the facts about transplantation, is important for donor, patient, and family whether or not the patient survives.

The donor's awareness that if it were not for him or her the patient would die, can bring feelings of importance and pride, but also fear: What if the procedure is not successful? Will I be responsible for my sibling's death? Will I get the same disease? These are frequent questions and/or fantasies that may be expressed. There are also numerous idiosyncratic fears of possible damage to the donor: Will I be able to walk? Will I be able to continue involvement in sports? One 22-year-old donor worried that she would jeopardize her chances of having children. A Puerto Rican family expressed the concern that the 14-year-old donor's pain following the procedure was genital pain and that her sexuality had been compromised in some way. A 13-year-old patient questioned whether he would remain small like the 8-year-old donor since he now had his blood.

In addition to the emotional reaction of child donors, in three of the families other early adolescent siblings expressed anger and distress at being left out of such an important process. They resented that all the attention was focused on the patient and the donor. One 12-year-old burst into tears on the unit, saying that she felt neglected and left out because she was unable to participate in her sister's recovery.

We found that giving specific information and maintaining an openness to these kinds of misconceptions and reactions can be helpful. However, especially with children and adolescents, this is not sufficient. It is not always easy for patients and siblings to reveal these kinds of thoughts and feelings, whose suppression can have a destructive effect. Consequently, we have found that a more active exploration of thoughts and feelings about the illness and the treatment provides relief to the patient and siblings as well as important information to the staff.

Coping Strategies of the Adolescent Patient with Aplastic Anemia

The physically ill adolescent struggles with needs to preserve independence, autonomy, identity, privacy, and approval of peers. We have been impressed with the rich diversity in adolescent patients' and their families' ways of adapting to this experience.

The adolescent's need to know the details of the disease and its treatment is a well-documented phenomenon. This mastery serves to protect against feelings of helplessness and fears of loss of control.

George, 16, exemplifies the use of control of the medical situation as both a defense and as a coping strategy. He quickly made efforts to take charge of his medical situation. He watched all indicators of his progress, such as blood count and bone marrow test results. He set goals for his improvement, for the change in his blood counts as well as for the date of his discharge. At times he would allow a visitor into his room, at other times he would not. The staff were helped by the social worker to realize the value of the patient's control of his situation. This was particularly hard because it threatened their own need to be in charge of such a dangerous medical treatment. Tensions were created by the conflict between his view and our view of the timing of his discharge.

In marked contrast, John, a 14-year-old Greek patient, demonstrated very little need to control his treatment. His parents remained in Greece, communicating daily by telephone. In addition to attending school, John had worked in Greece on the family farm with his father. We surmised that he was not so threatened by the separation and the medical procedures because he had already achieved a level of independence. While in isolation, he was pleasant and cooperative, although not passive. He consoled himself by singing songs about his home and about separation from loved ones. He developed collaborative relationships with the staff that were mutually satisfying.

All of the adolescents attempted to maintain privacy by keeping the lights off in their rooms, making it difficult for staff and visitors to see them. The patients complained at length about the use of masks and gowns by staff and family and often insisted that people stand outside the glass partition so they could observe their faces rather than the indistinct, masked figures. When feeling better, most of the adolescents insisted on wearing their adolescent garb instead of hospital clothing, enhancing the maintenance of previous identities.

The amount of contact that the adolescents maintained with peers varied. Where ongoing communication was possible, it became an important part of the adolescent's efforts to cope with both illness and isolation. When there are a number of adolescents on the unit, they spend much of their day on the telephone with each other discussing the details of the day's activities. The suggestion has been made that closed circuit television might be a way of providing group services to these patients. One 16-year-old boy ran up a $900 telephone bill during a 70-day stay on reverse isolation. He was athletically oriented and tended to rely heavily on peer acceptance for continued assurance of his worth and importance. In addition, his contact with peers shielded him from an overprotective mother whom he often refused to allow into his room.

Another moving example of peer support of the adolescent was provided by a patient on our pediatric oncology service. While he was undergoing chemotherapy and losing his hair, his three best friends accompanied him to the clinic, all with shaved heads. In this way they tried to protect him from being singled out as different from them in a crowd.

The Effect of the Family Coping Style on the Adolescent Patient

We were impressed with the impact of the families' ways of handling independence and dependence on the adolescent patients' adjustment to illness and isolation.

George's mother had become overly involved with him over the past several years because of his illness. Her extreme anxiety about him and her overprotective behavior seemed at times to promote excessively independent behavior on George's part as a reaction. This counterphobic, sometimes dangerous behavior in response to an overprotective, guilt-ridden parent was also described by Agle and Mattsson in their work on hemophiliacs.[8]

Vicky's family, on the other hand, had high expectations for her independent functioning. Both of her parents had worked outside the home for a number of years, and the children had become accustomed to accepting more responsibility. They visited Vicky regularly but infrequently. Vicky easily substituted her need for her parents' attention with the nurses, welcoming them into her room and forming close attachments with them. She was also a very studious person and independently involved herself in painting and other creative activities.

Mary was one of nine children in a family that had recently moved to New York from Puerto Rico. The family moved because the father had been unable to find employment. They did not understand English well, nor did they comprehend the disease and its treatment. They thought that such a severe treatment meant that Mary would die, although this was not initially verbalized. From their perspective it was more important for them to put their energies into the survival of the rest of the family than Mary's (in their view) hopeless treatment. In addition, they feared that the 18-year-old donor would lose his job if he participated. The mother could not visit because she was phobic about the subway. The family withdrew from treatment for a period of time until the social worker was able to work with them and correct some of these misconceptions. It was also important for her to help them with their very real social and economic needs. Mary became passive and compliant on the unit, watching television most of the time and asking few questions. She expressed fears of leaving the protection of the room and returning to the care of the family whom she was not sure she could trust.

These are examples of three different ways that families responded to the disease and its treatment which further contribute to the diversity of the adolescent's coping style. This interactive diversity includes the specific disease, its progress and its treatment, the personality structure of the patient and his or her past history, the social and cultural characteristics of the family, and current situational and environmental factors. The social worker's role is to assess the relative importance of each of these and to select the most salient issues for intervention. The social worker's task is to enhance the family's natural coping abilities in this most unusual and stressful experience in order to optimize the patient's and the family's utilization of these stressful but potentially life-saving medical procedures.

Stress on Patients and Families with Severe Combined Immunodeficiency Disease

Seven infants diagnosed with severe combined immunodeficiency were treated on the reverse isolation unit during this period (see Table 1). Five of these patients underwent fetal liver and thymus transplants. The other two had bone marrow transplants. The mean length of stay on the unit for these patients was 19.7 months. Five of the infants lived and are doing well. Two of them died of infections at ages 2 and 2½ years, underscoring the tremendous importance of the technique of isolation. What to a normal child is a mild infection is to these children a life-threatening illness.

In contrast to the diversity of adaptational responses observed in the adolescent patients and their families as described . . . two common themes were highlighted by the infants in reverse isolation: (a) the impact on the family of the fact of genetic transmission of the disease; and (b) the importance of the developmentally specific dyadic relationship between the mother and the infant.

The Impact of Genetic Transmission

There are multiple forms of SCID. Certain types are transmitted as a homozygous recessive disorder with a defective gene from both parents. There is also a sex-linked recessive form which is transmitted solely by the female parent. In our series of 8 patients, there were six males and two females. One of the males clearly had the sex-linked form of the disorder. The possibility of a sex-linked disorder was highly probable in two others.

The feelings about the genetic transmission of the disease are a most important stress on families of infants with SCID. Mattsson and Gross[9] reported from their study of hemophiliac children and their families that "a crucial factor determining the common positive adaptive outcome seemed to be the mother's ability to master her guilt over having transmitted the illness" (p. 1355). Mattsson's studies on hemophiliacs are the only parallel investigations on the impact of genetic transmission.

We found that parents had more difficulty coping with the feelings about having transmitted the illness when they had another child or relative who had died of the same disease. In these cases the parents knew prior to conception of the second child that there were high risks involved for the child's health. In our series, four of the eight families of children with SCID had lost another child or sibling to the same illness.

> *Mrs. K. had two previous children die of this disease. It became clear to the social workers that much of her anxiety about Mark related to unresolved guilt, anger, and sadness about these deaths and that she subsequently displaced these feelings onto Mark.*

This also agrees with Mattsson and Gross' finding[9] that each of the mothers of the eight poorly adjusted hemophiliacs "identified her hemophiliac boy with a deceased relative (usually a hemophiliac) and saw her son as unrealistically vulnerable at all times" (p. 1355). It was also true for our families, however, that the fact of having previous children die of this disease alerted the parents to the symptomatology, making possible early diagnosis and treatment.

Initially, all of the fathers tended to be less involved with the medical treatment than the mothers were. In addition, three of the fathers viewed their wives as primarily responsible for the birth of a sick child and therefore withdrew emotionally and physically, leaving most of the decisions and care to the mother. This placed an added burden on these mothers who had already felt guilty for having insisted on bearing a child even though the chances of the child's being ill were high. Clearly, the role of the father, especially in relation to his adjustment to the fact of genetic transmission, was an important factor in the overall adaptation of the family to the presence of illness and its treatment.

The Importance of the Dyadic Relationship between Mother and Infant

Because of the developmentally specific needs of the infant, the dyadic relationship with the mother is most important. For all the mothers, caring for their infant in this environment was a difficult task. The lack of privacy and freedom to come and go is quite different from that which is possible in one's own home. The two mothers who had great difficulty in allotting sufficient time to the infant, and in using the time appropriately once there, were the mothers who were viewed as immature by the staff and who gave the most evidence of psychopathology. Compounding factors were present in the history of these two mothers. One had two children die of this illness, and the other had two siblings die of the same disease. In addition, neither of these mothers had emotional or physical support from their husbands. Two other mothers who had experienced deaths in their families from this illness and yet were better adapted to their infants and to the treatment situation presented an interesting contrast. These latter mothers had more emotional and physical support from their spouses than did the more poorly functioning mothers, and they seemed to have worked through their grief over previous losses and subsequent guilts more completely. In addition, they did not give evidence of prior psychopathology.

All of the mothers made use of intellectualization and cognitive mastery as primary coping mechanisms. Several of the mothers came from rural areas with less than a high school education. After a year or more on the unit they demonstrated an extraordinary amount of knowledge of the disease and its treatment and a greater sophistication and knowledge about the world in general. In addition, they revealed life goal changes for themselves, especially desires for higher education and more challenging employment. This increase in knowledge with a consequent raising of self-esteem proved a powerful coping mechanism. This also highlights the growth potential in good adaptation to crises.

References

1. O'Reilly, R. J. Immunodeficiency, severe combined. In A. R. Liss (Ed.), *Birth defects atlas and compendium* (2nd ed.). New York: National Foundation, 1978.
2. O'Reilly, R. J., Pahwa, R., Dupont, B., & Good, R. A. Severe combined immunodeficiency: Transplantation approaches for patients lacking an HLA genotypically identical sibling. *Transplant Proceedings,* 1978, *10,* 187–199.
3. Thomas, E., Fefer, A., Buckner, C., & Storb, R. Current status of bone marrow transplantation for aplastic anemia and acute leukemia. *Blood,* 1977, *4*(5), 671–681.
4. Brown, H., & Kelly, M. Stages of bone marrow transplantation: A psychiatric perspective. *Psychosomatic Medicine,* 1976, *38*(6), 439–446.
5. Holland, J., Plumb, M., Yates, J., Harris, S., Tuttolomondo, A., Holmes, J., & Holland, F. Psychological response of patients with acute leukemia to germ-free environments. *American Journal of Psychiatry,* 1977, *134*(5), 563–564.
6. Pffeferbaum, B., Lindamood, M., & Wiley, F. Pediatric bone marrow transplantation: Psychological aspects. *American Journal of Psychiatry,* 1977, *134*(11), 1299–1301.
7. Holland, J., & Gerstenzang, M. *Bone marrow transplant in identical twins,* in press.
8. Agle, D., & Mattsson, A. Psychological complications of hemophilia. In M. Hilgartner (Ed.), *Hemophilia in children.* Littleton, Mass.: Publishing Sciences Group, 1976.
9. Mattsson, A., & Gross, S. Adaptional and defensive behavior in young hemophiliacs and their parents. *American Journal of Psychiatry,* 1966, *122,* 1349–1356.

VIII

The Crisis of Treatment
Kidney Dialysis and Transplantation

Technology and machinery are a growing part of modern medicine. Artificial hip joints, pacemakers, and dialysis machines are used routinely in treatment. Moroever, the pace of developments in biomedical engineering and human transplant methodology has made the concept of replacing worn-out or diseased human organs an everyday reality. As with specialized hospital environments (see Part VI), such advances create new coping tasks for patients and their families. In this section, we focus on patients with chronic renal disease, who must accept the use of an artificial kidney and possible long-term dependence on a machine in order to survive.

Dialysis patients need to make significant emotional adjustments to the technology that sustains their life. Unlike a colostomy, which requires a few extra hours for care and maintenance, or a pacemaker, which can almost be ignored between battery changes, chronic hemodialysis involves prominent changes in life-style and major psychological conflicts. Specific aspects of the treatment often prove troublesome, such as the strict dietary and fluid restrictions or the 12–24 hours a week needed for dialysis—time that often must be taken away from work or family activities. Care of the arteriovenous shunt is another source of concern for patients because of the ever-present threat of injury or infection and because of its cosmetic effect. Moreover, many patients are plagued by a sense of physical deterioration and chronic fatigue.[1]

267

In the first article, Denton C. Buchanan and Harry S. Abram describe stages of adaptation and some of the tasks confronting dialysis patients. When dialysis begins, patients are hopeful that they will eventually get better and tend to downplay the difficult aspects of treatment. Gradually, however, hopefulness is replaced by fear as patients and their families begin to realize that dialysis is not a panacea and that they face an uncertain future. Some patients cope by adopting a stoic calm that helps them control their feelings. But depression and despair sometimes set in as patients move from acute to chronic adaptation and dialysis comes to be seen as a permanent way of life. Patients may see fistulas, shunts, and scars as symbols of their "bondage to the machine." Perhaps it is not surprising that one man shot his dialysis machine in a moment of intense frustration.[4]

Dialysis patients find it hard to preserve a satisfactory self-image and maintain a reasonable balance between autonomy and dependence. Most patients have experienced a period of severe, debilitating illness and have had to accept the status of a dependent invalid. Once they begin dialysis, patients are expected to resume independence and self-sufficiency outside the treatment setting as well as to accept their total dependence on a life-giving machine and the staff who maintain it. Buchanan and Abram point out that staff can facilitate the adaptation process by enabling patients to assume an active role in managing their treatment and by recognizing that both self-reliance and help seeking are viable coping styles.

Patients and their family members must also handle the financial strain caused by medical bills and reduced income and master the problems associated with filing insurance claims and coping with the welfare system. James and Anne Campbell have recounted the varied skills they used to deal with the economic aspects of Jim's dialysis and kidney transplant.[2] Medicare and private insurance did not cover expenses, and alternative sources of aid had to be identified. Consequently, the couple faced the tasks of searching out certain types of potential assistance, coordinating claims and benefits among insurance agencies, and meeting eligibility requirements that frequently involved disclosure of private financial data. They needed writing skills to maintain extensive records. Moreover, they had to contend with the sense of dependency and stigma aroused in the process of proving that they were "needy" enough to "deserve" financial assistance.

Home dialysis is an economical alternative to treatment in a hospital or a satellite dialysis center. It also affords patients more control over their lives because the treatment can be scheduled more flexibly. However, such benefits may be balanced by the responsibility placed on the shoulders of the partner (usually the spouse) who must help connect the patient to the machine and stand by in case of accidents or emergencies. In addition, partners often accept the task of providing comfort and strength and of coping with rapid changes in emotional balance that range from mutual sharing and pleasure to weariness and despair.[2,6]

The second article by Sally E. Palmer, Lino Canzona, and Lokky Wai examines family adaptation among patients and spouses involved in home dialysis. Family members who were successful in home dialysis shared responsibility for treatment procedures. They were flexible in their roles and able to convey their needs to each other and to staff. Moreover, such families provided an emotionally supportive environment that promoted the independence of individual family members while maintaining enough control to accomplish necessary treatment tasks. Patients and their spouses often experienced an increase in marital closeness, though strain was aroused when spouses overlooked their own needs in an effort to accommodate to the patient. Spouses and children who were able to take an active role in coping with the stress of home dialysis may experience pride in their accomplishments and develop a deeper sense of competence and personal maturity.[5]

As the only treatment option that frees end-stage renal disease patients from dialysis, transplantation is an emotion-laden experience for recipients and donors. In addition to the general problems patients encounter in the period of serious illness that generally precedes an organ transplant, there are specific problems associated with transplantation itself. These include the side effects of immunosuppressive drugs, the uncertainty of rejection episodes, and the efforts to resume self-reliance after a time of chronic illness and dependence. Transplant patients must learn to adjust to a sense of mutilation when the diseased organ is removed and to alter their body image and accept the donor's organ as their own. Recipients may also identify with the donor and believe that a transplanted organ endows them with the donor's personal qualities. Consequently, a man can feel threatened when receiving a kidney from a woman.[3]

Because only one kidney is necessary to maintain good health, one encounters the situation in which a healthy person may volunteer to give up a kidney to save someone else. In the third article, Elaine M. Musial highlights the issues that confront patients and prospective living-related donors in this situation. Patients are torn between the desire for a transplant and their fear of rejection and understandable reluctance to ask a family member to make such a significant sacrifice. One way patients cope with this problem is to convey their concern to a confidant who then informs other family members about the need for a donor. An active search and selection process ensues in an effort to balance many competing considerations and to identify a suitable donor. The family may want to exclude members who have special responsibilities, whereas those who have been involved in family disputes may see an opportunity to reestablish their family ties. (For a more detailed discussion, see the book by Simmons, Klein, and Simmons[7].)

The author illustrates some of these issues by presenting a case study of a young woman who needed a transplant. Each of Donna's family members expressed a willingness to donate, but the family thought that her brother might use his role as donor to manipulate Donna. Although the brother was a suitable donor, the physicians obliged the family by offering a medical excuse for rejecting him. Similarly, some physicians will provide a medical excuse for a prospective donor who changes his mind about donating. Although such actions can be effective in avoiding immediate family disputes, they also lead to family "secrets" that may have a lasting effect on family adaptation. Moreover, they are inconsistent with the current trend toward direct and honest interchange between patients and health care staff.

In general, there is a rapidly shifting pattern of emotions among all participants during the surgery and recovery process. Donors' uneasiness prior to surgery may be mitigated by a belief in the value of what they are doing, a good relationship with the physician, and emotional support from family and friends. When the donor experiences postsurgical turmoil and pain, anger may be aroused, and family members may regret their part in encouraging the donor. Donors also worry about the functioning of the kidney; they may feel guilty about prolonging the recipient's suffering and blame themselves if the kidney is rejected. With reassurance both before and after the transplant, donors and their families tend to feel that their basically altruistic act was deeply meaningful and worthwhile both for themselves and the recipient.

References

1. Baldree, K. S., Murphy, S. P., & Powers, M. J. Stress identification and coping patterns in patients on hemodialysis. *Nursing Research,* 1982, *31,* 107–112.
2. Campbell, J. D., & Campbell, A. R. The social and economic costs of end-stage renal disease: A patient's perspective. *New England Journal of Medicine,* 1978, *299,* 386–392.
3. Castelnuovo-Tedesco, P. Transplantation: Psychological implications of changes in body image. In N. B. Levy (Ed.), *Psychonephrology I: Psychological factors in hemodialysis and transplantation.* New York: Plenum Press, 1981.
4. Galloway, A. L. Emotional aspects of dialysis and transplantation. *Critical Care Quarterly,* 1978, *1,* 75–85.
5. Goldman, R., Cohn, G., & Longnecker, R. The family and home hemodialysis: Adolescents' reactions to a father on home dialysis. *International Journal of Psychiatry in Medicine,* 1980–1981, *10,* 235–254.
6. McGee, M. G. Familial response to chronic illness: The impact of home versus hospital dialysis. *The American Association of Nephrology Nurses and Technicians Journal,* 1981, *8,* 9–12.
7. Simmons, R. G., Klein, S. D., & Simmons, R. L. *Gift of life: The social and psychological impact of organ transplantation.* New York: Wiley, 1977.

19

Psychological Adaptation to Hemodialysis

DENTON C. BUCHANAN and HARRY S. ABRAM

After studying patients' adaptation to chronic hemodialysis in the late 1960s, Abram[1] described a series of stages through which a dialysand passed. When entering dialysis the patient was at death's door and much too numb to care about his future. Apathy was the general attitude in this initial stage. A period of euphoria followed when the patient realized he had "returned from the dead" and was joyous over his fresh start. After a few weeks of dialysis, a state of anxiety developed as the patient became more and more aware of the life-maintaining equipment and procedures. The final stage described by Abram was the struggle for normalcy the patient undertook in coping with his illness.

These stages are not seen as frequently today. In the 1960s there was a serious shortage of dialysis centers and much to be learned about dialysis procedures. Thus, patients were often moribund, manifesting the symptoms of end-stage renal failure at the time they began dialysis. Although this is still true occasionally,

Reprinted and updated from *Dialysis and Transplantation*, 1976, 5, 36, 41–42, 84.

DENTON C. BUCHANAN • Director of Psychology, Royal Ottawa Regional Rehabilitation Center, Ottawa, Ontario, Canada K1H8M2. **HARRY S. ABRAM,** deceased • Former Professor, Department of Psychiatry, Vanderbilt University Medical School, Nashville, Tennessee 37232.

273

patients more often are accepted into a hemodialysis program at an earlier phase in their renal failure. Consequently, the dramatic recovery "from the dead" and the euphoric return are not as common today.

As patients enter dialysis in a less life-threatening situation, it is more useful to view the adjustment process as composed of two general stages. These stages overlap, and reactions ebb and flow as stressors appear or disappear. However, the stages serve a heuristic purpose and also have been described among families of patients with chronic illness.[6] The initial stage represents the acute psychological responses of dialysands. A second and permanent stage follows in which the long-term adaptational process sets in, challenging all of the patient's resources.

Acute Adaptation

With the exception of the initial trial on the machine, most patients accept dialysis well. Their early reactions are hope for future well-being and anticipated benefits from increased efficiency. The family tends to be overly protective and concerned, taking on many of the patient's duties to allow him time to "get better." The concept of hemodialysis as a chronic lifelong treatment has not yet established itself.

Gradually, however, the hope for future benefits from dialysis changes to fear of an unknown future. As the patient and his family begin to realize that his activity away from the machine is reduced and that he may never feel completely well again, anxiety becomes a pervasive emotional response.

In moderation, anxiety is adaptive and useful to the patient. Anxiety may represent the patient's concern about his health, motivating him to comply with his regimen. However, when this vague and diffuse fear of the future continues unabated, the reaction can become serious. Tension, insomnia, and conditions such as tachycardia and hyperventilation can occur. Sudden panic may overcome the patient, and he may try to flee from an unknown fear. A more common response is withdrawal and reclusion from social contact. Occasionally patients will masturbate while being dialyzed. This can be interpreted as an attempt to cope with anxiety by inducing a pleasurable and distracting sensation. The treatment staff are usually puzzled by these coping mechanisms. After an apparently good adjustment, what went wrong? Often the staff will attempt to aid the patient on an educational basis, instructing him about the machine's function and the nature of his illness. Unfortunately, this only feeds the patient's fears. A better response is to encourage the patient to ventilate his feelings and explore his problems *as he sees them.*

Chronic Adaptation

The chronic adaptation stage occurs when anxiety over the unknown future changes to a realization that dialysis is a way of life. Despair and doubt replace an overly optimistic expectation of the treatment. The principal psychological reactions in this stage are regression and/or depression, although a variety of symptoms may be present. The patient may adopt a stoic calm that masks inner despair. Vague somatic complaints are common. The patient may project his despair by becoming suspicious of the staff. It is important to note that the defensive maneuvers utilized by the patient are unconscious and not employed voluntarily, though they may be annoying to treatment staff.

Regression

The patient may adopt earlier modes of behavior which he found comforting at one time. The demanding or overdependent patient has regressed to a childlike state, providing him with a sense of security and gratification. Thus, the dialysand gives up adult responsibilities in order to be cared for, just as the sick child is allowed to stay home with mother and miss school.

The extended family often plays a prominent role in encouraging the patient to utilize regression. They are concerned about his fate and feel helpless in aiding him. They often unwittingly encourage the patient to adopt a variety of illness behaviors, since caring for him allows the family some active involvement in the patient's well-being. The staff can be most effective in dealing with regression if they look for the environmental events that perpetuate the behavior.

Depression

Dialysands often experience feelings of hopelessness, sadness, and bleakness in their outlook on life. Much has been written of the multiple losses sustained by the patient, the continued reminder of his chronically ill status, and feelings of resentment related to changes in body image and decreasing self-concept—all of which increase the prevalence of depression.

Shunts can serve as a symbolic target for the patient's depression. Blood clots at the shunt site are not infrequent, and their occurrence is stressful. Patients can have the misconception that such clotting causes emboli to float through the body, perhaps striking the heart or brain. Reichsman and Levy[9] even suggested that as feelings of helplessness and hopelessness increased, medical complications occurred, especially clotting at the shunt site. Shunts also serve as a visual reminder and stigma. Levy[7] has reported that switching from an external, bandaged shunt to an internal fistula causes a significant elevation in the dialysand's mood. One of his patients stated, "With the shunt I was bandaged and I was different and always reminded of being different from other people. Now it's like I'm not branded anymore."

Staff members who routinely stick needles into this symbolic object generally are unaware of its hidden meaning. Such thoughtlessness (as perceived by the patient) is translated into the belief that the perpetrator is uncaring. If possible, the patient should be involved in the procedure to reduce his passive role and to remove staff from the "administrator" role. A recent suggestion that depression also may be reduced with lower B.U.N. [blood urea nitrogen] levels and shorter dialysis runs warrants further study.[8]

Conflicts in Adaptation

Independence

In adjusting to hemodialysis, the patient must cope with contradictory messages concerning his autonomy. He must passively accept the dialysis regimen imposed upon him by treatment staff as well as remain dependent upon a machine for the rest of his life. At the same time he is urged to lead an independent life away from the dialysis program. Despite his fatigue, lethargy, anemia, sporadic nausea, and fluctuating mental alertness, the dialysand is expected by the treatment staff to assume the responsibilities of a normal, healthy person—being employed, supporting a family, having an active social life, and so on. Understanding, establishing, and maintaining this split personality is a major accomplishment for the patient in adapting to his illness.

It is extremely difficult, however, to live a life with such duality of purpose. It is much more common to adopt one of the two extremes, either of which is considered by us [to be] maladaptive and "uncooperative."[2] One extreme is to become excessively dependent, submissive, and to adopt the sick role completely. Such an attitude of helplessness throws the total burden of care upon the medical and nursing personnel and places a heavy demand for support upon the patient's family. The opposite extreme consists of a patient's excessive independence. He may rebelliously refuse to accept the program's restrictions and be labeled "hostile" or "destructive" by the treatment staff. In its ultimate form, such personal independence is exemplified by the patient who purposely, deliberately, and thoughtfully removes himself from the program to die. Patients may react to their decreased independence by demonstrating their control in inappropriate ways. For example, we have a male patient who deliberately is late by several hours for his home dialysis treatment at least once or twice a week. He states that *he* wants to be the one to decide when to start dialysis, not his wife or a posted schedule.

Identification

Adjustment to hemodialysis involves a process in which the patient decides to what extent he will identify with his illness. Most patients eventually reach a mental attitude of tolerance without enthusiasm. They show up for treatment regularly, maintain their diet to a reasonable degree, and tolerate the program. However, they do not like to talk about their illness and, in general, avoid any "extracurricular" attention to their disease.

One extreme of the process is the identifier who becomes

totally absorbed in hemodialysis. Such a person may be employed by the Kidney Foundation in fund raising, may give speeches at local church groups, or organize tours and vacations for patients through other dialysis centers. The identifier is a pleasure to treatment staff and is considered totally adapted to hemodialysis. After all, he places his values in the same cart as we do—increased activity and benefits for patients. Such an adaptive skill does represent an extremely healthy defense mechanism, simply stated as, "If you can't beat 'em, join 'em." Identifiers receive enormous reinforcement and secondary gain from the approving communications and encouragement of the staff. "He is like us!"

The converse of the identification conflict is presented by the total avoider or denier. This person denies the severity or even the existence of his illness. He behaves in such a way as to avoid confrontation with his illness and fails to comply with his dietary and medication regimen. In its ultimate form such denial results in suicide. Clearly, this extreme in the identification process in "uncooperative" and "nonadaptive."

Expectations

A third conflict is the difference between the dialysand's expectations of his life and the expectations of the dialysis staff. In the extreme case this conflict changes its course in an interesting manner. In the acute stage of adaptation the patient may hope for a reprieve from his uremic-induced lethargy. He expects a metamorphosis to occur, resulting in total physical well-being. Staff members present a contrary expectation, emphasizing the aspects of the illness, diet, and the operation of the machine. Their attention is upon the restrictions of the illness; the patient's concentration is upon the benefits to be gained. As the patient moves from the acute to the chronic stage of adaptation, his enthusiasm wanes, and his expectation for normalcy dwindles. Perhaps triggered by this changing attitude, staff members begin to make known their contrary expectation, that of the patient becoming an active, responsible citizen. Essentially, the dialysand perceives the staff as constantly being at cross-purposes to him. The staff's expectations always seem to be opposed to his.

Role of the Treatment Staff

Several references have been made to the staff's involvement in the patient's adaptational process. Some summary thoughts are presented here.

The influence of the treatment staff upon psychological adaptation occurs in both a conceptual and interpersonal fashion. The conceptual influence is really a matter of definition. A patient is not "adapted" until the staff declares him so. It is the staff and not the patient who establish the criteria for adaptation. If the dialysand succumbs to the emotional distress of his illness, he is considered "unadapted." If he allows his many problems to overcome him, or if he grows weary of the constant repetitive treatments, he is judged "unproductive" or "uncooperative." In essence, adaptation is partly a matter of whether the patient measures up to a standard that we establish for him, not what *he* judges he is able to do. The challenge for us is to consider whether the patient has failed to adapt or is encountering one of the many hazards in the *continuing process* of adaptation to hemodialysis.

The interpersonal influence occurs in the communications directed toward the patient by the staff that encourage or impede his progress in adapting to his illness. As care givers, the staff has an investment in the patient. His failure to get well or to progress is seen by staff as its failure. Often the frustration felt in caring for a slowly progressing patient is translated into increased staff expectations or demands which may mask hostility toward the ungratifying patient.

Acting-out behavior or the expression of anger and frustration by the patient is difficult for the staff to handle. Yet anger and frustration are normal emotional reactions to an illness that produces such psychological stresses. Development of coping skills on the part of the patient is increased when the patient is allowed to ventilate his fears and anger without reprisal. However, if the staff communicates "a good patient is one who behaves himself," then the patient's means of expression is suppressed.

A third problem area is that of the staff's defenses. In particular, denial allows a means of warding off the reality of the patient's condition. After an intellectual and emotional investment in a patient's treatment, it is very difficult for treatment staff to tolerate the failure of a patient to improve. Some patients can have a full recovery and return to a productive life, but some cannot. Our job is to expect only what is possible and to aid the patient in being satisfied with his own level of adaptation.

Kaplan De-Nour[5] has demonstrated the influence of staff attitudes upon patients' adjustment to hemodialysis. She found that on units where there was a common expectation and team attitude among the nurses, the patients fulfilled their potential for adjustment. On those wards that lacked a team opinion or held unrealistic expectations, the patients did less well than would be expected by "objective rates." Furthermore, Kaplan De-Nour states that "the ability of the team to form a realistic team opinion seems to be directly linked to the physicians' ability to assess correctly their patient's condition." A physician's tendency to overestimate the level of a patient's status or to deny the reality of a patient's physical condition seems to cause the lack of consensus in the nursing team.

In closing, quotations from two physicians who are suffering from end-stage renal failure are pertinent:

Patients on dialysis are accustomed to being told by the doctor, 'You are doing fine'—usually after the latest measurements of electrolytes and creatinine. The patient then thinks to himself, 'If I'm doing fine, why do I feel so rotten?' After undergoing correction of several days' accumulation of metabolites in a few hours, who could feel well with the resultant cerebral edema? Who, with a hematocrit of 17 percent, feels well enough to function when he cannot climb his own stairway because of dyspnea?[3]

I would like to stress the following points: In the final analysis of the evaluation of dialysis . . . the main considerations must be the quality of life and the length of life a patient may enjoy as a result of treatment; the total spectrum of a patient's life should be considered. The degree of rehabilitation, indicating a patient's ability to return to work, does not necessarily reflect quality of life; a patient who is dependent on maintenance dialysis cannot lead a normal life.[4]

References

1. Abram, H. S. The psychiatrist, the treatment of chronic renal failure, and the prolongation of life: II. *American Journal of Psychiatry*, 1969, *124*, 157–167.
2. Abram, H. S. The 'uncooperative' dialysis patient: A psychiatrist's viewpoint and a patient's commentary. In N. B. Levy (Ed.), *Living and dying: Adaptation to hemodialysis.* Springfield: Charles C Thomas, 1974.
3. Calland, C. H. Patrogenic problems in end-stage renal failure. *New England Journal of Medicine*, 1972, *287*, 334–336.
4. Eady, R. A. J. Why I have not had a kidney transplant after nine and one-half years as a hemodialysis patient. *Transactions Proceedings*, 1973, *5*, 1115–1117.
5. Kaplan De-Nour, A. Prediction of adjustment to chronic hemodialysis. In N. B. Levy (Ed.), *Psychonephrology I: Psychological factors in hemodialysis and transplantation*. New York: Plenum Press, 1981.
6. Kessler, J. W. Parenting the handicapped child. *Pediatric Annals*, 1977, *6*, 654–661.
7. Levy, N. B. Coping with maintenance hemodialysis: Psychological considerations in the care of patients. In S. G. Massry & A. L. Seller (Eds.), *Clinical aspects of uremia and hemodialysis*. Springfield: Charles C Thomas, 1975.
8. Maher, B. A., Lamping, D. L., Dickinson, C. A., Murawski, B. J., Olivier, D. C., & Santiago, G. C. Psychosocial aspects of chronic hemodialysis: The national co-operative dialysis study. *Kidney International*, 1983, *23* (Supplement 13), S50–S57.
9. Reichsman, F., Levy, N. V. Problems in adaptation to maintenance hemodialysis: A four-year study of 25 patients. *Archives of Internal Medicine*, 1972, *130*, 859–865.

20

Helping Families Respond Effectively to Chronic Illness
Home Dialysis as a Case Example

SALLY E. PALMER, LINO CANZONA, and LOKKY WAI

Introduction

The importance of the family as a treatment resource in chronic illness is being increasingly recognized. The dramatic rise in health care costs has precipitated a move toward home care and the training of patients and their families to perform treatment previously assigned only to professional staff. Home dialysis is probably the prime example of this, as it involves complicated medical procedures, including access to the patient's circulatory system with the danger of contamination or machine failure. An emotionally stable home environment has been recognized for many years as an essential prerequisite for successful adaptation to long-term dialysis therapy.[1]

The purpose of this paper is to analyze further the family functioning patterns of home dialysis patients and their partners,

Reprinted in abridged form from *Social Work in Health Care,* Fall 1982, *8,* 1–14.

SALLY E. PALMER • Lecturer in Social Work, Faculty of Continuing Studies, University of Western Ontario, London, Ontario, Canada. **LINO CANZONA** • Department of Social Work, King's College, London, Ontario, Canada. **LOKKY WAI** • Department of Social Work, University of Western Ontario, London, Ontario, Canada.

as well as how they feel about their marriages. Based on the [previously mentioned] research, it will be hypothesized that families with more flexible, open patterns of interaction will be more successful with home dialysis. Beyond this, no hypotheses will be formulated: Much remains to be learned about family interaction in chronic illness, so this study will be exploratory. It is hoped that some tentative conclusions can be reached which have relevance for treatment staff, especially social workers.

Methodology

Two approaches are used in this paper. The first is an in-depth assessment of a small group of families (20) with whom one of the authors worked closely over a two-year period; in these families the patient's marriage partner was also the dialysis partner. The findings are based on the clinical assessment of a professional social worker. The second approach is a statistical analysis of a study which originated from this social worker's experience, a retrospective study of 291 home dialysis families covering sixteen centers in Ontario, Canada including the 20 original families. The clinical impressions were obtained from personal interviews, for a minimum of five and a maximum of 20 hours, with each family. These contacts included the original assessment of families for home dialysis training, regular weekly sessions with them during their training, counseling sessions on referral from medical staff for specific social problems, and routine home visits with a nurse from the training center. The families who were seen least frequently had already been trained before the social worker became involved with the unit, but much background knowledge was gained about them from the regular interdisciplinary meetings by which patient progress was monitored.

The clinical impressions of the families obtained from these contacts were measured against a [process] model of family functioning developed for clinical use.[2] The model identifies the significant aspects of family functioning as task accomplishment, role performance, communication, affective involvement, and control, noting that these aspects are interdependent and begin with observable behavior, moving toward abstract concepts.[2] The model also involves interdependence between the aspects. . . .

The retrospective study of 291 patients included all those who commenced home dialysis training in 16 Ontario centers between June 1975 and December 1978 and were still on home dialysis in 1979. As the focus of this paper is the family, we are only concerned with patients who were married and had their spouse as a dialysis assistant, 126 families. They range in age from 21 to 74 years (mean = 48 years), and 66 percent are males. Their average elementary and secondary school education is grade 10; 30 percent went beyond secondary school, 14 percent to university (mean = 3 years), and 16 percent elsewhere. Their country of origin is most frequently Canada (76 percent), then Britain (6 percent), and Italy (3 percent). The majority of families (59 percent) still have children living at home; 25 percent have one child; 34 percent have two or more.

The data reported in this paper was collected by an interview schedule administered by trained interviewers and a brief self-administered questionnaire on sexual satisfaction. Data was obtained on patients' and partners' respective feelings about various aspects of the marital relationship, including changes during home dialysis, and about the help given by the partner with dialysis tasks.

Findings

Task Accomplishment

Family tasks are defined . . . as the provision of basic necessities, allowing and supporting the development of the family and its members, and meeting family crisis. The major family task relevant to this study is the management of dialysis in the home, usually three times weekly, for four to five hours each time. The families who were able to sustain the physical and emotional demands of home dialysis over a prolonged time (two to three years) were observed to have some common characteristics in their approach to the task.

Generally, the successful families shared the responsibility for the treatment regimen. This does not mean they shared dialysis tasks, but each felt responsible for his/her own part of the job to be done.

Mrs. C. took a serious approach to her part in the dialysis routine, and her husband respected her growing expertise with such tasks as inserting the needles which tapped his blood supply. Together they monitored the progress of each dialysis in terms of his blood pressure and weight loss. When any malfunction of the machine or unusual occurrence took place, they conferred before deciding how to respond. They suffered the average number of setbacks on dialysis, but seemed able to absorb these because of their mutually supportive approach to the task. Mr. and Mrs. I. were observed, from the beginning of their training, to have a dominance/submission relationship. He issued the orders and she obeyed. Although the policy of the training unit was to encourage shared responsibility, in case of the patient's incapacity, it appeared that the I.'s marriage was based on this unequal balance. Thus, no attempt was made to change their pattern, as it was thought that beginning dialysis was already a traumatic experience for the I.'s. Several months after they commenced treatment at home, an accident occurred with the machine; a large leak in the plastic dialyzer developed near the end of the dialysis period when it would be least expected. Mr. I., being already weak from several hours of dialysis, became unconscious from the loss of blood; his wife, without his leadership, was unable to respond quickly. Although she called for help, by the time relief arrived from the hospital, Mr. I. had died from loss of blood.

The main difference between the C. and I. families was the clarity of task assignments. Mrs. I. had the responsibility for providing emergency backup to her husband, but he would not allow her the appropriate autonomy so she lacked knowledge and confidence in a crisis. Although not all couples experience such tragic consequences as the I.'s from the failure to share responsibility appropriately, many examples could be given of couples who were unclear about their tasks. A common pattern was for partners to become more concerned about dietary restrictions than were the patients, with the result that the latter "cheated" when the partner was absent, rather than taking responsibility for the restrictions themselves.

Role Performance

Role is a broader concept than task, as it includes attitudes toward self and others, which in turn affect task accomplishment.

The more successful families were those who were flexible enough in their role performance to adapt to the new expectations of a home dialysis regime. They had generally evolved reciprocal roles which were clear and satisfying to them before the advent of illness, so the prospect of having to modify their roles was not as threatening to them. Some families, on the other hand, were newly formed and still uncertain of their roles; or their mutual expectations were so rigidly structured that any change was resisted as a threat to the precarious balance of the family structure.

The R. family was able to adapt to home dialysis roles with minimum of trauma, even though a number of stressful events occurred during the five years Mrs. R. was dialyzing at home. They were a middle-aged couple with two children at university, still living at home; they had evolved a comfortable and flexible relationship over their twenty-odd years of marriage. During the five years of home dialysis, Mr. R. developed a chronic illness which eventually prevented him from helping with dialysis. One of their sons inherited his mother's condition, and the family was faced with the prospect of his commencing dialysis in the next few years. Nevertheless, the family maintained its stability, responding with a sense of loss to these stressful events, but managing to integrate them without hurting each other or breaking down, either individually or as a group.

The B.'s were about the same age as the R.'s in the previous case and had one child in high school. Mrs. B. was her husband's assistant and also had a chronic medical condition which deteriorated during the four years she was helping him to dialyze at home. The family roles had always been somewhat imbalanced, with Mary the teenaged daughter taking a great deal of responsibility for housekeeping, even though Mrs. B. seemed physically capable of doing more of the work herself.

Eventually it developed that Mary's behavior outside the home was becoming increasingly irresponsible, and she was charged with shoplifting. Neither parent seemed concerned about this. Mrs. B. was more like a dependent child than a mother to her daughter. Mr. B. functioned well in his work role, but was unable to take his wife's place as a parent. It may be that the B.'s would have had difficulty with Mary without the onset of chronic illness, but the addition of home dialysis to a family whose roles were already strained resulted in a poor environment for Mary, who was both overburdened and neglected.

The [preceding] cases illustrate the importance of assessing the effect of chronic illness and its treatment on the whole family, not just the patient and spouse. In systems terms, if there is a weak link in the system, like Mrs. B., the stress will be passed on and may lead to breakdown in another part of the system. The rigidity of the B.'s role performance made it impossible for them to expand to encompass additional demands, so they partially abdicated their roles as parents.

Communication

In the process model of family functioning, the characteristics of effective communication are given as: clarity, directness and sufficiency (of information) on the part of the sender, and availability/openness on the part of the receiver. This is consistent with the findings of Pentecost, Zwerenz, and Manuel.[3] In that study a family's communication pattern was considered good to the degree that members expressed their ideas clearly and took responsibility for their own feelings, e.g., using the first person "I think," "I want," to preface their statements.

Along the spectrum of good to poor communication across the 20 families under consideration, it could be generalized that younger couples tended to have better communication patterns. This probably relates to the cultural norms to which our present middle-aged couples have been socialized during their formative years, whereas younger couples tend to place less value on polite behavior and more on open expression of feeling. A comparison of the L. and S. families will illustrate this point.

The L.'s were a young couple in their mid-twenties who had contended with Mr. L.'s dialysis since the early days of their marriage, with the additional hardships of low income and difficulty in conceiving children. Their open communication patterns became evident in their approach to two important issues during the two years the social worker knew them.

Firstly, they let the dialysis staff know when they were feeling unsupported around problems in Mr. L.'s treatment. They lived over fifty miles from the dialysis center, and at one point experienced repeated difficulties with a malfunctioning machine. On their next clinic visit, the L.'s told the dialysis staff, in clear terms, that they were not satisfied with the staff's response to their telephone calls about difficulties with the machine. The L.'s were also open and secure enough in their relationship to introduce the topic of their apparent infertility with the nephrologist and social worker during a home visit. They described without difficulty their pattern of sexual relations, and the nephrologist was able to suggest a modification which resulted in Mrs. L. becoming pregnant a few months later.

The L.'s openness was in contrast to several older families who complained to other patients or to the social worker about lack of staff support; the latter said they were afraid of repercussions if they criticized the nurses.

In contrast, Mr. and Mrs. S. were a retired couple in their sixties, who treated each other and those outside their family with the utmost courtesy, showing the strain of Mrs. S.'s condition only through their behavior. Mrs. S. found the task of inserting needles into her husband almost impossible, but continued to attempt this for many months before finally expressing her strong aversive reaction and asking that Mr. S. be dialyzed in the hospital.

Meanwhile, Mr. S. kept up his reputation as a jovial man who never let his inner fears and depression show through his cheerful exterior. He continued to joke with the staff at his local country store, at the same time as they reported to his wife that they knew his condition was worsening. They noticed his footsteps as he approached the store becoming slower and heavier over time, and realized he was presenting an unreal self to them when he joked and laughed. Mrs. S. did not share this knowledge with her husband, but told the dialysis staff. Mr. S. died within a year of his unsuccessful experience with home dialysis.

Mr. S. died from a heart condition, which was very likely aggravated by the repression of his negative feelings, and by the lack of communication within the marriage. He must have felt the strain of his wife's anxiety about her part in treatment for many months before she expressed this openly and asked for relief, but he never commented on this to the staff. Similarly, Mrs. S. did not tell her husband that she or the staff at the country store were concerned about his deteriorating conditon; had she done so, this might have opened the door to him to express his fears.

Although the principle that repressed fear, hostility, and discouragement can contribute to diseases such as hypertension was well known to the treatment staff dealing with the S.'s and similar families, they were inhibited from attemtping to change such well-established communication habits. The consensus of the staff was that a long-term marriage based on overt politeness and satisfaction, despite hidden negative feelings, should not be disturbed at a time of crisis brought on by a worsening medical condition.

Affective Involvement

As defined in the model, optimal affective involvement is characterized by a family environment which provides emotional security as well as a sense of being valued and supported for all family members. At the same time involvement should allow for a degree of autonomy in thought and behavior for individual family members. In a number of families in the patient group, affective involvement appeared to meet both these conditions, and the families did well on home dialysis. The following examples demonstrate over-involvement and under-involvement respectively, and their effects on the management of a dialysis regimen.

Mrs. E., in her fifties, had not been well for most of the thirty years of her marriage, and had been unable to conceive children. Mr. E. was a high-energy, perfectionist man who devoted his life, outside working hours, to the care of his wife. He took on his role as a dialysis assistant with such zeal that he referred to the machine and equipment as "my machine" and "my supplies." Mrs. E. appeared to love and appreciate her husband, but she became a passive participant in her treatment. Although she adhered to the regimen, she showed little interest in any treatment innovations or even in her own medical crises and periodic infections requiring hospitalization. She gradually became worn down, and died of heart failure after four years on home dialysis.

It appeared that Mrs. E. gradually lost her will to live; although her husband devoted himself to keeping her alive, his will for her to live could not be transferred to her. In effect, Mrs. E. was deprived of her autonomy because her husband was, in a sense, living her life for her.

Mr. J. was an emotionally isolated man who had been very successful in his chosen career. He seemed to lack the capacity to develop close emotional bonds with his wife and children, having lost his own parents when he was a child. Mrs. J. was very lonely and longed for a more intimate marital relationship; she welcomed the opportunity to assist her husband on dialysis, hoping it would bring them closer. Mr. J. appeared to be threatened, howev-

er, by the prospect of more intimacy with his wife and tended to withdraw from their mutual activities around treatment. The trouble she took with his diet was undermined by Mr. J.'s resistance to following the rules of his regime. His condition steadily deteriorated, but he failed to show concern about the effects of his careless life-style.

In the J.'s marriage it could be said that the absence of emotional involvement and the defenses Mr. J. built up to support his isolation were counterproductive to the dialysis treatment. To avoid involvement with his wife in their mutual tasks around dialysis, he failed to carry out his own role, thereby making it impossible for her to keep him well. In these two families we have examples of too much emotional involvement by the partner, resulting in withdrawal by the patient, apparently because of encroachment on his or her personal autonomy.

Control

This is defined in the model as the process by which family members influence each others' behavior. When controls are lacking, tasks do not get done, because some degree of control and acceptance of control are essential to make the minor shifts required to meet ongoing demands.

The G. family had always been marginally stable because of Mr. G.'s irresponsibility when he went drinking after work "with the boys." He was not an alcoholic, but enjoyed drinking with his co-workers and tended to ignore the feelings of his wife waiting at home. Mrs. G. was fairly tolerant of her husband's behavior until she began dialysis and found herself, occasionally, waiting hours for her husband when she was supposed to start dialysis. Each time this happened, Mrs. G. would tell the staff about it, and they would reprimand Mr. G. but the pattern continued until eventually Mrs. G. was given a transplant.

Families with an inadequate control mechanism are difficult to identify prior to training, because both partners tend to contribute to the situation. Partners who suffer from their spouse's irresponsible behavior seem to be ineffective in producing any change, moreover, they tend to cover up for their delinquent spouse, presenting a united front to outsiders. Three of the 20 families had problems with control which interfered with home dialysis, and the difficulty always appeared briefly in the training period. In retrospect, it is important to recognize that the more responsible partner will rationalize or minimize the irresponsible behavior, so the behavior should be judged on its merits, not on the interpretation given by the partner.

General Effect of Home Dialysis on Family Functioning

A thread running through all the families in relation to the [preceding] aspects of functioning is that functioning suffers to the extent that illness controls the family. In these cases, patients allowed their disease and its treatment regimen to take over their lives to some extent; other family members were drawn in or neglected. In the successful families, however, such as the C.'s and the R.'s, the patients controlled their conditions and were supported in their efforts by the other members.

Discussion and Implications for Social Work Treatment

The clinical assessment of a small group of families on home dialysis demonstrates the importance of a family structure with flexible roles and open communication. Families who could not adapt to new roles by sharing responsibility and authority or could not communicate their fears and frustration were less successful on long-term home dialysis. The larger study, in which feelings and perceptions of patients and partners were sought, complements the [preceding] findings by suggesting some specific areas of strain. The actual work of dialysis does not seem to be a problem for partners: Their involvement in dialysis tasks is not associated with their feelings of closeness or satisfaction with their marriages. Strain on partners seems to come more from their sense of lack of understanding and emotional support from the patient, as these two aspects showed the greatest discrepancy between patients' and partners' perceptions.

The increase in marital closeness noted by both partners and patients in the larger study may have detrimental aspects, as their mutual concern for the patient's health may cause partners to give up some of their autonomy and submerge their needs in favor of the patient's. These accommodations lead to closeness but not necessarily to satisfaction for the spouse who makes them. From these points which are beginning to emerge from the study of home dialysis families, some treatment approaches may be suggested. The indication that more attention should be given to partners' needs is in accord with a program reported some years ago, in which dialysis spouses met in a small group over a period of months.[4] They initially denied having problems, but gradually began to share their feelings and concurrently gained an increasing sense of emotional separateness from their patient spouses. The findings discussed . . . suggest that the members of dialysis families should be helped, individually or in groups, to identify their own needs, to communicate these within the family, and to expect more emotional support from the patient rather than focusing on the illness. Patients may require a great deal of help from their families, but they still have something to give. From [these] findings, it seems that understanding and emotional support are the areas of greatest partner need. An open, flexible family, which controls the patient's illness, rather than being controlled by it, is likely to provide the best environment for ensuring that the needs of all family members are recognized. Such a situation is most likely to lead to long-term success with home dialysis and other forms of chronic illness.

The finding in the larger study that decreasing sexual satisfaction was a greater problem for patients than for their partners may be related in part to the patients' concern about family unhappiness, mentioned at the outset. Although the patients' own diminishing physical satisfaction cannot be discounted, it is generally accepted that one's self-image as a sexual being is partly based on the ability to satisfy a partner. In view of this, some of the patients' dissatisfaction may come from a fear of their partner's reactions. It may then be useful for patients to know that partners feel better about the sexual aspect of their marriage than do patients. Discussion between the partners may also help to diminish their mutual concerns about satisfying each other sexually.

A final conclusion, which may be drawn from the findings in the small group, relates to staff reticence to interfere with an established marital relationship even when it is counterproductive to home dialysis. Our knowledge of crisis tells us that this may be the best point for intervention to produce change in a system. Despite the staff's reticence, it is apparent that a poorly functioning family can contribute to patient deterioration and even death. Thus, we have a responsibility to attempt to change families which are not functioning well.

References

1. Meldrum, M. W., Wolfram, J. G., & Rubini, M. E. The impact of chronic hemodialysis upon the socio-economics of a veteran patient group. *Journal of Chronic Diseases,* 1968, *21,* 37–52.
2. Santa-Barbara, J., Steinhauer, P. D., & Skinner, H. *Process model of family functioning.* Toronto: University of Toronto Press, 1981.
3. Pentecost, R. L., Zwerenz, B., & Manuel, J. W. Intrafamily identity and home dialysis success. *Nephron,* 1976, *17,* 88–103.
4. Shambaugh, P. W., & Kanter, S. S. Spouses under stress: Group meetings with spouses of patients on hemodialysis. *American Journal of Psychiatry,* 1969, *126,* 928–936.

21

An Unsung Hero
The Living Related Kidney Donor

ELAINE M. MUSIAL

Over the past fifteen years, renal transplantation has become the most acceptable treatment of end-stage renal disease. Because transplantation returns the patient to a normal physiological state by restoring normal renal function, it is more acceptable than hemodialysis or peritoneal dialysis which, although prolonging survival in these patients, cannot adequately compensate for all of the complications of the uremic state.

At the present time, kidneys used for transplantation are acquired from two sources: the cadaver donor and the living related donor. A living related donor kidney is preferred because of the more favorable prognosis associated with this type of transplant.[1] However, for someone who does not have any potential donors within his family, cadaver transplantation is an alternative.

Because of the better prognosis associated with living related donor transplantation, efforts are made to secure a kidney from this source in all possible cases. This places tremendous pressure on the patient and his family to select a donor from among themselves.

Reprinted from *Nephrology Nurse*, 1980, 2, 21–22, 60–62.

ELAINE M. MUSIAL • Nephrology Nurse Clinician, Duke University Medical Center, Durham, North Carolina 27706.

What factors are considered in making the selection and what is the effect of donation on the donor before, during, and after he has made the decision to donate his kidney? Recently, much interest in these questions has been generated, and much has been learned about the effects of the donation on the donor. In order to better understand how the decision to donate is made and how the donor reacts to the situation, it might be helpful to follow a family through this process in order to view the dynamics of the situation.

Selecting a Donor

I first met Donna when she came to tour the dialysis unit prior to beginning her treatments. She was so young; it didn't seem fair that her life should be complicated by illness, but it was. She had end-stage renal disease secondary to chronic glomerulonephritis. She hadn't even known that she was sick; she was just feeling a little more tired than usual. Her renal disease was discovered during a preemployment physical for her first job after finishing high school.

The medical plan was to stabilize her on hemodialysis initially and to provide a renal transplant as soon as possible. Donna was the youngest child in her family and had three sisters and a brother who were all considered potential donors. Her parents were also considered. The doctors felt sure they would be able to get a "good match" from one of these and were anxious to select a donor.

Although the physicians play a major role in donor selection, actual donor selection takes place within the family itself.[25]

Physicians usually tell the patient that a living related donor transplant yields the most favorable result, but that if one is not available, a cadaver donor will be found and other methods of treatment will remain available to them, e.g., hemodialysis or peritoneal dialysis. This places the burden of presenting the situation to his family on the patient himself.

To be forced to ask his family members to donate a kidney so that he may return to a state of well-being may be a traumatic experience for the patient. The patient may fear that his request will be rejected or he may be fearful of the consequences of his request on a family member.[6] Frequently, the patient will contact a family member in whom he feels able to confide and will present the situation to him. This person will, in turn, present the situation to the remaining family members. In other cases, the patient's spouse may contact the family to discuss the situation.[5]

In both cases, the spouse or the "confidant" in the family plays a significant role in the selection process. This person can apply pressure on other family members without jeopardizing family cohesion. This person is also helpful in that he allows family members to verbalize their feelings regarding their participation without being embarrassed or feeling that they are letting down the potential recipient.

Like the potential recipient, family members experience stress during this period.[5,7] Whether or not to donate a kidney is a difficult decision to make. Individual family members share the fears of the potential recipient regarding the consequences of the surgery for the donor. Conflicts may arise within the family with regard to who should or should not be considered as a potential donor. The basis for these conflicts arises from several sources within the family. There may be concern over the personal and family responsibilities of a particular family member and the family may hesitate to allow that person to be the donor.[3,4] Previous family disagreement and/or ill feelings toward a particular family member may also be the basis for exclusion from consideration as a potential donor.[3] Families may also wish to exclude a member who has, for one reason or another, become the "black sheep" of the family. The other family members may be fearful that such a recipient may use his donation for his own purposes, thereby placing further strain on the family relationship and possibly causing the recipient discomfort and guilt in the future.[2] If the potential donor is married, the recipient may actively oppose his or her consideration as a donor because of concern and fear for the spouse.[5] In addition to the above considerations, potential donor willingness is another aspect of the preselection process which deserves careful consideration.

Family members who are willing to donate a kidney are motivated by various forces. Many see the donation as a family responsibility or are motivated by a "do unto others as you would have them do unto you" philosophy.[8] Other potential donors may see this as an opportunity to repay the potential recipient for a past favor. Others, like the "black sheep" type previously mentioned, may see this as an opportunity to reestablish themselves as a respectable family member.[9] Religious beliefs, guilt over past relationships, and altruism are other possible motivations. Whatever the reasons and whatever the method which the family uses in preselection, all family members who express willingness to donate progress to immunological screening.

In Donna's case, she chose to inform her sister, Cathy, of the situation with which she was faced. Cathy then served as the catalyst for determining who would serve as potential kidney donors. All family members were informed by Cathy of the situation and after discussion, all expressed willingness to donate. The family did express concern about Donna's brother being considered because they felt that if he should be selected as the donor he might use this to manipulate Donna and other family members in the future. However, they also felt uncomfortable excluding him from immunological screening, especially since all other family members were participating. The physicians, after hearing how the family felt, decided to include him in the screening but assured the family that they would offer a suitable excuse for rejecting him as a donor.

The initial screening included determination of ABO compatibility. Two of Donna's sisters and her father were found to be ABO incompatible and were thus removed from consideration. Tissue typing was then done on her sister and brother and her mother. It was found that both her sister and brother were HLA identical to Donna. Her mother was a two antigen match. Because of the previously mentioned concern about Donna's brother, the doctors informed him that although he was not an unsuitable donor, Donna's sister, Cathy, was a more suitable match. The doctor's reasoning for not telling him that he was unsuitable arose from a concern that if the transplant from Cathy was unsuccessful, there would be a chance for a second transplant. The family concurred with this reasoning.

Cathy was enthusiastic about the prospect of donating her kidney for Donna. She had always been very close to Donna, in spite of their age difference (Donna was 18 and Cathy was 33) and wanted Donna to have the best chance possible. She was anxious, as was the rest of the family, to have Donna well again. Before the final decision was made, Cathy was carefully informed of the risks of surgery and the prospects, both positive and negative, of the surgery for Donna. Cathy was also informed that if she should change her mind about donation, the physicians would give some medical reason so that she could withdraw with dignity.

Donor Risks and Fears

The risks of transplantation to the donor include a 0.05% mortality from the surgery itself and a possible long-term risk from possible trauma, neoplasm, or surgery to the remaining kidney which has been estimated at 0.07%.[11] A complication rate of 15%, consisting primarily of respiratory, wound, and urinary tract complications, has been reported.[12] The surgery itself may cause other problems for the prospective donor. It usually requires a four to six week recuperation period which may be a problem if the prospective donor is employed. Child care will also have to be arranged during this period if the donor is usually responsible for this.[5]

The prospect of surgery causes anxiety in the donor. In fact, anxiety increases as the surgery approaches. This anxiety may be lessened by the tendency, which families demonstrate, to provide concern and support to the prospective donor during the pretransplant period.[2] In addition, four factors have been identified which aid the potential donor in dealing with anxiety. They are: a firm belief in the good they feel they are doing by their donation, the positive relationship which they have formed with their physicians, the emotional reinforcement they receive from both the recipient and their family, and the attention they receive from friends.[13] The fact that the patient is informed that if he or she decides against donating, the physicians will provide some medical or immunological reason so that the donor may withdraw without losing face,[14] can also help in decreasing the anxiety in the pretransplant period.

Although Cathy admitted being fearful about the experience she was undergoing, she still wanted to donate her kidney. She underwent a comprehensive evaluation which included a complete history and physical examination, hematological work-up, determination of chemical regulatory function, urinalysis and urine culture, immunological work-up, EKG, chest x-ray, IVP, renal arteriograms, bilateral venograms, and a glucose tolerance test. No abnormalities were found and transplantation was scheduled.

Donna was admitted about three days before the scheduled surgery in order to get her in optimum condition. Cathy was admitted on the day before surgery. The surgery went well; the transplanted kidney began to function almost immediately. Postoperatively, both recipient and donor were doing well.

Postoperative Reactions

After surgery, the donor is treated just as any other patient undergoing unilateral nephrectomy. Because the surgery usually involves some rib resectioning, coughing and deep breathing may be painful. However, it should be encouraged in order to prevent pulmonary complications.[15] Medications to control pain should be used as needed. The function of the remaining kidney should be monitored closely. An increase in renal mass known as compensatory hypertrophy is expected to occur in the remaining kidney. This adaptive phenomenon usually occurs within seven days of surgery, although it may take longer in an older donor, and is monitored closely by creatinine clearances, blood urea nitrogen, and serum creatinine levels.[12]

> *After surgery, Cathy became very angry. She was very uncomfortable and verbalized that she felt poorly prepared for the experience, even though it had been explained to her very carefully. Cathy had never had surgery before the nephrectomy, and she could not deal with the pain she felt, even though she knew that she would experience it. Her family had informed her that Donna was doing wonderfully. She didn't seem to have any pain and was up and about in her room on the day after surgery. Cathy, on the other hand, was in such pain that she couldn't even turn by herself. Cathy's husband, who had not seemed to play an important role in the process until now, also expressed a great deal of anger during this time. He hated to see Cathy suffer so much while Donna "was sitting upstairs like a queen on her throne with the rest of the doting family clustered around her." He apparently, although he had never said anything about it before, was against Cathy's being considered as a donor from the beginning. Because of his anger during this time, he could not be very supportive of Cathy.*
> *During this period, the hospital staff remained supportive of Cathy. After the first few days, Cathy began to improve physically. Her pain was lessened, and her outlook began to improve. The big boost came when Cathy was finally allowed to see Donna for herself. She related later that seeing Donna doing so well and knowing that the kidney was functioning well was the biggest factor in improving her feelings regarding her situation. Months later, Cathy could recall few negative aspects of her experience. She ex-*

pressed that "knowing that Donna is better is enough to overshadow any painful memories of the experience."

Donors often experience a great deal of turmoil after the surgery. The donor who has considered himself to be basically healthy is placed into a sick role for which he is not well prepared.[6] He may feel more uncomfortable than he ever anticipated. The donor's family and even the hospital staff may be unsympathetic to the donor's feelings at this time.[2] After all, the donor isn't really sick. He is still considered healthy even though he has been subjected to major surgery. An interesting thing also happens within the family during this time. While the family was very concerned and supportive of the donor before the surgery, this interest shifts to the recipient after the surgery and may contribute to the lack of support which has been described.[2] This may result in a feeling of loneliness and frustration for the donor.

The family's reaction to the donor's situation may arise from guilt or anxiety over encouraging the donor to submit to the surgery. Their denial of the donor's suffering may be their attempt to resolve these guilt feelings, i.e., if the donor is not really suffering, there is no reason for the family to feel guilty about the surgery.

The donor needs a great deal of support during this period, and this support is not often forthcoming from the family or the hospital staff. The donor is the "unsung hero" of this story. His importance diminishes tremendously from the point of transplant and onward. This leads to a feeling in the donor that he is unappreciated and unimportant. Prior to the actual surgery, the donor received a great deal of attention from staff and family. However, after surgery and during the period of recuperation, this attention decreases. This may be disappointing to the donor. Recipients continue to have this attention, which in a few cases causes resentment in the donor. In the long run, this feeling of resentment and anger is resolved and lasting effects are uncommon. Many donors feel that the act of donating a kidney was the most meaningful experience of their lives. The self-satisfaction gained from the experience is enough to make it worthwhile. In fact, the role of the hospital staff should be to assist the donor to realize this self-satisfaction, even if the transplant is unsuccessful.

Another factor which may contribute to the turmoil experienced by the donor in the posttransplant period is the effect of the surgery on the recipient. The donor will be concerned about the functioning of the transplanted kidney. If the kidney works well, the donor may be relieved. However, if the kidney does not function immediately, he may feel personally responsible for prolonging the suffering of the patient.[16]

In order to avert some of the problems which have been identified in relation to the selection of a donor and the turmoil he experiences as a result of his donation, several actions should be taken.

1. Support for the donor should be provided throughout the experience, and more especially from the point of final selection and onward. The donor needs an outlet for his many fears which he will not ventilate to his family. Ideally, the person who assumes the role as a support person for the donor should not be one who is also involved in the care of the transplant recipient. The donor will not easily verbalize his feelings to someone who is closely involved in the care of the recipient for fear that the staff member will feel badly about them for having these feelings and may inadvertently transmit these feelings to the recipient.

2. Support should also be provided to the spouse of the donor. He is likely to share many of the feelings of the donor and needs to be able to verbalize these feelings without fear of recrimination.

3. All potential risks should be carefully discussed with the donor. He should also be informed about what he can expect, both intellectually and experientially, following the surgery. He should also be made aware of the possibility of rejection in the recipient. If this does occur, he should receive continued support because there is a tendency for transplant donors to blame themselves if the kidney fails.

4. The donor should receive adequate follow-up of their medical as well as their emotional status. Ideally, the support person who has worked with the donor prior to surgery and during the hospital experience would continue to follow the patient after discharge. This person should remain available to the donor in order to answer questions that may arise and to provide continuing support.

The decision to donate a body organ to another is a difficult one, loaded with physical and emotional repercussions. The staff caring for this patient has a tremendous responsibility to the donor; they should assist the donor in achieving a positive outcome from what may be a very difficult and painful experience.

References

1. Dougherty, J., & Bannayan, G. Renal transplantation. In M. Forland (Ed.), *Nephrology*. Flushing, N.Y.: Medical Examination Company, 1977.
2. Kemph, J., Bermann, E., & Cappolillo, H. Kidney transplant and shifts in family dynamics. *American Journal of Psychiatry*, 1969, *125*, 1485–1490.
3. Eisendrath, R., Guttman, R., & Murray, J. Psychological considerations in the selection of kidney transplant donors. *Surgery, Gynecology and Obstetrics*, 1969, *129*, 243–248.
4. Fellner, C., & Marshall, J. Kidney donors—The myth of informed consent. *American Journal of Psychiatry*, 1970, *126*, 1245–1251.
5. Simmons, R., Hickey, K., Kjellstrand, C., & Simmons, R. Family tension in the search for a kidney donor. *Journal of the American Medical Association*, 1971, *215*, 909–912.
6. Schumann, D. The renal donor. *American Journal of Nursing*, 1974, *74*, 105–110.
7. Harrison, J., & Bennett, A. The familial living donor in renal transplantation. *Journal of Urology*, 1977, *118*, 166–168.
8. Wilson, W., Stickel, D., Hayes, C., & Harris, N. Psychiatric considerations of renal transplantation. *Archives of Internal Medicine*, 1968, *122*, 502–506.
9. Bernstein, D., & Simmons, R. The adolescent kidney donor . . . the right to give. *American Journal of Psychiatry*, 1974, *131*, 1338–1342.
10. Kemph, J. Observation of the effects of kidney transplant on donors and recipients. *Diseases of the Nervous System*, 1970, *31*, 323–325.
11. Hamburger, J., & Crosnier, J. Moral and ethical problems in transplantation. In L. Rapaport & J. Dausset (Eds.), *Human transplantation*. New York: Grune & Stratton, 1968.
12. Uehling, D., Malek, G., & Wear, B. Complications of donor nephrectomy. *Journal of Urology*, 1974, *111*, 745–746.
13. Fellner, C., & Marshall, J. Twelve kidney donors. *Journal of the American Medical Association*, 1968, *206*, 2703–2707.
14. Fellner, C. Organ donation: For whose sake? *Annals of Internal Medicine*, 1973, *79*, 589–592.

IX

The Crisis of Treatment
Total Parenteral Nutrition

Total parenteral nutrition (TPN) is a relatively new and increasingly valuable treatment that can have a major psychological impact on patients and their families. Patients on TPN obtain most or all of their nutrients via a catheter inserted into a major vein rather than by mouth. This therapy is useful for patients who suffer from poorly nourished states or loss of bowel function due to cancer, severe injuries, or kidney, liver, or bowel disease. Although TPN may be a temporary treatment lasting between a few days and several months, many patients have their lives maintained indefinitely by the procedure.[4] Living with TPN is especially hard because patients are deprived of the pleasure associated with two basic human functions—eating and drinking. A major task confronting such patients is to integrate the life-sustaining technology into a new identity.

Many of the adjustments TPN patients must make are similar to those of home dialysis patients (see Part VIII). Patients confront the task of grieving for the loss of body function and maintaining self-esteem in the face of somatic changes and an ever-present protruding catheter. Patients and their families must become proficient in self-care of the TPN apparatus, restructure their lives to accommodate the demanding schedule required for infusion of TPN solutions, and come to grips with fears about equipment failure and their ability to handle potential medical emergencies. Finally, patients and their families must cope with the financial burden of this expensive treatment.[2,4] The impact of these problems is less for patients on partial parenteral nutrition who can eat small meals and those on temporary parenteral nutrition who may look forward to a return of body function.

Successful adaptation to TPN is linked to patient characteristics and coping styles. MacRitchie[3] found that TPN therapy was especially turbulent for patients who experienced a sudden loss of bowel function and for whom eating was a significant source of pleasure. One such patient went on food binges, whereas another craved food and became "nutritionally promiscuous" by frequenting restaurants and fast food establishments. A second group of patients saw TPN as a task to be mastered. They took responsibility for their lives and tried to keep the therapy from controlling their activities. Some patients coped by minimizing the negative impact of TPN, whereas others needed help and sought reassurance from staff. Effective coping depended on personal resources such as flexibility as well as on family support and continuing contact and aid from hospital staff following discharge.

The articles in this section depict the impact of TPN on patients' lives and their resilience in adapting to this radical life-sustaining technology. In the first selection, Beth S. Price and Eleanor L. Levine examine the psychological problems produced by TPN and patients' early emotional reactions to it. The patients uniformly experienced some realistic depression as they grieved over their inability to eat. They saw themselves as abnormal and were concerned that others might reject them. Patients coped by trying to modify their body image to incorporate the extensive surgery, scars, and catheter tubing taped to their chest. Patients also tried to mentally prepare themselves to manage the TPN apparatus alone at home. Veteran TPN patients who were managing successfully were able to encourage neophytes and to identify unique ways of handling practical tasks. Prior to hospital discharge, patients often had mixed feelings about TPN therapy and about the quality of their lives. Patients recognized their dependence on the TPN apparatus but found it hard to adapt to necessary restrictions such as the limit on strenuous exercise because of the danger of disturbing the catheter.

The impact of TPN therapy initially disrupted normal activities and reverberated throughout patients' lives. Nutrient solutions ran in at night and caused patients to void every two hours.

For some patients, full-time employment was difficult due to fatigue and the problem of scheduling the 10 to 12 hours of daily TPN therapy. Marital relationships and family dynamics were also affected. While patients were hospitalized, family members reassigned tasks and established a new family equilibrium. Patients thus had to struggle to regain their former roles when they returned home. Despite all these hardships in the early phase of adaptation, within a year most patients were able to accept their limitations and to reestablish most of their normal routines. Healthy adaptation was promoted by ego strength, personal determination, and strong family support. In general, adaptation was better among patients with chronic bowel disease because the relief from disabling symptoms balanced the inconvenience of TPN.

Building on the first article, which considers early adaptation, the second selection by Mark Perl and his associates describes the psychological aspects of long-term home intravenous hyperalimentation (HIVH; for discussions of home parenteral nutrition, see Heimburger[1] and Pressel[5]). Many of the responses to TPN reported here are similar to those noted earlier. For example, the authors found that depression was common in the three to four months after the initiation of HIVH. Depression was occasionally accompanied by denial of illness and noncompliance with treatment regimens, such as when patients went swimming, "forgot" to hang IV bags on time, or failed to maintain sterile technique when changing dressings. In general, though, patients managed their self-care and no major life-threatening medical incidents occurred.

Especially in the early months of treatment, patients were bothered by realistic fears that their catheter might become infected or that the pump could malfunction and they would die. These fears were intensified when potentially dangerous incidents actually occurred, such as catheter tubing becoming disconnected or a blood clot forming in the catheter. Several patients who lived alone coped with the fear that something would go wrong and endanger their life by being especially attentive to the care of their equipment. Staff responded to patients by answering questions when problems arose, giving needed emotional support, and offering "refresher" courses on care of the TPN equipment. Patients' fears lessened over time as they gained confidence in their ability to handle the procedures.

Family life and sexual functioning also underwent changes. Martial relationships were strained by TPN, especially in those cases in which problems already existed. Some spouses coped by becoming actively engaged in the management of the TPN equipment, whereas others shied away from any direct involvement. The majority of patients experienced changes in their sexual relationship. Factors such as altered body image, embarrassment about the pump and tubing, and spouses' fears of hurting the patient all contributed to sexual problems, though improvements were noted after the first few months of TPN treatment. An encouraging aspect of TPN is that most patients are able to resume active and productive lives even though they must cope with such a radical life-sustaining treatment.[2]

References

1. Heimburger, D. C. Home parenteral nutrition. *The Alabama Journal of Medical Sciences,* 1982, *19,* 377–380.
2. Johnston, J. E. Home parenteral nutrition: The "costs" of patient and family participation. *Social Work in Health Care,* 1981, 7, 49–66.
3. MacRitchie, K. J. Parenteral nutrition outside hospital: Psychosocial styles of adaptation. *Canadian Journal of Psychiatry,* 1980, *25,* 308–313.
4. Malcolm, R., Robson, J. R. K., Vanderveen, T. W., & O'Neil, P. M. Psychosocial aspects of total parenteral nutrition. *Psychosomatics,* 1980, *21,* 115–125.
5. Pressel, P. Total parenteral nutrition: Physician and lifeliner. *Journal of Enterostomal Therapy,* 1982, *9,* 27–29.

22

Permanent Total Parenteral Nutrition
Psychological and Social Responses of the Early Stages

BETH S. PRICE and ELEANOR L. LEVINE

Permanent total parenteral nutrition (TPN) is a new form of life-sustaining therapy.[1,2] This treatment is indicated in situations where the disease results in a state in which the small bowel is no longer able to perform its normal absorptive functions to support life.[2,3] Initiating this type of therapy requires the operative insertion of a permanent silastic catheter into the subclavian vein through which essential nutrients are infused into the body to meet the daily requirements for growth and metabolism. TPN is an artificial and unnatural source of feeding and nurturance which demands major adjustments in life-style. Patients must learn the intricacies of the entire TPN system and become totally self-sufficient in its use. For this, patients undergo a period of training during which they learn to operate this complicated apparatus independently. This highly complex and completely sterile procedure is repeated 365 days a year!

The medical team must be cognizant of the psychological and

Reprinted in abridged form from the *Journal of Parenteral and Enteral Nutrition,* 1979, *3,* 48–52. Copyright 1979. Reproduced by permission.

BETH S. PRICE and ELEANOR L. LEVINE • Social Service Department, Toronto General Hospital, Toronto, Ontario, Canada M5G1L7.

social effects of this technology and help the patients come to terms with them. Only in this way will the patients benefit maximally from the use of TPN.[4]

Method

This report is based on the authors' observations and experience with 19 consecutive permanent TPN patients at Toronto General Hospital from April 1975 to April 1977, each of whom was referred for social work assessment and counseling. Information for this study was obtained by serial in-depth interviews. The method of eliciting data in the interviews was through the counseling process, which involved both direct and open-ended questions. The patients were not aware of their participation in a study because the primary role of the authors was originally entirely clinical. The study evolved in the form of a retrospective analysis and assessment of the psychosocial problems of patients on TPN.

The period of contact varied from 1 to 19 months, with an average exposure of 7.4 months. The age range of these patients was from 17 to 60 years, with 10 males and 9 females in the group. The majority (12) were married, 4 single, 1 divorced, 1 separated, and 1 widowed. All socioeconomic classes were represented as well as a variety of professions and jobs. The major focus of our study is the time during hospitalization and the initial six months following discharge (this early stage is the most traumatic).

Results

TPN patients experience a diverse range of feelings and emotions because of their new way of living; however, the temporal sequence of reactions is often predictable. The patient goes through a series of stages, beginning with the initial reactions of numbness or disbelief, even denial. During this stage the patient often denies the likelihood of the permanence of this therapy, followed by a growing awareness of pain, sorrow, anger, and grief, a preoccupation with his losses, i.e., bowel, and the inability to eat or drink. Gradually, there is a period of reorganization in which the patient struggles to incorporate the loss, accept the limitations, adapt to a new way of living, and establish a new state of equilibrium.[5,6] The final stage is accelerated for many by the possibility that they may eat again, if only in a very limited sense, which results in a subjective feeling of hope.

Early Emotional Reactions

Depression

Clinical depression, the severe reactive type, was a common emotional response to the TPN procedure. This was seen in every situation and, in most cases, was moderate to severe in intensity, albeit short lived in some. This despondency related to the loss of a natural and meaningful source of personal pleasure and human interaction—eating. Every patient misses and craves food. They read advertisements, feel hungry, and never lose hope of eating again, often bargaining for even a "cup of tea." They are obsessed with food and the lack of oral intake—to bite, taste, chew, swallow. "How does one describe the horror of losing the ability to eat?" said Mr. K. after 4 months.

Every patient misses demarcations of the day which mealtime has always provided. This sameness of routine deprives them of a diversion that human beings universally depend upon. They can also no longer turn to the refrigerator to relieve boredom, anger, frustration, and, especially, hunger! Eating is a normal function of everyday life and a major aspect of the socialization process. Many of our daily human encounters have their basis in food— coffee breaks, eating in restaurants, holiday rituals (Christmas, Thanksgiving, Passover). This form of normal interaction and behavior is taken away from TPN patients. In the early stages, depression is omnipresent but diminishes as patients and their families learn to cope adaptively.

Body Image

There are well described and documented alterations of body image attributable to any chronic illness and surgery.[4,5,7−9] These were corroborated by our patients. Superimposed, however, are the effects specific for TPN patients who have usually undergone extensive surgery and who experience a severely altered and negative body image. For some, partial or complete removal of the bowel signified not being a "whole person." They were often repulsed by their own bodies and had difficulty accepting their mutilated forms, i.e., multiple scars, emaciation, or cushingoid features as a result of prednisone therapy.

The cosmetic effect of multiple surgical procedure and the actual location of the silastic catheter was a constant source of concern. Patients felt self-conscious about a foreign object protruding from the body, with 30 inches of plastic tubing coiled and taped to the chest. Each person tended to have a strong interest in their physical appearance but now perceived themselves as unattractive or repulsive, i.e., there was the aggravation of an already distorted body image. This physical insult was a tremendous assault of the feelings of self-respect and self-esteem. In our population, these feelings were universal and were easily elicited as soon as trust was established.

Anxiety

There was a high degree of anxiety and fear of the unknown. Patients were initially overwhelmed by the various TPN procedures they were learning and questioned how they would cope with the complex sterile protocol and home training program in order to care for their own "life lines." They were uncertain as to what the future held for them: "Will I ever be healthy again?" To alleviate this anxiety, every patient while still in the hospital was introduced to other neophyte TPN patients as well as to some of our veterans. It was reassuring for them to see how well the home patients looked and to have the opportunity to discuss their unique ways of managing, i.e., traveling, sexual functioning, etc.

Period of Adaptation

As patients adapted to a new way of life, several other significant emotions and behaviors became operant. All initially felt very different and unique, even "freaky." They did not see themselves as "normal" and equated non-eating with an abnormal state. Along with these feelings were fears of the attitudes of others, i.e., spouse, children, friends, people in the community, and employers. Patients wondered if they would be accepted or rejected, discriminated against, and ridiculed. They experienced a strong sense of social embarrassment.

As the time of discharge drew close, a "love-hate" (life death) relationship developed with the TPN apparatus, a process similar to that reported by dialysis patients.[10] The patients realized that this incredible technology was keeping them alive, yet every day of their lives they would have to "hook up" to be fed. This created a dilemma. The formerly independent person struggled with feelings of complete dependence, the lack of control over his own body functioning, and reliance on the mechanical apparatus to be sustained. Extreme feelings of frustration and ambivalence were common.

Freedom to choose and the power to make simple decisions of daily living were sharply curtailed. Because of the insertion of the catheter, patients had to restrict many of their usual activities. While improved new dressings eliminated many former concerns, swimming, showers, and water sports still have to be excluded. Athletics, a healthy outlet for expressing emotions, were limited, and such contact sports as football were impossible because of dangers to the line. Parties, holidays, and rituals, all which traditionally include food and drink, provided less enjoyment and meant a decrease in social contact and interaction; thus, many of the "pleasures" in life were removed or altered. Patients felt grateful to be alive yet questioned the worth or quality of life in view of the multiple restrictions and complexities it now entailed.

Resumption of Normal Activities

Employment

Return to a fairly normal life-style was a goal of the home training TPN program. Patients were encouraged to return to work as soon as their physical and emotional condition permitted.

If a patient worked a regular day, he had to learn to schedule his employment hours around being "hooked up" to feedings (work 8 hours, travel to and from employment for approximately 2 hours, and run the TPN apparatus for 10 to 12 hours). This highly restrictive schedule left little time for any other family or leisure time activities. Because the solutions run through the night and disrupt sleep, the patients sometimes feel weak and tired during the day.

Of our 10 patients who were the main breadwinners of their families, only 2 were working full time. These prime earners fit into two categories: self-employed and employee. The self-employed patients had greater potential to return to work because of the flexibility they could build into their working hours. Two of our 3 self-employed patients were, in fact, working much less than even half time. Only 2 of the remaining 7 in an employee status were able to handle the demands of a full-time position and are still working. This sample of employables includes not only 5 recent patients but also 5 who have been on TPN from 6 to 18 months.

Sleep

Because of the large volume of solutions being absorbed by their bodies throughout the night, these patients were awakened by the urge to void approximately every 2 hours. In addition, they felt tense because of a continual concern about whether the equipment was functioning properly, i.e., speed of running solutions, tube placement, etc. This sleep disturbance caused fatigue and often necessitated a nap during the day, which also contributed significantly to emotional vulnerability.

Marital Relationships and Sexual Functioning

We found that the state of the marriage and its own inherent support systems prior to TPN correlated with the patient's desire to live and the strength to fight for health. Where stress and strife existed in the relationship, both partners felt angry, fearful, and confined by the initiation of permanent TPN. Those couples with stable, happy marriages, exemplified by mutual sharing and empathy, made a better adjustment although even they experiened some difficulties in their efforts to adapt to TPN.

Sexual functioning was a major concern. Chronically ill patients married over 15 years had already experienced a diminished sex drive and, therefore, had infrequent or nonexistent sexual relationships with their spouses. Patients married for less than 15 years, while seriously affected in their sexual relationships because of disease, had at least sporadic sexual satisfaction. Single, separated, divorced, and widowed patients with long-term bowel disease had been severely deprived of both sexual activity and social interaction.

After discharge, the problem pattern for all the above mentioned categories, except in 2 patients, continued or intensified. Those married for many years never reverted to a more normal marital relationship. Those married fewer than 15 years viewed TPN as a further imposition to their already restricted sex lives and experienced anxieties and fears related to dislodging the catheter with vigorous motion or varied positions. Because of the demands of family responsibility and the TPN protocol, patients felt that lovemaking had to be timed and, therefore, lacked a great deal of spontaneity. One exception in this category was noteworthy. One patient had been married for 12 years and was the mother of two children. For the first time in her marriage, this patient with Crohn's disease had little pain and was out of the hospital for 10 consecutive months; her sexual relationship with her husband improved significantly.

Single persons, toward the time of discharge, became increasingly anxious because they had spent most of their lives as patients either at home or in the hospital. They had been isolated, lost friends, and finally lost confidence in performing simple social skills. TPN intensified these fears because they had to learn to face the world as healthy people without having the usual crutch and often retreated into their shy, withdrawn world. Our 4 chronically ill single patients were inexperienced sexually and unattached. They realized that the disfigurement caused by the tubing taped to the chest minimized their chances of any casual sexual contacts. They anticipated that intercourse would be unlikely, unless it was preceded by an established caring relationship. This was a discouraging prospect for them.

The 4 patients who had sudden bowel catastrophes all had normal sexual relations prior to this trauma. Three of them were single, 1 married (now deceased). After discharge, the married patient became impotent, a situation which was psychologically induced. The 3 other patients allowed themselves time to convalesce and feel more relaxed with the TPN system, but then expected to resume an active sex life.

Family Involvement

TPN has major implications for family functioning. Classically, when one member of a family suffers from long-term illness or the disease requires special routines and procedures, the relationships within that unit are altered. In our sample, when the patients no longer participated in eating, the dynamics of family interaction changed. The capacity to cope with these major changes was an essential requirement of both the patients and their families. Meal preparation was a prime example. The female patients quite comfortably continued to cook for their families; male patients often assumed many of the cooking responsibilities while they were temporarily unemployed and thus relieved the spouses of their traditional and primary task. The alternative to this type of role reversal was loss of a role. One patient's wife regretfully and angrily surrendered her domain in the kitchen; after 35 years of marriage there was no one but herself to cook for and she was robbed of her raison d'être.

Despite the fact that TPN patients cannot eat, they view mealtime as an essential and valued family event. Sixteen of 19 patients continued to sit with their families during dinner.

While every patient was eager to return home from the hospital, they were extremely anxious. They feared being totally responsible for their own apparatus, not having the professional staff to turn to if problems arose. To reduce this fear, we insisted that one family member learn the TPN procedure prior to the patient's discharge. Many of the "back-up" people expressed similar concerns; nevertheless, they participated and took pride in contributing to their partner's health. Armed with the knowledge and security of available assistance, every patient returned home with his or her confidence bolstered.

Because of the prolonged hospitalization, the family often had been forced to assume all the patient's traditional duties, so that the patients worried about how they would fit in or whether they would be needed. The sharing of responsibilities was in a state of flux. Family members were reluctant to relinquish their new roles for two reasons: (1) they did not want to overtax the patient physically and emotionally; (2) they were not willing to risk another reshuffle should the patient resume his duties and it be only temporary. The patient's reintroduction into the family, therefore, created a disturbance in the family balance which they had been forced to find in the interim.

Communication also became skewed. Most of our families and patients denied or repressed their emotions in order to "protect" each other. While the motives were genuine, this mechanism was dangerous in that it stifled open and honest expression and sharing of feelings. In the long run, it caused major emotional outbursts because of pent-up frustration, resentment, or hostility. Our patients were urged to communicate their need to be reinstated in their former family roles, and the families were encouraged to share their anxieties about the patient's ability to fulfill these assigned roles. Another new equilibrium had to be worked out within the system.

One practical problem with which TPN families have to contend is storage space for supplies. Patients receive their supplies from the hospital pharmacy on a one-month basis. The volume of supplies is so great that it fills a standard large-size refrigerator, which makes it impossible to share one with the family. This necessitates the purchase of a second refrigerator, which is an added burden in terms of storage and cost.

Coping Patterns

We observed a pattern in the different coping mechanisms of those patients who had long-term gastrointestinal problems, compared with those who had a sudden bowel catastrophe. Patients with chronic bowel disease seemed to cope more effectively, at least initially. They were usually so grateful to have fewer symptoms that their compliance and adjustment was less fraught with turmoil. From their long years of suffering, they were more emotionally prepared for the trauma they now faced. Patients with acute problems, however, may never have been seriously ill, so that their long-term hospitalization with totally foreign procedures was devastating. Their fears were enormous. Often, with such a first-time illness, the patient grieved and mourned for the loss of functioning. We believe that the long-term patients made an initial adjustment with somewhat less stress because of a "trade-off" between two different life-styles, both involving chronicity. The "new" life on TPN, while still hospital- and apparatus-dependent, had greater rewards. The possibility of being pain free and leading a more normal life was preferable to chronic suffering. The patients with acute illness perceived only the multiple losses.

Discussion

Two major themes emerge for TPN patients and their families. One is the question of the *quality versus quantity of life*. Because of total food deprivation, patients experience grief (reaction) over the loss of a major function, eating, which is of particular pleasure and importance to them. Therefore, they see little purpose in undergoing the long and arduous task of learning to maintain themselves on TPN unless there is some meaning in life and the potential for self-realization. The issue becomes *how* one will live rather than *how long* one will live.

The other issue is that of *chronicity*. Although these patients are not chronically ill in the strictest sense, there are definite elements of chronicity attached to the permanency of TPN. Chronically they have (1) little or no absorption in their bowels; (2) a foreign object in their bodies; (3) lack of ability to eat normally; (4) a chronic dependence on the hospital for supplies; and (5) repeated hospital admissions. Although most of our patients thought and talked about death as an alternative, each exhibited a strong will to live by making a concerted effort to attain a healthy state.

With TPN, a major advancement of medical technology, there are now reported survivals for over five years in otherwise hopeless medical situations;[11,12] however, this type of medical progress has created new psychological stresses for patients and their families. Since the patients' lives depend upon the TPN apparatus, (they must accept not only the use of this mechanical device to survive but must adapt to the loss of normal body function and face the reality that they are permanently dependent on it as a substitute.

Our study indicated that the early stages of adapting to TPN are the most traumatic for the patients. Once they attained a maximal degree of physical health on TPN and the critical psychosocial demands and issues of this phase were addressed, they could lead relatively independent and satisfying lives within one year. In the final analysis, it is the patient's ego strength, determination, and family support system that make the difference between a mentally healthy adaptation and a life of chronic dysfunction that plagues all family members. It is, therefore, mandatory that every member of the health care team be aware and alert not only to the patient's practical ability to run the apparatus but also to their psychological adjustment as well as that of the family.[13,14] In this way there can be a high correlation between physical restoration and optimal social-emotional functioning.[15]

While ours has been an impressionistic study based on a relatively small sample, with no controls, these patients do share some feelings common to many other chronically ill individuals. The TPN procedure confers a unique and potentially devastating experience on them. Obviously, more work must be done.

ACKNOWLEDGEMENTS

The authors thank Dr. Kursheed N. Jeejeebhoy for access to his patients and for his helpful criticism of the manuscript.

References

1. Dudrick, S. J., Wilmore, D. W., Vars, H. M., & Rhoads, J. E. Long-term total parenteral nutrition with growth, development, and positive nitrogen balance. *Surgery,* 1968, *64,* 134–142.
2. Dudrick, S. J., & Rubert, P. L. Principles and practices of parenteral nutrition. *Gastroenterology,* 1971, *61,* 910–910.

3. Jeejeebhoy, K. N., & Anderson, G. H., Sanderson, I., & Bryan, M. H. Total parenteral nutrition: Nutrient needs and technical tips. *Modern Medicine in Canada.* 1974, *29*, 832–841, 944–947.

4. Moos, R. H. The crisis of treatment: Survival by machine. In R. H. Moos (Ed.), *Coping with physical illness* (Vol. 1). New York: Plenum Medical, 1977.

5. Moos, R. H., & Tsu, V. D. The crisis of physical illness: An overview. In R. H. Moos (Ed.), *Coping with physical illness* (Vol. 1). New York: Plenum Medical, 1977.

6. Kübler-Ross, E. *On death and dying.* New York: Macmillan, 1969.

7. Adler, M. L. Kidney transplantation and coping mechanisms. *Psychosomatics,* 1972, *13*, 337–341.

8. Andreasen, N. J. C., & Norris, A. S. Long-term adjustment and adaptation mechanisms in severely burned adults. *Journal of Nervous and Mental Disease,* 1972, *154*, 352–362.

9. Williams, C. D. The CCU nurse has a pacemaker. *American Journal of Nursing,* 1972, *72*, 900–902.

10. Abram, H. S. Survival by machine. The psychological stress of chronic hemodialysis. In R. H. Moos (Ed.), *Coping with physical illness* (Vol. 1). New York: Plenum Medical, 1977.

11. Jeejeebhoy, K. N., Langer, B., Tsallas, G., Chu, R. C., Kuksis, A., & Anderson, G. H. Total parenteral nutrition at home: Studies in patients surviving 4 months to 5 years. *Gastroenterology,* 1976, *71*, 943–953.

12. Heitzer, W. D., & Orringer, E. P. Parenteral nutrition at home for 5 years via arteriovenous fistulae. *Gastroenterology,* 1977, *72*, 527–532.

13. Lipowski, Z. J. Physical illness, the individual and the coping process. *Psychiatry in Medicine,* 1970, *1*, 91–102.

14. Adams, J. E., & Lindemann, E. Coping with long-term disability. In G. C. Coehlo, D. A. Hamburg, & J. E. Adams (Eds.), *Coping and adaptation.* New York: Basic Books, 1974.

15. Langer, B., McHattie, J. D., Zohrab, W. J., & Jeejeebhoy, K. N. Prolonged survival after complete small bowel resection using intravenous alimentation at home. *Journal of Surgical Research,* 1973, *15*, 226–233.

23

Psychological Aspects of Long-Term Home Hyperalimentation

MARK PERL, RICHARD C. W. HALL,
STANLEY J. DUDRICK, DeANN M. ENGLERT,
SONDRA K. STICKNEY, and EARL R. GARDNER

Total parenteral nutrition (TPN) is still in a growth phase in this country. Although it has been only 12 years [now 16] since the technique was first described by Dudrick and his co-workers,[1] it is estimated that 2,400,000 units of TPN solution—a standard unit containing 1 liter of TPN solution were administered in 1977, and by 1979 this rose to 4,300,000 units.[2] Ambulatory home intravenous hyperalimentation (HIVH) maintenance, on a semipermanent or permanent basis, has become an increasingly viable option for patients with severely compromised bowel [function]

Reprinted in abridged form from the *Journal of Parenteral and Enteral Nutrition*, 1980, *4*, 554–560. Copyright 1980. Reproduced by permission.

MARK PERL • Department of Psychiatry, University of California Service, San Francisco General Hospital, San Francisco, California 94110. RICHARD C. W. HALL • Chief of Staff, Veterans Administration Medical Center, Memphis, Tennessee 38104. STANLEY J. DUDRICK • St. Luke's Episcopal Hospital, Houston, Texas 77025. DeANN M. ENGLERT • Nutritional Support Nurse Consultant, Denver, Colorado. SONDRA K. STICKNEY • Hermann Hospital, Houston, Texas 77025. EARL R. GARDNER • deceased, formerly of Department of Psychiatry, the University of Texas Medical School, Houston, Texas 77025.

and/or nutritional status. These patients, who formerly may not have survived, or at best would have needed continuous hospital care, now can live at home and lead active lives.[3] In 1977–1978, 167 patients were registered on HIVH in the United States,[4] but we estimate the true figure at between 600 and 1000 because many patients are short-term cases and are not listed.

The advent of HIVH has necessitated the setting up and training of highly skilled medical teams and elaborately equipped treatment centers. The technology in this field is still very much in an evolutionary phase. Along with the nutritional and surgical challenges an entirely new spectrum of psychological and social problems has emerged in these patients. Our knowledge and techniques for dealing with these situations have had to be flexible and adaptive.

This Study

This report emerged from a program of psychological assessment and followup of patients and their families in our ambulatory HIVH clinic. Our aims were (1) to make an initial evaluation of patients entering the HIVH program with regard to their coping skills, presence of psychopathology, level of cognitive functioning, sexual and marital adjustment, and overall activity; (2) to follow patients and their families longitudinally and to elucidate their specific emotional reactions to HIVH; and (3) to devise methods for the staff to manage the psychological aspects of these patients.

Review of Literature

Since HIVH is a new technique, it is not surprising that there are very few published reports on its psychological aspects. In a fairly brief report MacRitchie[5] described the responses of 9 patients who had been on HIVH (intermittent infusion) for periods of 3 to 58 months. The patients were described as passing through stages of disbelief and hopelessness in the initial stages, followed by a period of adaptation while being instructed in HIVH techniques. MacRitchie emphasized the physical and social impact of the loss of the eating function. Other effects, such as changes in sexual activity level and ambivalent feelings toward the HIVH machinery, were pointed out. No mention was made of long-term activity level and social adaptation in these patients.

Price and Levine[6] (see Chapter 22) described the early responses of 19 adult patients and their families during the inpatient phase and in the first few months of outpatient care. They reported that anxiety, depression, and body image problems were common; that patients experienced a "grief" reaction to the loss of their eating function; and that, in general, those who had had chronic bowel disease coped better with HIVH than those who had a sudden bowel catastrophe. Progress seemed to correlate well with pre-HIVH family adjustment and support.

Malcolm et al.[2] evaluated 59 patients placed on HIVH in the hospital, three of whom were long-term cases. In the very early stages (0–48 hr) the authors observed a 20% incidence of transient delirium, depression, or even hypomania. They ascribed these reactions to biological causes affecting brain function (organic brain disorders). During the next 1 to 12 weeks, anxiety and depression occurred frequently, and paranoid reactions were seen in a few patients. In the long-term group, stresses affected functioning in many areas, including work, family life, and sexuality.

There is an extensive literature on patients' reactions to chronic illness, and in a general way these findings may apply to patients on HIVH.[7–10] For example, Moos and Tsu[9] point out that ill patients must master 7 separate "tasks": pain and incapacitation, the hospital environment, the professional staff, their own anxiety and depression, body image and self-image changes, relationships with significant others, and preparation for an uncertain future. Hinton[10] describes common sources of stress in patients diagnosed with cancer: pain, disfigurement, concern over the future, loss of work role, dependency on others, alienation from loved ones. Depression and anxiety states are very prevalent in these patients, while paranoid and hypomanic symptoms are seen occasionally. Those facing death[7,8] must contend with anxiety and feelings of mourning and often experience guilt or anger or minimize and deny their illness.

There are some similarities between the situation of HIVH

patients and those on long-term hemodialysis. Abram's classic paper[11] points out the fundamental dilemma faced by patients whose life is prolonged by mechanical means, i.e., is this life worth living? This author elucidates 5 areas of conflict which dialysis patients encounter: dependency (and compliance) requirements versus the need to be independent and lead a "normal" life; relating to an inanimate object, the dialysis machinery, with the consequent disturbances in body-image; ambivalence over life and death, the latter being an ever-present and ominous possibility; denial of illness as a major psychological defense; and interpersonal conflicts related to the dialysis unit personnel and the patient's spouse. Czaczkes and De-Nour's[12] monograph gives a more complete account and draws conclusions similar to those of Abram regarding the psychological processes in dialysis patients. There are, however, major differences between hemodialysis and HIVH, which make the latter a unique situation in medicine. Patients must maintain a high level of medical "know-how": connecting up infusion solutions, monitoring the pump-catheter system, and keeping it infection free. They are more dependent on technology for survival on a day-to-day basis, yet are able to lead more active and independent lives than dialysis patients.[2] The treatment does not imply a deteriorating course and prognosis as does hemodialysis.

The HIVH Clinic

Patients enter our HIVH clinic[3] after a period of hospitalization and treatment for their primary condition. They undergo a rigorous training program related to catheter care, with spouses and parents of child patients often participating. Most patients can change their own dressings, and some even mix their own solutions at home. Patients are generally on a continuous (24-hr) infusion schedule, and the use of portable vests is common during waking hours. Some patients have become adept at the use of a heparin lock for occasions when they want to turn off the infusion. Patients living [near the clinic] in Houston are seen at weekly or biweekly intervals; those living out of town are seen every 2 to 3 mo, and strict liaison is maintained with their local physicians.

Over a 12-mo period, all adult patients in the ambulatory HIVH clinic were assessed by a staff psychiatrist and a psychiatric nurse, working in close connection with the other members of the IVH team. Patients already established on HIVH and new admissions to the clinic were assessed to a total of 22. Only those (N = 10) maintained continuously on HIVH for 6 mo or more were included in the present study. There were 6 males and 4 females, from 24–66 years of age; 8 had diseases leading to the "short bowel syndrome," 7 of whom were expected to require TPN indefinitely. Their diagnoses were: Crohn's disease (4); Gardner's syndrome (2); metastatic carcinoid (1); stab wound (1); anorexia nervosa (1); and non-specific bowel inflammation with adhesions (1). All socioeconomic classes and a variety of occupations were represented in the sample . . . . Based on our interviews as well as nursing staff reports, the behavioral trends in these patients are presented in a number of areas of functioning.

Depression

Eight patients displayed clinical evidence of at least mild depression when first assessed, with dysphoric mood, crying spells, insominia, and/or feelings of hopelessness; 2 patients seemed not to have been troubled by these feelings. There was evidence of a pre-existing personality disorder (maladaptive behavior patterns) in 2 of the depressed patients. Nonetheless, most of the depression could be related to obvious and severe current life stresses: the underlying illness, the need for TPN, the loss of eating function, marital and family difficulties, financial hardship, etc. Typically, depression was marked in the 3–4 mo following instigation of HIVH. The course of the depression then waxed and waned; exacerbations characteristically occurred in response to increased stress, and were not long lasting (days or weeks rather than months). Three patients experienced brief but intense bouts of suicidal despair, although no suicide attempts were made.

A patient making good adjustment at home became severely depressed on three separate occasions when readmitted to the hospital for exacerbations of his underlying chronic illness, for which in one admission abdominal surgery was required. He expressed feelings of hopelessness and questioned the need for "all this treatment" and the HIVH. Despite definite suicidal ideation, he stated that he "wouldn't go through with suicide" because of the distress it would cause his family. He was seen daily by the team psychiatrist for supportive interviews to which he showed a positive response: The depression abated, as did the suicidality. During one hospitalization antidepressants were used (amitriptyline, up to 100 milligrams, orally at night), but it is unclear that this contributed to the improvement; the patient may have intestinally absorbed little of the medication, and the duration of treatment was short lived (1 week). Following each discharge home and the resumption of his usual activities, the patient's mood improved markedly, though the depression never totally left him.

The degree of depression seemed also to be related to the prospects of recovery of gastrointestinal function.

A patient with Crohn's disease had some remaining bowel function, but was led to believe that he would require permanent TPN. He was markedly depressed for a prolonged period. He was then given a revised, more optimistic prognosis, i.e., that within several months he might not require parenteral feeding. His mood recovered dramatically within a few days.

Depression at times presented as partial denial of illness and poor compliance with the staff's instructions regarding catheter care:

A patient who was living alone and feeling depressed "forgot" to hang HIVH bags at the correct times and became mildly dehydrated.

Another depressed patient "experimented" with the equipment by riding upside down in an amusement park ride to see if the pump would "defy gravity." Fortunately no damage was done.

Patients occasionally presented with catheter-tip infections following deviations from sterile technique in dressing changes. In the past in some of our clinic patients, infections followed swimming or showering, in defiance of staff instructions.

Such slippages in self-care can, of course, lead to extreme consequences, through metabolic imbalance or septicemia; Abram has termed such neglect "passive suicide."[11] Remarkably, the incidence of self-neglect has been extremely low, considering the ever-present potential for harm in this population. During the survey period, there were no instances of major "disaster" (death, septicemia, irreversible metabolic damage) due to such neglect. Nursing staff vigilance and availability played a crucial preventive role.

Specific psychiatric intervention was sometimes requested in response to a patient's sudden decompensation following new stresses. The mainstay of treatment was supportive psychotherapy, ventilation of feelings by the patient, and reassurance and encouragement by the staff. Nonpsychiatric staff participated in this process.

Fear—A Response to Technology

Fear was almost universal in our patient group, especially in the early months of HIVH. Fears were related to realistic dangers, such as catheter infection, pump malfunction, and air embolism and were not conceptualized by us as "free-floating" or "neurotic" anxiety. At times fear approached terror that life-sustaining equipment was about to fail and they would soon die.

> *Patients made it very clear what their feelings were about being dependent on the pump-catheter system, in [such] statements as: "You play with your own life day by day." "You go to bed not knowing if you'll wake up the next morning." "You never know what to expect next."*

Almost all the patients could relate several "horror stories" of incidents where some potentially dangerous event occurred outside the hospital.

> *A patient, while traveling in an airplane, noticed that his HIVH pump had stopped. He installed a simple substitute pump which he happened to be carrying, until he could get his original pump replaced.*
> *A patient observed that her HIVH catheter had clotted off. She injected what she thought was heparin to clear the line, but found it was xylocaine instead. Fortunately, there were no sequelae.*
> *The catheter tubing of a patient living alone was jolted and became disconnected. Blood backed up in the catheter and spilled onto the floor. The patient, though frightened, had the presence of mind to reconnect and tape the tubing. No negative results ensued.*

In each of these and other similar incidents, the patient

would telephone the central clinic for advice. If there was any question as to the functioning of the system or safety, the patient was immediately brought into the clinic, by air ambulance if needed. Though costly at times, such prompt action was deemed necessary, worthwhile, and effective in heading off dangerous sequelae. Psychologically, such action, or the potential for action, was immensely reassuring. Patient fears, though realistic, sometimes became exaggerated and interfered with daily functioning.

> *During the first 3 months of HIVH, a patient found his sleep severely troubled by dreams of the tubing breaking. He kept waking up periodically, fearing that he would bleed to death by morning.*
>
> *Several patients who lived in outlying areas worried that something might go wrong with the HIVH system while they were alone and that no one would be available to help, not even the local doctor. They became fastidious about averting kinks and air bubbles in the tubing, sepsis, fever, etc., and were at times preoccupied to the exclusion of other activities.*

The fears responded to nursing staff interventions; the availability and accessibility of nurses to patients at all times; willingness to have the patient return to the clinic for catheter problems, fevers, etc., "refresher" courses in catheter and nutritional management, and intense emotional support and reassurance. Psychiatric intervention was seldom requested or needed in these cases; likewise, the use of antianxiety agents, such as diazepam, or antipsychotics, such as chlorpromazine, was eschewed. With the passage of time, patients became less fearful of being overtaken by a "catastrophe" and more confident that they could handle a crisis. As the level of fear became manageable, overall functioning and activity improved.

Body Image Changes

In our outpatient group, we did not observe true somatic delusional thinking, although other authors[2] have reported its presence in the early stages. Almost all our patients, however, reported the feeling that they looked "weird" or deformed because of their indwelling catheters.

> *A patient, professionally employed, stated that he was aware of the*

HIVH equipment through every waking moment, both at work and socially, and felt uncomfortable and embarrassed much of the time.

A male patient tried (by wearing heavy outer clothing) to hide the fluid bags, pump, and catheter. He felt as though the fluid bags made him appear to have breasts.

Several patients were troubled by members of the public staring and asking questions—especially when children did so.

Some body-image distortions were more pronounced:

Patients made statements like: "I feel I am a machine, not just hooked up to one." "I feel the catheter will pierce my heart." "The HIVH causes my body to malfunction." "If I connect the pump wrong I'll pump myself back into the bottle."

No psychotic episodes occurred, and patient reality-testing was otherwise intact. Such feelings occurred mainly early in the course of HIVH and seemed related to the fears already mentioned. They responded to the educational processes outlined above, and no psychotropic drugs were used.

Loss of Eating Function

In the first 2–3 months of HIVH, almost all patients were distressed by not being able to eat. They reported feeling painfully aware of the barrage of TV and newspaper advertisements inducing people to eat and drink, and felt excluded from daily rituals (meals, coffee breaks, social drinking) and festive occasions (birthdays, holidays) in which food played a major role.

A patient was totally restricted from any oral intake because he developed massive diarrhea after eating. On his birthday he was thoughtlessly sent a huge, luscious-looking cake by a family friend.

At Thanksgiving a patient wistfully requested that a turkey be hung up inside the HIVH bag.

In our group, all the patients eventually regained some eating function, though they derived little nutriment from it and their diet was necessarily restricted. Many reported craving "a real meal" at times; two described almost continuous hunger pangs, despite good nutritional balance.

A patient oscillated between sticking to a bland diet and going on "eating binges" usually on social occasions. Defying medical advice, she ate spicy and irritative foods; she knew that she would "pay the price" later on in symptoms of abdominal pain and diarrhea.

Patients were encouraged by the staff to spend mealtimes in the usual way, eating what they could. Those not living alone did so, continuing to derive social and family satisfaction from meals. Cooking for others became important for at least 4 of our group, and being on HIVH did not usually dull patients' awareness of or sensitivity to the smells and tastes of food. (Two patients reported a temporary diminution of the sense of taste for the first 3 mo of HIVH, though no physiological cause for this was found.)

Family Life and Sexual Functioning

TPN seemed to add significantly to the stresses on marital relationships, already under strain from the patient's pre-existing illness. In 4 families, the spouses were emotionally supportive and helped with dressing changes and the management of HIVH solutions. In 3 others, the spouses seemed overwhelmed by the patient's new needs, distanced themselves emotionally, and refused to become involved in catheter care. We found, as did Price and Levine,[6] that where there was a previously stable relationship, couples continued to exhibit sharing and empathy when one partner began HIVH. Where the relationship was already dysfunctional, TPN added significantly to the discord.

Even in the most stable families [the] advent of TPN had a profound effect on the life-style of couples.

Following a long-standing chronic illness, a patient commenced home TPN. The patient's spouse was initially both caring and supportive and quit work to spend time with the patient. Because of health-related debts, they sold their car and house and moved into an apartment closer to the HIVH clinic. Though they had been emotionally close, they now became less involved with each other; their sexual activity also diminished.

In some male patients on long-term HIVH, zinc deficiency could cause secondary impotence, which could be reversed by the addition of adequate amounts of this trace metal to the solution.[13] In our survey, however, we did not encounter sexual difficulties related to this cause. Six of the patients reported diminished frequency and reduced enjoyment of sexual relations, especially in the early months of HIVH. Psychological factors were adduced, relating mainly to the patient's altered body image and feelings of embarrassment and discomfort at being connected to a clicking pump, bags, tubing, etc.

A patient feeling sexually inhibited humorously noted: "When I try to make love, there are three of us, me, my partner, and the clicking machine." This patient subsequently learned to disconnect the tubing using a heparin lock and successfully engaged in sexual activities.

Emotional depression also reduced sexual desire. Another inhibitory factor was the partner's fear of harming the patient. Sexual relations tended to improve after the first few months on HIVH, especially in those families in which we had characterized the spouse as supportive and empathic.

Parent–child relationships, too underwent changes following the initiation of HIVH. Several patients reported feeling inhibited in the presence of their children, and vice versa.

A parent of two young children was afraid to play actively and "roughhouse" with them, lest they damage his HIVH catheter and pump.

A patient's teenage children had reluctantly undergone training in the rudiments of catheter care and what to do in an emergency (e.g., clamping the catheter if hemorrhaging). The children expressed anxiety and revulsion at the "tube coming out of your stomach" and refused to be nearby during routine dressing changes.

Other instances were reported where previously involved relatives became anxious in the presence of the HIVH equipment and began avoiding the patient; understandably, this was a source of distress to the patient.

Finances

Extreme financial difficulties dogged all our patients through the course of their illness and became more pronounced after starting HIVH. Englert and Dudrick[3] reported the costs of HIVH maintenance in 1978; the cost of maintaining a patient on HIVH for 1 year at our center [in 1980 was] $30,000. Patients with adequate health insurance find that most of their fluid and equipment costs are covered, though they still bear many hidden costs —e.g., travel and transportation, the cost of storage refrigerator for HIVH bags. Those without sufficient health insurance have had to rely on grants from pharmaceutical manufacturers, hospitals, and even charitable funds set up by their churches or communities. Attempts [have been] made at the national legislative level to obtain Medicare or similar benefits for HIVH patients.

Activity Level and Employment

Perhaps the most striking feature of the HIVH patient group was the high level of activity and employability. Three patients were judged more active after the institution of HIVH than previously, 5 maintained previous activity levels, and 2 became less active. Patients were encouraged to resume full-time employment whenever possible following adjustment to HIVH. Of the 5 patients who had previously been salaried or self-employed workers, 3 continued their occupations (2 full time and 1 part time) following HIVH; in addition, 2 patients who had been part- or full-time homemakers continued this activity. One patient who had been almost totally inactive and bedridden took up part-time college studies once on HIVH; another became very active in a church group. The 2 patients who became less active than previously gave up their full-time jobs and remained at home but retained some family and homemaking activities.

Leisure and structured social activities occupied an important place for at least 4 patients:

A patient on continuous HIVH infusion plays golf regularly, at times finding it more convenient to carry the solution bags on his back rather than in front. He likes rodeo sports and is able to ride horses and rope steers while using a heparin-lock arrangement to temporarily disconnect the infusion.

A patient bowls regularly once a week and is captain of the local bowling team.

> *Two patients have become very active in the affairs of their local churches since commencing HIVH, one being asked to preach on occasions.*

Some activities were necessarily curtailed or restricted, for example, swimming and showers which could cause catheter contamination, body contact sports which could interfere with catheter placement and pump function. Such restrictions were regarded as no more than inconveniences by most patients. Of more concern were the logistics of travel and the necessity of carrying adequate supplies of nutrient fluid and equipment. Despite this, patients frequently made road and air trips, at times having supplies sent to their destinations.

Several patients complained of varying degrees of fatigue, and even the fully employed persons occasionally needed to take time off work to rest. The primary illness seemed implicated here, as fatigue and weakness had been present prior to HIVH in all these cases.

The Patient and the Public

As with all major medical advances, HIVH has brought publicity and even fame to its first patients. Some proudly display scrapbooks of interviews with the press and photographers. Two patients have given public lectures based on their experiences.

HIVH elicits a mixture of amazement, disbelief, incredulity, and admiration from the general public. It also provokes fear and even anger, which seem to be rooted in ignorance. Thus, patients going out in the street, supermarket, church, and even among relatives face a steady barrage of searching questions. The interrogation usually reduces to a single puzzlement: How can a person survive without eating? All patients are aware of being "different," and at times resent the curiosity and the inquiries. Two patients have reported encountering anger and hostility from anonymous members of the public.

> *A patient received a life-threatening letter, accompanied by the statement that "HIVH is against God's will; you shouldn't be alive." Another patient was similarly confronted by an angry individual who categorized HIVH as "the work of the devil."*

Ignorance about HIVH is not confined to nonmedical persons.

A patient visiting a rural town ran out of HIVH fluid. She encountered a "stonewall" when she requested a bag a dextrose water from the local hospital, to tide her over the next day. None of the staff had heard of HIVH, and no one believed her story.

Patient–Staff Interactions

Patient interaction with surgeons, nurses, and dietitians was that of admiration, respect, and gratitude for the skills which had kept them alive. On the other hand, patients sometimes felt powerless, helpless, and at the staff's mercy. Statements like "they run my life" were typical.

During the process of treatment and patient education about HIVH, conflicts occasionally arose between a patient and the staff; in 3 cases the psychiatric team were asked to intervene. Our interviews suggested that underlying the anger and hostility of the patients there often were unexpressed feelings of depression about the illness and the need for TPN and resentment at being dependent on a machine for survival.

A patient, rehospitalized with an exacerbation of his bowel condition, became angry over what he perceived as neglect and lack of caring by the medical and nursing staff. He demanded narcotic analgesics and refused to deal with certain of the staff members, calling them incompetent. He stated that he would leave and seek help elsewhere. After several discussions with the psychiatrist, he recognized the feelings of frustration and depression underlying his anger.

Patients sometimes did, of course, have legitimate reasons for criticizing members of the staff. Often, disagreement arose over points of technique. Having managed their own catheter care and nturition for periods of months or years, patients were keenly aware of the technical aspects; a staff member's deviations from "the right way" provoked fear and ire.

A rehospitalized patient argued vehemently for 30 min with a nurse who was changing her catheter dressing. The patient had been independent and managing very well at home. The argument, over the correct way to clamp the catheter, became heated, and eventually the chief HIVH nurse was called in. The senior nurse vindicated the patient's technique; the staff person was in error.

Organic Brain Disease Screen

Three patients showed some evidence of mild or moderate encephalopathy (organic brain syndrome) at initial assessment. This was manifested by impairment of abstraction ability, concentration, or immediate or long-term memory. Two of the patients were taking narcotic analgesics at the time of assessment. No other evidence of specific disease (such as localizing neurological signs, EEG changes) was found. Follow-up psychological tests were not included in our survey.

Discussion

The application of the technique of long-term HIVH can significantly reduce morbidity and mortality in patients with compromised bowel function and nutritional status; only by the coordinated efforts of a highly specialized and motivated multidisciplinary team can these results be achieved. In order to be maintained as an active outpatient on HIVH, it is necessary that emotional needs be understood and that the psychological problems be handled in as enthusiastic and competent a manner as the physical problems are handled. Thus, the basic hyperalimentation team, consisting of the physician/surgeon, nurse, pharmacist, and dietitian, must now be augmented to include the psychiatrist and the psychiatric nurse.

Our preliminary study arose from the psychiatric professionals' first year with the HIVH team. The sample size was small, and control groups were not used, but the following tentative conclusions seem reasonable, based on our clinical findings. Of course, many of these hypotheses will need validation using rigorous instruments in a controlled situation.

Emotional depression is very common in HIVH patients; 8 of our 10 patients experienced at least mild depression, as noted by others.[2,5,6] It is not clear, however, how much depression is present before the start of HIVH, i.e., how much the underlying illness is responsible. Depression was most pronounced in the first 3–6 mo of HIVH treatment, and seemed to be, in part, related to the issue of whether the patient would ever regain normal eating function. Apart from this loss, other severe intercurrent life stresses seemed operative also. However, we have no reason to think that there is any biological depressive effect of HIVH per se, although this has been suggested.[2,5] Occasionally, some medical cause may have been implicated, e.g., if the patient were on a course of steroid medications. Most of the depression, however, occurred in the absence of such factors and was thought to be reactive to life stress.

Three patients experienced [episodes of increased suicidal feelings]. This, then, is not an uncommon occurrence. Depression of this severity tends to be transient and reactive to an increase in stress. Despite the availability of methods of self-harm, depressed patients tend not to actively pursue this route; rather, they neglect their care and risk passively harming themselves. Patients who are depressed, even those who are suicidal, do not necessarily require inpatient psychiatric care. The mainstay of treatment seems to be supportive interviewing by the HIVH staff and/or the psychiatric personnel. Tricyclic antidepressants are indicated occasionally.

Fear surrounding the workings of the pump-catheter system is pervasive; the sense of vulnerability and danger is, of course, reality based. Fears are worse during the early stages of HIVH and in those who live farthest from the clinic. Some body-image distortion occurs during the initial adjustment phase; however, nursing staff support and patient education, rather than psychiatric counseling, form the basis of management, and the fears abate as the patient becomes more confident in knowledge of HIVH.

The finding of *mild organic brain syndrome* in 3 patients requires further investigation. The source of this dysfunction may have been the primary illness but may also have been due to the HIVH treatment per se, metabolic aberrations (such as trace metal deficiency), or drug effects. Malcolm *et al.*[2] have raised the possibility of an effect of HIVH on neurotransmitter metabolism.

Once the patient has adjusted to HIVH (after 3–6 mo), activity and productive employment can be maintained and even enhanced. This is perhaps the most noteworthy finding of our study. There is some embarrassment at carrying or wearing the vest, pump, and bags in public as well as social discomfort at the curiosity and questioning which are elicited. Overall, however, patients are extremely gratified with the new lease on life afforded by HIVH and seem to put up with the inconveniences with a good sense of humor. HIVH allows patients to be independent and functional in other areas too, e.g., sexual activity, family life, recreation, social activity, and travel. Patients can and do take part in the social pleasures of food-related activities, despite their dietary restrictions. The primary illness, rather than the presence of HIVH, governs the level of activity which the patient may attain.

The public and the medical profession are still largely ignorant of HIVH. A campaign of education is needed to publicize the contribution that HIVH can make to the care of the nutritionally impaired, but funding for HIVH maintenance must be secured if all who need treatment are to obtain it. A nationwide patient support organization ("Lifeline"[14]) is now in existence.

The basis for the success of an HIVH program is the clinic nursing staff. A highly trained HIVH nurse, available 24 hr a day to deal with emergencies, not only is important for the patients' physical care but for emotional support as well, to prevent and alleviate fear and depression. Likewise, the HIVH education program and refresher courses can bolster the patient psychologically; ambivalent feelings must be recognized and allowed verbal expression. Clear lines of authority should be laid down, so that staff and patients know who is to be called in a crisis. To minimize staff members being pitted against one another, i.e., team "splitting" and/or "burnout" we suggest frequent team discussions of difficult cases.[15]

The psychiatric professional's role in the HIVH team is (a) to make initial and followup evaluations of patients' mental state and coping mechanisms, (b) to provide counseling and/or pharmacological interventions to patients and their relatives during crisis, (c) to advise the other team members regarding the ongoing management of stress in their patients.

ACKNOWLEDGEMENTS

Many thanks are due to Mrs. Dorothy M. Manley and Ms. Mindy Leifer for their patient help in the preparation of this paper.

References

1. Dudrick, S. J., Wilmore, D. W., Vars, H. M., & Rhoads, J. E. Long-term total parenteral nutrition with growth, development, and positive nitrogen balance. *Surgery*, 1968, *64*, 134–142.
2. Malcolm, R., Robson, J. R. K., Vanderveen, T. W., & O'Neil, P. M. Psychosocial aspects of total parenteral nutrition. *Psychosomatics*, 1980, *21*, 115–125.
3. Englert, D. M., & Dudrick, S. J. Principles of ambulatory home hyperalimentation. *American Journal of IV Therapy*, 1978, *5*, 11–28.
4. The New York Academy of Medicine. Registry of patients on home total parenteral nutrition (Memo). December 14, 1978.
5. MacRitchie, K. J. Life without eating or drinking. Total parenteral nutrition outside hospital. *Canadian Psychiatric Association Journal*, 1978, *23*, 373–379.
6. Price, B. S., & Levine, E. L. Permanent total parenteral nutrition: Psychological and social responses of the early stages. *Journal of Parenteral and Enteral Nutrition*, 1979, *3*, 48–52.
7. Moos, R. H. (Ed.). *Coping with physical illness*. New York: Plenum Press, 1977.
8. Kübler-Ross, E. *On death and dying*. New York: Macmillan, 1969.
9. Moos, R. H., & Tsu, V. D. The crisis of physical illness: An overview. In R. H. Moos (Ed.), *Coping with physical illness* (Vol. 1). New York: Plenum Press, 1977.
10. Hinton, J. Bearing cancer. In R. H. Moos (Ed.), *Coping with physical illness*. New York, Plenum Press, 1977.
11. Abram, H. S. Survival by machine: The psychological stress of chronic hemodialysis. *Psychiatry in Medicine*, 1970, *1*, 37–51.
12. Czaczkes, J. W., & De-Nour, A. K. *Chronic hemodialysis as a way of life*. New York: Brunner/Mazel, 1978.
13. Dudrick, S. J., & Englert, D. M. Total care of the patient receiving total parenteral nutrition. *Psychosomatics*, 1980, *21*, 109–110.
14. Lifeline Foundation Incorporated, 30 East Chestnut Street, Sharon, Massachusetts 02067. Marshall Koonin, President. Phone: (617) 784-3250.
15. Hall, R. C. W., Gardner, E. R., Perl, M., Stickney, S. K., & Pfefferbaum, B. The Professional Burnout Syndrome. *Psychiatric Opinion*, 1979, *16*, 12–17.

X

The Crisis of Treatment:

Stresses on Staff

Health care settings provide a work environment for staff as well as a treatment setting for patients. Although these two aspects of the environment serve different functions, they are closely related. For instance, staff who feel little support from peers or supervisors may find it hard to create a supportive and clear treatment setting. The press of required activities can lead staff to use less time-consuming methods of care that encourage patients to be passive and dependent. Conversely, staff attention and expectation are powerful resources that can promote patient compliance and recovery. In this section, we examine the special stressors health care staff encounter, how they cope with them, and the implications for patient care (for an overview of these issues, see Cartwright[2]).

The problems faced by health care staff stem from the nature of the tasks they perform and the way in which hospitals are organized.[5] Problems of excessive workload and understaffing are especially prevalent in intensive care and other specialized treatment units in which nursing staff are rushed and subjected to continual stimulation. These units provide little opportunity for reflection, and staff members typically lack control over the pace and organization of their daily activities. The repetitive routine of close observation (such as taking vital signs every 15 minutes), the alertness required to handle complex machinery and procedures, and frequent acute emergencies make the nurse's job especially demanding. The threat and incessant reality of death and the need to continue full nursing care and involvement with patients who have no hope of surviving or who are in an unconcious limbo where life is maintained only by machines force nurses to confront their feelings about death on a daily basis.

In the interpersonal realm, nurses act as mediators and coordinators in maintaining smooth relations among the many people who come into a unit. They deal with distraught families, frightened patients, and doctors who often cope with their own distress at losing a patient by directing their anger and frustration at the nearest nurse or by abdicating their responsibility and leaving the nurse to take charge and inform the family. On cancer units that serve patients who no longer have much hope of remission or cure, doctors and nurses often feel a sense of failure and inadequacy. Doctors may deal with these feelings by retreating from the patient, limiting their visits, and focusing on their research interests where they can find intellectual rewards and some emotional immunity. When doctors use distancing as their main coping strategy, they shift responsibility for the patient's emotional health to the attending nurses.

In the first article, Avery D. Weisman emphasizes that caregivers may be as distressed by their patients' predicament as are patients themselves. In his view, health care staff are vulnerable to "caregiver's plight," which includes such diverse reactions as aversion and abhorrence of patients, ill-founded optimism, and profound anxiety and emotional overresponsivity. To avoid progressive demoralization and impairment of professional self-esteem, Weisman recommends that caregivers practice self-management skills, try to understand the value of small contributions to a patient's welfare, share concerns and learn from each other, and use former patients as "absent witnesses" in an imaginary self-monitoring review. More generally, Weisman points out that comprehensive care requires a combination of protocol (medical treatment of the illness), plight (knowledge about the nonmedical or psychosocial ramifications of the illness), and promise (the caregiver's effort to contribute to good management and provide humanitarian patient care).

To give humanitarian care, staff must come to grips with some natural but often guilt-provoking reactions to patients. Kafka's *The Metamorphosis* describes the frightening transformation of

Gregor Samsa from a man into a giant cockroach. As the story unfolds, Gregor is insidiously and eventually totally rejected by his family. This rejection, or "Gregor effect," occurs because human beings are dominated by a drive for self-orientation. We must defend ourselves against the implications of human ambiguity and thus are driven to reject "ambiguous men" (that is, seriously ill and dying persons).[6] Such reactions help to explain why nurses who are provided with more free time typically do not intensify their contact with more "ambiguous" patients. By understanding the tendency to avoid and withdraw from some patients as a natural coping strategy, staff can accept these feelings and moderate their influence on patient care.

The importance of confronting such issues is highlighted by descriptions of how unresolved staff anger can affect the quality of health care. For instance, "uncooperative" patients may be subjected to subtly cruel treatments channeled through the details of nurses' daily work: painfully administered injections, forcing a patient to wait for medications, and delays in answering call lights. More direct forms of "punishment," which are sometimes "justified" by medical rationale, include administration of placebos (to avoid potentially harmful medications), isolation of patients in a treatment room (so as not to disturb other patients), secretly adding weights to a patient's traction (so she would not feel the pain), and mouthing words without sounds when addressing a patient who is worried about deafness.[3] One reason for such reactions is that staff are taught not to express anger at patients, whereas their daily work stimulates anger and other emotional reactions without providing channels for appropriate expression of these emotions.

How can health professionals avoid "caregiver's plight" and cope with the stressors they experience? Individual and organizational approaches are both helpful in the coping process. In regard to individual approaches, staff employ many of the same types of coping skills used by patients and their families. They learn to use denial constructively (for example, to ignore permanent disfigurement and concentrate on a patient's assets), to derive satisfaction from having met the challenge of a difficult job, to employ humor to ease the tension, to accept their own feelings (such as temporary depression or anger) as natural human reactions, and to find support among their peers.[1] Staff involved in the treatment of severely ill patients develop a combination of such coping strategies to handle the emotional upset their work involves and to define their contribution in an acceptable way.[4]

Health care professionals often generate a common fund of knowledge about typical stressors and effective coping strategies. Mutual support groups provide an organizational arena in which this information can be shared, feelings can be ventilated and understood, and the staff team can be strengthened as a source of emotional support.[7] In the second article, William Beardslee and David Ray DeMaso describe their experience leading staff groups that focus on the work-related issues aroused by caring for seriously ill children. Nurses discussed their guilt and frustration at temporary negative effects of treatment (such as pain and nausea), the strain of constantly dealing with children in medical crises, and the difficulty of maintaining satisfaction while caring for a dying or chronically ill patient. Other themes arose from the nature of the hospital social system and involved staff miscommunication, inconsistency or conflict over treatment orders, and the hectic pace and constant work pressure. Staff dealt with these issues by identifying and learning about specific sources of stress, emphasizing such coping skills as altruism and the use of humor, and sharing their feelings and experiences to gain support and information from one another.

Mutual support groups are important in that they focus primarily on sharing problems and learning individual coping strategies. But staff stress can also be tempered by improving hospital structures and policies. Staffing patterns in critical care areas can be altered to allow nurses some respite, for example, by scheduling four 10-hour days followed by three consecutive days off or by temporarily rotating full-time staff out of such areas. The predictability of hospital settings and the consistency and continuity of care can also be promoted by structured orientation programs for nursing and house staff, policy guidelines that offer clear expectations about hospital routines, and the use of nurse educators to organize ongoing in-service education programs.

In the third selection, Lorrin M. Koran and his colleagues describe their effort to improve the work environment in a burn unit. They were invited to conduct an intervention because unit staff were showing mild depression and physical and emotional withdrawal from patients that seemed to be attributable to work pressure, confusion about unit policies, and lack of personal autonomy and support from supervisors. Staff were assessed and provided with feedback on their actual and preferred work milieu. Target areas for change were identified, and Koran worked with unit staff to plan and implement specific modifications. The staff felt that the changes had a beneficial impact on their work setting. Day shift staff were most affected and reported more involvement and staff cohesion as well as increases in program clarity and autonomy and decreases in work pressure. By improving the work environments of health care professionals, such intervention procedures can promote staff morale and the quality of patient care.

References

1. Caldwell, T., & Weiner, M. Stresses and coping in ICU nursing. I. A review. *General Hospital Psychiatry*, 1981, *3*, 119–127.
2. Cartwright, L. Sources and effects of stress in health careers. In G. Stone, F. Cohen, & N. Adler (Eds.), *Health psychology: A handbook*. San Francisco: Jossey-Bass, 1979.
3. Geist, R. Consultation on a pediatric surgical ward: Creating an empathic climate. – American Journal of Orthopsychiatry, 1979, *47*, 432–444.
4. Koocher, G. Adjustment and coping strategies among the caretakers of cancer patients. *Social Work in Health Care*, 1979, *5*, 145–150.
5. Moll, P., Denny, N., Mote, T., & Coldwater, C. Hospital unit stressors that affect nurses: Primary task versus social factors. *Psychosomatics*, 1982, *23*, 366–374.
6. Preston, R. *The dilemmas of care: Social and nursing adaptations to the deformed, the disabled, and the aged*. New York: Elsevier, 1979.
7. Weiner, M., & Caldwell, T. Stresses and coping in ICU nursing. II. Nurse support groups on intensive care units. *General Hospital Psychiatry*, 1981, *3*, 129–134.

24

Understanding the Cancer Patient

The Syndrome of Caregiver's Plight

AVERY D. WEISMAN

What is it about cancer and the cancer patient that seems to mobilize more distress among patients, caregivers, and people at large than almost any other disease? Despite its unknown origin, erratic course, unpredictable treatment, and uncertain outcome, cancer is appalling to contemplate, as if it could confer a death sentence on anyone unfortunate enough to acquire it. A recent American Cancer Society (ACS) survey,[1] for example, showed that the general public tends to underestimate both the incidence of cancer and the effectiveness of treatment. This suggests that people want to think cancer is less common that it actually is, because they believe treatment is so ineffective. Furthermore, when asked to report reasons for fearing cancer, many people cite the prospect of unremitting pain, especially near death, prolonged invalidism, unchecked invasion, progressive helplessness, deterioration, and even decay. But reasons for fearing cancer are almost always iden-

AVERY D. WEISMAN • Project Omega and Department of Psychiatry, Massachusetts General Hospital and Harvard Medical School, Boston, Massachusetts 02178.

tical with reasons for fearing death.[2] It seems apparent that education alone does not eradicate these frightening and largely inaccurate emotional expectations.

The severity of psychosocial problems during the course of cancer is apt to change with transitions in treatment. Patients differ greatly in their tolerance of physical symptoms, therapy, and demonstrable emotional distress.[3] Emotional distress is not wholly determined by the number, kind, and extent of physical problems. While patients with advanced cancer and severe pain are likely to have more psychosocial distress, the stage of illness is only one of several risk factors that predict impaired coping with nonmedical problems.[4]

It is a mistake to think that all cancer patients face similar problems or that they are equally distressed at the same time. There are transitions which merit recognition as indicating separate psychosocial phases in the life of a cancer patient (see Chapter 8).[5] For example, someone who after diagnosis has finished treatment, gone into remission, recurred, then failed to benefit, passed into nontreatment limbo, and from there has undergone progressive deterioration and decline has had manifestly different degrees and types of distress at each of these phases, which demand appropriate coping behavior.[5,6] However, these changes occur not just because of cancer treatment but as a result of being a vulnerable cancer patient.

Stressful responses of cancer caregivers, a term including any professional engaged regularly in cancer care, have obviously been around for a long time. Only recently, however, have psychosocial investigators[7] begun to study these reactions systematically. Vachon,[8] for example, has pointed out that certain personal and professional problems which caregivers develop in terminal care settings may be traced to their motivations and frustrations. Closer examination indicates that what is here called "caregiver's plight" refers to much more than the familiar "burnout." It is wholly possible that some of the distress suffered by patients might be iatrogenic, namely, the result of emotional burdens felt by caregivers and secondarily placed on patients. A caregiver who feels exhausted and truculent can hardly be expected to carry out still other unrewarding duties with forbearance and understanding. Sooner or later, the patient will be blamed for being needy and sick, and as a result, will hesitate to ask for needed medication, nursing care, or even for information.

A Few Common Observations

Cancer care involves many more people than just the patient and the physician. Distress may actually be more severe among caregivers than patients. Expectable problems and anticipated distress among patients are usually more pronounced at recurrence than at diagnosis or nearing death. However, among caregivers, distress increases according to nearness of death.

There are no typical cancer patients, only people with cancer. It is easier to generalize about a mythical cancer patient than to examine ourselves and our reactions to patients as individuals.

The cancer predicament is more extensive than simply receiving treatment, because cancer is almost never just a biological event. How patients feel is as much at stake in cancer as their fate. Since thier actual time in treatment is far less than the total duration of illness, psychosocial issues are therefore uppermost and more prominent for a longer period than are medical issues.

Understanding the cancer patient is based on an assumption that another person can be understood and empathized with, even though he or she undergoes an experience that is difficult to share and often evokes a measure of aversion. Consequently, assessment of cancer patients requires vigorous, uncompromising, persistent, and candid self-monitoring on the part of caregivers.

Protocol, Plight, and Promise

The cancer predicament involves three interrelated concepts: protocol, plight, and promise. While the distinction between them is often confused, or just ignored, closer analysis shows that practices and ideas which are appropriate for one will influence what is thought and done about the others.

Protocol is not just the outline of treatment but a set of rules, roles, and behavior assigned to patients and caregivers. Patients are asked only to cooperate; they do not need to be understood as individuals. The only function of a protocol caregiver is to supervise and administer treatment with a central aim of completing the course without serious side effects or incidents. The only real issue is compliance and effectiveness, not a doctor–patient relationship. All treatments might as well be given by the same person.

The importance of protocol should not, of course, be minimized. It represents the organic tradition in medicine, which has given us so much. Protocol simplifies and standardizes treatment, avoiding imponderables, putting aside other aspects of care, and doing what we trust will, one day, provide the greatest good for the largest number of cancer patients. Plight and promise mean protocol plus, namely, therapeutic factors that make formal treatment more comprehensive and comprehending.

Plight is that part of living with cancer which is largely nonmedical. It includes problems, expectations, deficits, readjustments, hopes, and concerns—whatever is covered by the awkward term psychosocial. The basic distinction between plight and protocol is the difference between the patient and the cancer. Medicine in general seems to be working toward a conception of illness beyond that circumscribed by disease and protocols of treatment. The buzz word today is "holistic." In its best sense, this means that patients contribute to their own well-being and at least put a signature on the degree and direction of their sickness and suffering.

Promise is a less familiar concept. It is that side of cancer care which personalizes the plight of the caregiver. Not every caregiver who has contact with a cancer patient promises anything or expects something in return. But any caregiver who has a sustained relationship with a patient implicitly promises to fulfill or contribute something to good management and care. If a patient expects something of a caregiver, then the caregiver expects something in exchange. As a rule, the caregiver's contribution to management is a pledge to offer safe conduct in one form or another beyond treatment itself.

A colleague may object, "I don't promise patients anything. I am very careful to explain choices and tell patients just that we'll do the best we can." This objection, however, refers only to promise for cure. Offering information, choices, and the doctor's availability to the limit of competence are also parts of safe conduct and involve promises including a pledge—the caretaker can be counted on. "I will take care of you in this way, to this extent. In return, please, I do not expect you to construe this as a promise for cure."

Other promises pledge safe conduct through support services and exact more specific responses from patients, such as gratitude, cooperation, remuneration, recovery, and so forth. There are also idiosyncratic promises which reflect the caregiver's personal plight and emotional needs, but these are expressions of countertransference, deserving more attention in their own right than can be given here.

Two Vignettes

A 38-year-old mother of four was admitted to the hospital because of inflammatory carcinoma of the breast. About nine months before, she had noticed a lump but had done nothing until the breast became noticeably misshapen and painful. She was tearful, tense, depressed, and somewhat apologetic. Her husband was dismayed, angry, very protective, and somewhat condescending. He seemed domineering and close to panic, while she was more defeated and submissive.

As she recounted symptoms during the past nine months, her brother's death was repeatedly mentioned, almost as a point of orientation for the whole illness. It turned out that he had died of a heart attack about one month before the lump appeared. When I returned to talk with her the next day, she again spoke more about the brother than anything else. Finally, I called it to her attention because it seemed to me that mourning for her brother had been delayed until just a short time before she came to the hospital. Delayed mourning had got in the way of seeking medical care for the breast tumor, and she now seemed to weep more for him than about her cancer plight. I drew no other conclusions.

Before I could see the patient again, her physician, a most esteemed and compassionate oncologist, wrote a large, not very lengthy note on her chart, stating that I was not to talk with her again. The head nurse told me that the patient asked the doctor if she "needed to see me again, because every time she did, she cried, and she had trouble enough." From her viewpoint, I was the bearer of sad tidings, who by responding to her grief, reminded her of her brother's death. Of course, she didn't have to see me. There was nothing mandatory about it.

The order to cease and desist was not a crass rebuff, but a sympathetic act designed to help a very sad lady. While I would have preferred a private conversation, or, better, that the physician simply recognize intense weeping as a temporary phase in the course of mourning, I understood how my presence could be construed as needless. Protocol requires that treatment of the breast be uppermost; it does not obligate a patient to weep, feel worse, or even undergo a delayed bereavement. Thus, if Dr. Weisman makes you cry, you certainly don't need to see him.

Here was a confusion of plight (the patient's predicament) with protocol (management of the tumor). My colleague and I differed in our respective promises about the patient's plight. I would have facilitated mourning for the brother, believing that his death compounded the distress she felt. Her physician's promise was to treat the tumor and to ameliorate other distressing facts in the personal plight. While I would have talked or let the patient talk more about the dead brother, the physician's pledge was to take care of her without discussing the brother. Which alternative would have ensured the safest conduct, I shall never know.

> *A middle-aged married woman with advanced cancer of the ovary was operated on for a second-look procedure to see if further chemotherapy was feasible. It was not. Despite treatment, the tumor had not diminished. As a result, she was about to go home without further treatment beyond palliation. Within a few weeks, she was expected to decline and deteriorate as she passed into the terminal phase.*
>
> *The patient accepted discharge too easily, even eagerly, saying, "I'll go home, regain my strength, and then think about going back to work." While comments like this are common in the preterminal period, under these circumstances, considering the patient's previous attitude of acceptance, the ward staff thought that her "denial" was excessive. Certain death had been replaced with a favorable, nonlethal outcome. Her eagerness was out of keeping both with her plight and protocol.*
>
> *I was asked to consult because of the concern that denial would interfere with adaptation and might prevent appropriate planning for imminent demise. In this instance, caregivers thought that the patient really expected that all would be well and wasn't mourning enough.*

It turned out that the patient knew very well what the prognosis was and why protocol suspended further treatment. She had no illusions about going back to work. Imagining this was a form of coping with permanent inactivity. However, she was candid about her marriage, telling me about frequent separations, long-standing impatience with her husband's personality and temperament, her own infidelity, their threatened divorce, and now, at last, during the long illness, a newly found understanding and reconciliation which she eagerly anticipated. Actually, there was very little denial, and she gave many indications of having coped well. What seemed to be flagrant denial was in truth unusual optimism and enthusiasm about returning home and resuming her marriage under better circumstances, regardless of the cancer and impending terminality.

This example shows the difference between protocol, which meant doing nothing more for the tumor and her plight. But caregivers superimposed their interpretation of safe conduct (promise) on her perception of plight, which was one of an anticipated reunion with her husband. In both vignettes, caregivers acted in full accord with a promise to help, although, in my opinion, they misinterpreted the patients' responses. Their promises did not accord with the actual plight.

I cite these examples to show how the caregiver's expectations and values slant interpretations of a patient's behavior. In the first instance, the promise was, "I will take care of tumor treatment and help you feel as well as possible. Of course, you do not need to see anyone you don't want to, especially if he makes you feel worse." The second promise was, "We offered you the best treatment we knew. The treatment didn't work well enough. But we want you to live as long as as well as possible. If you say that you're going back to work, this is out of the question and bound to disappoint you." There was no disagreement in either case about the protocol, only about the interpretation of plight. Having construed the plight to match the therapeutic aim, instead of the reverse, the physician in the first vignette and the ward staff in the second accepted the surface interpretations of weeping and denial and responded compassionately but inaccurately.

The distinction between protocol, plight, and promise can be seen most directly in three different questions:

What treatment is required at this time? (protocol)

What problems does this patient face right now? (plight)
What is being asked of me? (promise)

Promise can be appropriate, inappropriate, or erroneous. Experience and continued observation are the only ways to settle differences of interpretation.

Common Distress Signals in Caregivers

Experienced caregivers are familiar with expectable behavior and emotional responses of cancer patients during psychosocial and treatment transitions. However, with some noteworthy exceptions, it is questionable how seriously they heed distress signals among themselves and in other professionals. In fact, the trajectory toward death is said to be more difficult for caregivers and survivors-to-be than for patients.[9] Occasionally, caregivers become impatient, irritable, and even antagonistic should a dying patient exceed predictions and live longer than anticipatory grief requires. It is a common observation that for many patients dying in the near future is much less disturbing than thoughts of being endlessly sick and unresponsive. Caregivers, however, may become so preoccupied with death and the patient's failure to thrive that, as a result, their distress may be shown by prolonged bereavement and profound misgivings about their own competence.

There is *no reaction among patients that cannot also occur in caregivers*. To care for someone means to feel something beyond professional duty.[10] While professionalization does shelter the caregiver and contributes much to the ability to manage more effectively, there are still many emotional reactions which exact incongruous penalties. I call these "distress signals."

Burnout

Whenever a caregiver gets weary, bleary, and dreary from trying to do too much for too long and feels defeated, victimized, or beleaguered by demands, the distress signal of burnout is unmistakable. But burnout should be understood as a late effect of distress, not unlike exhaustion. Different kinds of symptoms precede it.

Aversion, Abhorrence

Not every caregiver response, early or late, is burnout. When otherwise helpful professionals feel abhorrence and a desire to avoid patients and customary duties, a breather is certainly indicated. This common distress signal is one that often generates guilt, because we are taught to care for, not to feel revulsion for, our work and patients.

Phony Optimism

Unsolicited, ill-founded cheerfulness is not the same as hope. It is as unseemly in a caregiver as lugubrious melancholy. When dealing with a near-terminal patient, it is wholly possible to remain matter-of-fact and keep a healthy respect for the patient and oneself without distorting reality or lapsing into empty efforts to encourage. I recall a physician who refused to answer his patient's questions but kept woodenly reiterating, "We must always think positively!"

Second Look, Second Promise

Second-look disappointment occurs whenever a patient relapses and then after an exploratory operation is put on another protocol. In second look, second promise, caregivers usually feel hypocrisy, insincerity, and inconsistency of motive and promise. They dread the second observatory operation, because even if therapy has been moderately effective, they suspect that whatever is done will, sooner or later, end in despair, failure, and a sense of having conspired against the patient.

Meltdown

There is perhaps no more dramatic distress signal in cancer care than an unexpected surge of anxiety, depression, or tears in a caregiver, hitherto thought to be a very detached, even cold clinician. It is most commonly found among resident physicians who become acutely aware of a patient's plight and of their own disguised wish to be all powerful, an attitude which suddenly collapses into forlorn helplessness.

Death Watch Solemnity

Caring for a terminal patient whom one has known well is both saddening and frustrating. But there is no inherent reason why tending a patient in this situation should be regarded as a sacred, semireligious duty to be performed on tiptoes and in whispers. Extreme death-watch behavior may be no more appropriate than drawing the blinds. It can hint at more serious emotional problems than are readily apparent from the caregiver's expressed concern and sympathy.

Besides these few examples, there are other distress signals symptomatic of caregiver's plight (see Table 1). Familiar instances, such as needless guilt, unusual indecisiveness, pangs of sadness, flashes of antipathy, chronic hopelessness, unexpected weeping, conviction of being totally ineffective, and denial of fallibility combined with inflated self-opinion, are further indications that the caregiver needs help. But not every distress signal is ominous. Mostly, they mean only that caregivers are no less or more than human, resilient and vulnerable. In fact, distress signals may be a sign of unfolding adaptation that will ultimately

---

Table 1. Symptoms of Caregiver's Plight

Burnout
Aversion, abhorrence
Phony optimism
Second look, second promise
Meltdown
Death watch solemnity
Denial of fallibility
Blame and shame
Bitterness and remorse
Unabated dismay
Pangs and wipeouts
Magical expectation

---

prove to be helpful. However, extremes also include excessive affectless detachment or vicarious mourning and identification, neither of which is seen as desirable. Countertransference reactions deserve special study because they are so hard to get at.

Practical Consequences

For the patient, good coping has only one significant aim in the terminal phase, when many caregiver reactions tend to occur—to reach accommodation with the inevitable and find an appropriate death.[11] For the survivor-to-be, the aim is to shorten bereavement through anticipatory grief, and for the caregiver, it is self-management and maintenance of morale. With the help of patients and survivors-to-be, caregivers can participate in realizing all three.

Good coping is a combination of optimism, resourcefulness, flexibility, and pragmatism. Because self-management requires daily examination of outstanding commitments, a caregiver could well ask these questions: "Are my obligations real or self-imposed?" "Am I promising more than can be delivered?" "Have these commitments been thrust on me or do I ask for more than I can handle?" "If I were the patient, what would I expect?" Awareness of expectable problems and appraisal of what actually might be done tend to protect caregivers against the dangers of promising too much. However, when a caregiver's promises exceed his or her capacity to fulfill them and stem more from personal self-esteem than from what a patient really needs, distress signals can always be found. Futile promises usually give way to a response indicative of caregiver's plight. Vocational demoralization is far more common than burnout.

What can be done about this? Aside from taking a short holiday or leaving the field entirely, three major recommendations can be offered: (1) least possible contribution, (2) shared concern, and (3) absent witness.

Least Possible Contribution

A little goes a long way; the least possible contribution is the one with the least strain, but with the best chance of making a difference, however small. Having made this contribution, which may be very insignificant against the background of need, one can add another contribution and then still another, until something quite unanticipated but substantial results. Morale in everyone seems better, care is effective, plight is less painful. Least possible contribution does not, of course, mean doing as little as possible, but doing only a little bit beyond the ordinary, something that most closely reflects the caregiver at his or her best.

Shared Concern

There is no better therapy for vocational demoralization and acute caregiver's plight than sharing critical incidents with colleagues who just might have similar misgivings and concerns.[12] Coping well is aided by having something to measure our efforts against and someone to derive support from. Colleagues may have nothing more to offer than mutual concern and willing ears, but they can help us learn how to listen for echoes of disappointment and promises unkept. Patients who cope effectively usually seek information and share problems with others. This is also true of caregivers. Unfortunately, opportunities range from limited to nonexistent on many busy services where protocol predominates. If those in charge of such services truly believe in comprehensive cancer care, they will realize the hazards of working too hard, expecting too much, and getting too little recognition, and they will think about the plight of caregivers.

Absent Witness

Reconstruction of the psychosocial concomitants of terminal illness, such as cancer, is a productive exercise in behavioral medicine. While special conferences, such as a psychological autopsy[13] are somewhat difficult to arrange on a regular basis, a variation called the "absent witness" shows that the way in which we share concern may be useful, either for an individual caregiver or a companionable group. In this exercise, a former patient, perhaps one who has died, becomes the absent witness, who is called upon to evaluate care that he or she received in a hospital. The witness is specifically asked about the caregiver who is feeling down or demoralized. "What did you want that you did not get?" "What should have been done that wasn't?" "What advice do you have for this caregiver?" "How could your illness have been different and better, short of total recovery?" When couched in these pragmatic terms, the differences between "should" and "could" and between guilt and undue expectations become very clear. Did the caregiver promise too much? What interfered with optimal caregiving? While certain self-contained clinicians might be dubious about the absent witness exercise, it merely asks for more evaluation of what every conscientious physican reflects on from time to time, anyway. The absent witness is not a critic but a corrective for distress signals.

Understanding cancer patients will remain one-sided (protocol only) or two-sided (protocol plus patient's plight), unless caregivers recognize their own potential for distress, which is not always signaled by burnout. Whenever distress is suspected, caregivers should try to identify the sources of trouble by asking a few pertinent personal questions. "If I were the patient, what would I expect myself to do?" "I feel angry, frustrated, guilty, depressed. What does the patient do that makes me feel that way?" "What more do I expect of myself, anyway?"

Just by keeping the distinction beteen protocol, plight, and promise firmly in mind, certain symptoms of caregiver's plight may even be alleviated. If clinical demands are too great, plight too poignant, or promises excessive, any motivation may deteriorate so that morale decreases. The most beneficial instruction for caregivers is frequently ignored: We should not only monitor ourselves but also heed an admonition to care for ourselves. Comprehensive psychosocial cancer care is a frontier shared by comparatively few, and because its benefits are usually destined to fall short of what is desired and hoped for, it can be a paradoxical affair.

References

1. American Cancer Society. Public attitudes toward cancer and cancer tests. *CA-A Cancer Journal for Clinicians*, 1980, *30*, 92–98.
2. McFate, P. Ethical issues in treatment of cancer patients. In B. Cassileth (Ed.), *The cancer patient: Social and medical aspects of care*. Philadelphia: Lea & Febiger, 1979.

3. Weisman, A. D., & Worden, J. W. *Coping and vulnerability in cancer patients: A research report.* Boston: privately printed, 1977.
4. Weisman, A. D., Worden, J. W., & Sobel, H. J. *Psychosocial screening and intervention with cancer patients.* Boston: privately printed, 1980.
5. Weisman, A. D. A model for psychosocial phasing in cancer. *General Hospital Psychiatry,* 1979, *1*(3), 187–195.(a)
6. Weisman, A. D. *Coping with cancer.* New York: McGraw-Hill, 1979.
7. Cullen, J., Fox, B., & Ison, R. (Eds.). *Cancer: The behavioral dimensions.* New York: Raven Press, 1976.(b)
8. Vachon, M. Motivation and stress experienced by staff working with the terminally ill. *Death Education,* 1979, *2*, 113–122.
9. Glaser, B., & Strauss, A. L. *Time for dying.* Chicago: Aldine, 1968.
10. Newlin, N., & Wellisch, D. The oncology nurse: Life on an emotional roller coaster. *Cancer Nursing,* 1978, *1*, 447–450.
11. Garfield, C. (Ed.). *Psychosocial care of the dying patient.* New York: McGraw-Hill, 1978.
12. Bermosk, L., & Corsini, R. (Eds.). *Critical incidents in nursing.* Philadelphia: Saunders, 1973.
13. Weisman, A. D. *The realization of death: A guide for the psychological autopsy.* New York: Jason Aronson, 1974.

25

Staff Groups in a Pediatric Hospital
Content and Coping

WILLIAM R. BEARDSLEE and DAVID RAY DeMASO

Much has been written on the emotional stresses of physical illness and subsequent health care from the perspective of children and their families.[4,11,13–15] The stress upon staff in caring for children has received less attention. Several studies[7,9,16] have detailed stresses affecting staff in adult centers, such as long working hours, intensive involvement with families, rapidly changing technology in medical care, and emotional strain from long-term involvement with severely ill or dying patients. This has led to interest in methods that help staff cope with such stress.

Several authors have recommended regular ward meetings[1,7–10] focused on the stressful aspects of the work experience. Hay and Oken[9] reported that such discussions in an adult setting can encourage sharing of the experience, provide an opportunity for ventilation of feelings, allow for problem solving, and, in some instances, reduce the staff's sense of guilt. These processes are

Reprinted from the *American Journal of Orthopsychiatry*, 1982, 52, 712–718. Copyright 1982 the American Orthopsychiatric Association, Inc. Reproduced by permission.

WILLIAM R. BEARDSLEE and DAVID RAY DeMASO • Harvard Medical School and Children's Hospital Medical Center, Boston, Massachusetts 02115.

similar to Yalom's[18] curative factors in group process. Cassem and Hackett,[1] using a clinical example, presented evidence that suggested these meetings can facilitate acute reduction of staff anxiety. Simon and Whiteley[16] presented a detailed description of one such staff group in an adult intensive care setting, while Eisendrath[3] described the problems liaison support groups encounter. However, there are few details of the actual content of the group meetings or of the main staff concerns in this literature. Moreover, none addresses the problems of staff working with children in a pediatric hospital.

This paper reports the authors' experiences in running staff groups whose purpose has been to explore the stresses engendered by the work, and presents observations on how staff members cope successfully with these stresses.

Setting of the Groups

The hospital where these groups met is a large, tertiary care pediatric center. The hospital floors are divided by subspecialty (i.e., cardiology, medicine, surgery) with a range of 12 to 30 patient beds on each. There are two multidisciplinary intensive care units containing 18 beds each. Nursing staff ranges from 16 nurses on a general medicine floor to over 50 nurses in an intensive care unit. There is one head nurse on each floor. A "primary nursing" care model is used by the staff.[2] Typically, a staff physician and about four resident physicians provide medical coverage on a rotating month-long period. Each floor, additionally, has a child psychiatrist and social worker assigned on a permanent basis.

Group Structure

Within this setting, the authors have conducted staff groups on the following floors: oncology, cardiology, general medicine, neonatal intensive care, and medical/surgical intensive care. All groups are still meeting, with one year being the shortest interval for any group and four years the longest. The meetings occur for

60 to 90 minutes each week at a set time and place. Most frequent participants are nurses, although social workers, activity therapists, and physicians attend on some floors. Attendance in a group varies from week to week due to rotating shifts and ward circumstances (e.g., medical emergencies). Attendance by the ward leadership varies from floor to floor.

The groups have been initiated only on those floors on which the staff clearly has been receptive to the idea. Several wards requested such staff groups specifically. A critical component in establishing the groups has been the support and sanction of the ward leadership, particularly the head nurse. With such support, regular meetings with good attendance over a period of years have taken place on several wards.

The focus of the groups is work-related concerns of the staff, with some emphasis on the feelings evoked by the patients. A shared professional work experience is seen as the basis for membership and content. Work-engendered feelings and experiences, not individual personal ones, are the central topics. The groups are explicitly not therapy groups.

Consultant's Role

Within the hospital, the authors have served as the ward psychiatric consultants as well as group leaders, with one exception. In general, on the Psychiatry Consultation-Liaison Service, the consultants to a particular ward assess all patients and their families for whom a psychiatric consultation is requested, and also assist the staff in the management of difficult patients. The model of consultation employed is that described by Geist.[6] The authors view the staff groups as a natural adjunct to the consultant's role and, as mentioned, have initiated groups most often because of the staff requests.

The consultant's role within the group is to ensure the meetings occur regularly and to encourage the sharing of observations, feelings, and methods of dealing with difficult situations. No specific theme, content, or subject is planned by the consultant; rather, the staff is asked to discuss its concerns at the time of the meeting. The focus is on work issues, not psychodynamic interpretations of individual staff experience. Specific advice about a patient or problem may be provided when asked, but in general the role is to facilitate discussion in the meetings. There are usually other weekly meetings to discuss the management of specific cases from a psychological viewpoint.

Content of the Groups

In groups, members of different professional disciplines working in different settings expressed recurrent common concerns. These were related to the demands of the work, not to either individual personality or particular staff characteristics. The themes of the groups can best be conceptualized as occurring in three major interrelated areas: (1) disease-related issues; (2) emotional needs of the patients; and (3) interactions with the social system in which the care takes place.

Disease-Related Issues

In general, only the sickest children, those who cannot be managed on an outpatient basis, are admitted to the hospital. As soon as they recover, they are discharged. The staff has repeated contact with children who are critically ill and very little contact with children who are well or getting better. The strain of constantly dealing with children in medical crisis was frequently discussed in the groups.

Moreover, the effect of treatment itself on the child was a frequent topic. On the oncology floor, for example, the side effects of chemotherapy administered by the staff often transform seemingly well children into very sick ones. Feelings about causing the children pain, whatever the long-run benefits of treatment, was often a central topic. Whether in neonatology, cardiology, or oncology, the staff wondered about the value of its interventions when the prognosis is grim or uncertain but the medical intervention intensive.

Children who require prolonged hospitalization likewise caused concern among the staff. Multiple feelings were stimulated by these patients. An example was an adolescent boy hospitalized for months with a progressive cardiomyopathy:

> *During hospitalization, this boy went from excellent health to severe congestive heart failure, and finally died. Cardiopulmonary resuscitation was required for frequent life-threatening arrhythmias. At times a delirium secondary to hypoxia altered his mental status. His course required total bed rest, extensive nursing care, experimental drug trials, and a futile wait for a heart transplant. Within meetings, there was discussion about nursing plans to help this unfortunate youngster along with expression of both the sadness and anger engendered in the staff by his care.*

A frequent dilemma was how to obtain satisfaction and pride while caring for a dying or chronically ill patient. Staff members held high expectations of themselves and worked diligently to meet their goals. However, when a patient is dying or not improving, it is difficult for them to feel confident that all has been done or to take pride in their care. Within the groups, there was frequent discussion of the sense of frustration and failure when a child dies or fails to improve. Staff members repeatedly observed that when a number of children died in a short time span, there was a noticeable difference in the staff. The staff was sadder and more burdened, often taking longer to complete their work.

The Emotional Needs of Patients

The physical care of patients with debilitating illnesses inevitably brings an intense emotional intimacy with the patients and their families. How to deal with this intimacy was a frequent focus of group discussion. The staff members are the primary emotional caretakers for the patients and their families on a daily basis. The staff is constantly and repeatedly bombarded with requests for emotional support. With the presence of "primary nursing," the bond between the nurse and the patient is intensified. On most services, there is daily contact among the family, the primary nurse, and the responsible physician. The nurse or physician frequently becomes more than a caregiver, and the relationship often lasts beyond the hospitalization. When a close relationship fails to develop between a family and the staff, it can become a chronic concern.

The intimacy with the patients and their families is frequently reflected in the twin poles of overinvolvement and underinvolvement. New staff members often become overinvolved. Continued high levels of intense involvement appear to make it impossible to continue working. Repeated overinvolvement is a wrenching emotional experience and can detract from the worker's ability to give to other patients. On the other side, underinvolvement makes it impossible to provide good care to a child and a family. The staff often talked about feeling that other areas of their lives were neglected or threatened as their work spilled over into their personal lives. Many of the staff work as much as 60 to 70 hours a week, with the attendant conflicts in family life. They reported dreaming about their patients; some reported difficulty leaving when their work was done, and others told of telephoning on their days off to check on patients. They noted that many of their social contacts, even their families, were overwhelmed by the work they did and could not provide much support:

> One nurse described the situation clearly: "I'll be sitting there having dinner with my friends. They will describe what happened to them during the day . . . so-and-so said this and that . . . then they will ask me. I'll say Joey died or Richard died. It sort of stops the conversation."

Discussions about understanding and working with parents were a frequent part of the meetings. In general, the staff felt better able to understand and talk with a youngster than with the parents. Feelings engendered by the parents were frequently mentioned. Anger, often at "perceived" poor parental care, arose at many meetings. An example was a young women who had not come to the hospital to feed her poorly eating infant postcardiac surgery. Once the staff expressed its anger, realization of the mother's guilt and fear which stopped her from coming were soon accurately identified. A more supportive approach to the mother resulted in her coming to the hospital and, within one week, successfully feeding her child. Another example occurred in neonatology:

> A mother was very angry with the staff from the moment of admission for no apparent reason. One nurse made an effort to establish a relationship with

this woman. When the infant improved he was transferred to another hospital. The mother asked that her breast milk, which she had expressed and bottled for her premature infant, also be transferred. However, the milk arrived one hour later than the baby, causing the mother to become furious. The nurse felt devalued and unappreciated. Review of the situation revealed the mother had a child previously with a developmental impairment, possibly secondary to obstetrical error. A full discussion of the source of this parent's anger helped deal with the particular nurse's and staff's frustration.

Grieving is a universal experience for patients and their families, which they share with the staff. Whether or not a child is terminal, there is the threat of death and certainly the shock of lost possibilities and dashed hopes. The staff has no break or escape from that within its work. The group meetings in all settings were used by staff to deal with the thoughts and feelings engendered by the losses. Physician attendance in the meetings often occurred around these circumstances. For example, in the medical intensive care unit, five deaths occurred within 72 hours, resulting in the physicians' request for a special staff meeting.

The Social System

The content of the groups frequently reflected the interactions with the social system in which the care takes place. First, the staff, especially nurses and resident physicians, is best described by the sociologist's term "multiple subordination." That is, the staff members have several different leaders who may give conflicting orders. This can be true on even a well-organized and administered ward. Staff occasionally is caught in the middle. Miscommunication and inconsistent approaches did occur frequently when decisions were made by people not immediately on the floor. An example is the conflict over resuscitation orders on a terminally ill child. Anger at the multiple subordinate role was often discussed.

The area of communication between intradisciplinary and interdisciplinary personnel was frequently identified as a problem. For example, issues of how to learn to trust other nurses arose directly with the beginning of a new intensive care unit.

Nursing and physician communication was a frequent topic of discussion, especially the issue of changing residents with varied orientations.

Working conditions were also often discussed. As an example of the complexity of the tasks required, in a meeting on the oncology floor, staff nurses wrote down the different tasks they might be called upon to perform in the course of a day. Their list included 31 different tasks ranging from admission assessments to intravenous procedures to record keeping to cardiac resuscitation to follow-up referrals. There were often frustrated comments about long working hours, heavy workloads, repetitive job assignments, and inadequate leadership. For the nurses, issues and questions about their identity as nurses were common and were similar to those described by Oberst.[12]

Successful Coping Patterns

At times the combined influence of the disease-related issues, the emotional demands of the patients, and the staff's social system lead to feelings of being overwhelmed. The term "burn-out"[5] used to describe these feelings, has received much recent attention. Nurses within the surgical intensive care unit brought to one group a listing of "how they felt," which contained many of the symptoms described in a depressive disorder, including insomnia, low energy, self-depreciation, decreased productivity, poor concentration, irritability, crying, and anhedonia. However, for the most part, staff seemed to cope very successfully with the demands of the work. As so little has been written about this side of the picture, we have chosen to concentrate on the successful coping patterns observed and supported within the staff groups.

Identifying Sources of Stress. It was important for the staff to know what was causing its subjective sense of difficulty, and either to do something about it or be able to accept it as inherent in the situation. Much group time was spent in articulating what the stresses were, whether they had to do with the scheduling and organization of the work to be done during the day, with disturbances within the families of patients, with communication on the ward, or with pain and sadness about the patients themselves. For example, as the work demands and the technological complexity increased on one service, the nurses constantly found themselves tired and overworked. Upon discussion, they realized that indeed there had been a quantitative increase in the amount of work required because of the new methods of care being delivered on the floor. They were able to convey this point successfully to the head nurse and to the nursing hierarchy and to have an effect on staffing patterns.

Stress as a Learning Experience. Work with ill patients provides an opportunity as well as a stress. An important way some of the staff coped was through learning. There was curiosity, both about new medical treatments and about their own emotional reactions, which allowed staff members to remain interested in difficult patients.

Inner Coping Mechanisms. Several inner coping mechanisms were observed to be successful and are similar to the mature choices of ego defense described by Vaillant.[17] Use of humor was common and helpful. Altruism, obtaining real satisfaction for oneself through helping others, was certainly evident on the floors. Suppression, the conscious decision to postpone gratification and to put certain things out of one's awareness, was another important coping mechanism. A corollary of this is that those staff members who stayed satisfied and at work the longest were those who were able to leave work-related matters at work. That is, they were able to put work concerns in perspective and out of their minds at times.

Sharing Feelings. Through the sharing of feelings and experiences aroused by taking care of the patients, staff members were able to realize that they were not alone and to gain support from one another. This sharing provided opportunities for clarification and validation of feelings by the staff, that is, of clearly defining what individuals were feeling with the help of their peers. Through modeling, certain staff members learned how others handled stresses on the ward and applied that to their own stressful situations. This sharing was particularly valuable in relation to the emotional aspects of caring for the dying or chronically ill patient. It was simply impossible to perform that work alone or to keep the myriad feelings and thoughts of doing this kind of work to oneself. Thus, this sharing of experiences was necessary to deal with the emotional pressures of working in this setting. *Staff Groups.* Finally, the role of the staff group in the coping pattern deserves attention. Certainly, sharing of feelings engendered by working occurs in other places and in other ways than in a staff group. The authors are convinced that such sharing is essential to counteract the stresses of the work, that it can and does occur in staff groups such as have been described, and that the presence of such groups increases the likelihood of the staff's successful coping and resultant enhancement of patient care.

References

1. Cassem, L., & Hackett, T. The setting of intensive care: In T. Hackett & N. Cassem (Eds.), *Massachusetts General Hospital of General Psychiatry.* St. Louis: C. V. Mosby, 1978.
2. Ciske, K. Accountability: The essence of primary nursing. *American Journal of Nursing,* 1979, *79,* 891–894.
3. Eisendrath, S. Psychiatric liaison support groups for general hospital staffs. *Psychosomatics,* 1981, *22,* 685–694.
4. Freud, A. The role of bodily illness in the mental life of a child. *Psychoanalytic Study of the Child,* 1951, *7,* 69–81.
5. Freudenberger, H. Staff burnout. *Journal of Social Issues,* 1974, *30,* 159–165.
6. Geist, R. Consultation on a pediatric surgical ward: Creating an empathic climate. *American Journal of Orthopsychiatry,* 1977, *47,* 432–444.
7. Gentry, W., Foster, S., & Froehung, S. Psychologic response to situational stress in intensive and nonintensive nursing. *Heart Lung,* 1972, *1,* 793–796.
8. Glaser, J., & Horvath, K. A tool for dealing with nursing problems. *Supervisor Nurse,* April 1979, pp. 46–52.
9. Hay, D., & Oken, D. The psychological stresses of intensive care unit nursing. *Psychosomatic Medicine,* 1972, *34,* 109–118.
10. Klagsbrun, S. Cancer, emotions, and nurses. *American Journal of Psychiatry,* 1970, *126,* 1236–1244.
11. Kornfeld, O. The hospital environment: Its impact on the patient. In R. Moos (Ed.), *Coping with physical illness* (Vol. 1). New York: Plenum Press, 1977.
12. Oberst, M. The crisis-prone staff nurse. *American Journal of Nursing,* 1973, *73,* 1917–1921.
13. Prugh, D., & Eckhardt, L. Children's reaction to illness, hospitalization and surgery. In H. Kaplan, A. Freeman, & B. Sadock (Eds.), *Comprehensive textbook of psychiatry* (Vol. 3). Baltimore: Williams & Wilkins, 1980.
14. Richmond, J. The pediatric patient in illness. In M. Hollender (Ed.), *The psychology of medical practise.* Philadelphia: W. B. Saunders, 1958.
15. Schowalter, J. Psychological reactions to physical illness in adolescence. *Journal of the American Academy of Child Psychiatry,* 1977, *16,* 500–516.

16. Simon, N., & Whiteley, S. Psychiatric consultation with MICU nurses: The consultation conference as a working group. *Heart Lung,* 1977, *6,* 497–504.
17. Vaillant, G. Theoretical hierarchy of adaptive ego mechanisms, *Archives of General Psychiatry,* 1971, *24,* 107–118.
18. Yalom, I. *The theory and practice of group psychotherapy.* New York: Basic Books.

26

Changing Hospital Work Environments
An Example of a Burn Unit

LORRIN M. KORAN, RUDOLF H. MOOS,
BERNICE MOOS, and MILFORD ZASSLOW

. . . Work stress . . . on patient care units in general hospitals is a pressing health care issue. Work-related stressors have been linked to lowered morale, impaired performance, and high rates of absenteeism and turnover among nursing and other health care staff.[1,2] In a cogent review, Cartwright noted that the responsibility for acutely ill patients, the emotional climate surrounding illness, and the often perfectionistic expectation of health care staff are all implicated in staff distress.[3] Moreover, recent studies have shown how stressful work settings can affect the quality of health care by lowering motivation and contributing to staff "burnout."[4,5]

Liaison psychiatrists have attempted to deal with these stressors using several different interventions, including attending team meetings and work rounds, establishing regular meetings to

Reprinted by permission of the publisher from *General Hospital Psychiatry*, 1983, 5, 7–13. Copyright 1983 by Elsevier Science Publishing Co., Inc.

LORRIN M. KORAN, RUDOLF H. MOOS, BERNICE MOOS, and MILFORD ZASSLOW • Department of Psychiatry and Behavioral Sciences, Stanford University and Veterans Administration Medical Center, Palo Alto, California 94304.

discuss the psychosocial aspects of patients' care, conducting didactic seminars, and formulating ward-based consultation programs.[6-8] Studies suggest that these interventions contribute to effective patient care by allowing staff to cope with their feelings and by improving the organization and clarity of ward policies and procedures.[7,9-12] Liaison psychiatrists may be able to enhance the effectiveness of these interventions by applying standardized assessments of the work environments of medical units and by adapting systematic feedback and change strategies that have proven successful in other settings. This paper reports an attempt to improve the work environment on a burn unit by providing nursing staff with feedback about the characteristics of their work setting and by helping them use this information to formulate and implement desired changes.

Setting and Method

The Burn Unit

The study was performed in the burn unit of a 425-bed county general hospital affiliated with a medical school. The full- and part-time staff of the burn unit included 18 nurses, three burn technicians, 11 attendants/orderlies, and two unit clerks to care for approximately five acute patients and six patients recovering from plastic and reconstructive surgery. A plastic surgeon supervised the medical care provided by two plastic surgery residents. Physical therapy, dietary, and social work services were available to the patients and staff on a consultative basis. The average length of stay in the unit was approximately 20 days, although some patients stayed more than 60 days.

Like many intensive care settings, the burn unit imposed severe emotional stress upon its staff. As Quinby and Bernstein note, burn unit staff are torn between their self-image as relievers of pain and the necessity of inflicting pain during dressing changes and debridement.[13] Patients reject staff for inflicting pain and become hostile and uncooperative during debridement. These patient reactions elicit anger and guilt among nursing staff. Furthermore, distraught family members often make unreasonable emotional demands on the staff. The psychiatric disorders that frequently precede or accompany severe burns add to the difficulty of caring for burn patients.[14-16] In addition to experiencing the stresses characteristic of burn units, staff are subject to the problems common to intensive care settings: heavy lifting of patients, exposure to affect-laden stimuli such as mutilated bodies and genitalia, conflicts with nursing administration over staffing and scheduling, lack of emotional support from physicians, guilt over inevitable mistakes, and anguish when patients die.[9,11,17]

Planning and Intervention Procedure

The head nurse of the burn unit invited the liaison psychiatrist to meet with the staff to explore problems affecting morale and patient care. A contract similar to those reported elsewhere[10,12] was designed at the first meeting with the staff. The liaison psychiatrist agreed to meet with the staff for an hour once every two weeks to attempt to resolve issues affecting the quality of patient care. Patient problems, administrative and staffing problems, difficulties with the burn unit physicians, and other matters impairing patient care were defined as appropriate topics for the group. Personal feelings and interpersonal conflicts could be explored if they related to patient care but not otherwise. No staff member was to be discussed if he or she was not present.

The liaison psychiatrist requested the staff's permission to employ a new technique that required staff members to complete a questionnaire (the Work Environment Scale [WES]) that elicited their perceptions of the burn unit's work environment and their preferences for an ideal work environment. The staff group would be given feedback about the results to help guide change efforts. The psychiatrist agreed that individuals' scores would remain confidential and that the overall results for the staff would not be revealed to staff of other units in the hospital. The burn unit staff agreed to complete the questionnaire before and after the series of liaison meetings as one measure of their impact.

These intervention procedures were adapted from earlier studies in which four steps were used to facilitate and evaluate environmental change: (1) systematic assessment of the work environment; (2) feedback to staff emphasizing real-ideal setting differences; (3) planning and instituting specific changes; and (4) reassessment. These procedures have helped stimulate positive changes in hospital-based and community-based psychiatric treatment programs,[18–20] and in educational and family settings.[21]

The Work Environment Scale

The Work Environment Scale (WES) is composed of 90 true/false items that measure ten dimensions of the social environments of work settings. These ten dimensions fall into three broad groups: relationship dimensions; personal growth or goal orientation dimensions; and system maintenance and change dimensions. The *relationship dimensions* (involvement, peer cohesion, supervisor support) assess how involved people feel in the work setting and how much they help and support one another. The *goal orientation dimensions* measure how strongly people are encouraged to make their own decisions (autonomy); how strongly the social milieu emphasizes good planning and efficiency (task orientation); and how intensely the press of work and time urgency permeate the work milieu (work pressure). The *system maintenance and change dimensions* evaluate the clarity and explicitness of rules and policies (clarity); the extent to which supervisors use regulations to maintain control (control); the emphasis on change and new approaches (innovation); and the pleasantness of the physical surroundings (physical comfort).

The WES has been applied to over 1,400 employees in general work settings and over 1,600 employees in health care settings. This scale has been used to compare health care settings, to contrast actual and preferred work environments, to test theories about expected differences among work environments, and to study the adaptation of individuals to work environments with different characteristics. Several studies have employed the WES to explore work environment influence on employee dissatisfaction and burnout. Detailed information about this body of research and the normative and psychometric aspects of the WES is provided elsewhere.[21–23]

To quantify their perceptions of the current work environment, the burn unit staff completed the WES Form R (real). To describe their preferred or ideal work setting, they completed the WES Form I (ideal). The staff were given the results of these assessments at the second meeting with the liaison psychiatrist, and the subsequent discussion was used to stimulate the group problem-solving process. The two forms of the WES were completed again six months later to assess staff perceptions of changes in their real and ideal work setting.

Results

The Preintervention Work Environment

Figure 1 shows the burn unit's real and ideal WES profiles at the beginning of the liaison meetings. Response rates were 72% for R.N.'s and 75% for all other staff. The subscale scores are compared to average scores (shown by a line at the standard score 50) of over 1,600 staff from a wide range of health care settings. Compared to these staff, burn unit staff noted above average emphasis on autonomy, about average emphasis on involvement and supervisor support, and below average emphasis on peer cohesion and on all four system maintenance and change dimensions. The figure also portrays the consistent and relatively large difference between the current situation and the staff's vision of an ideal work environment. Staff wanted much more development of all aspects of the work environment except supervisor control and work pressure.

The problems enumerated by staff prior to the first meeting corroborated the WES findings. Staff members complained of poor cooperation with one another. They noted that poor communication in managing difficult patients was creating intrastaff anger and conflict. Nurses felt that they were unable to deal with important patient care problems because they could not confront each other directly. These problems illustrate the specific issues underlying the relative lack of involvement, peer cohesion, and supervisor support shown by the WES profile.

Staff also expressed the need to increase autonomy and clarity by defining roles and clarifying expectations for each shift and for specific staff members. Several staff members expressed sen-

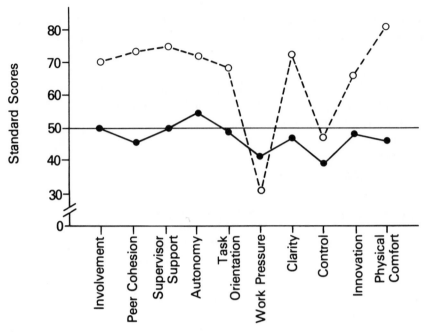

Figure 1. Preintervention WES profiles for burn unit staff (●—● = Real, o- - -o = Ideal).

sitivity because of critical comments about their work, frustration in dealing with patients' and families' intense and hostile feelings, and anger at resident physicians who were frequently unavailable when decisions had to be made about patient care. Finally, the staff felt that new and flexible approaches to these problems were needed (that is, an increase in innovation).

The Intervention Procedure

When staff received the WES profiles, they felt the discrepancies between their actual and preferred work environments validated their subjective impressions. The profiles of work settings outside the hospital were used to provide perspective. During the 11 subsequent meetings (two on the day shift, eight at the change between day and evening shift, and two during the night shift), the psychiatrist used the WES profiles to focus the discussion and to guide staff in developing solutions to work-environment problems affecting patient care.

The psychiatrist employed many well-known techniques to enhance the group problem-solving process.[11,12,24] Staff members were helped to ventilate their feelings about individual patient problems, staff communication gaps, and conflicts among staff and between staff and physicians. The group process was guided to enable disagreements to be explored and resolved in a manner enhancing the intrastaff cohesion. The psychiatrist helped staff members moderate their tendencies to be perfectionists and suppress anger and guilt. He attempted to increase autonomy and clarity by helping staff to develop clearer definitions of the responsibilities of physicians, nurses, and burn technicians. Finally, he met with the unit's head nurse and medical director to facilitate their exploration of conflict-laden nurse–physician communication problems. Undoubtedly, the liaison psychiatrist's physician status increased his ability to secure cooperation from the unit's physicians.

Shortly after the group meetings were initiated, the psychiatrist began to receive requests to consult about specific patients. These requests were used to teach staff about the nature and treatment of acute and chronic pain, specific management plans for patients with antisocial or other personality disorders, and management of delirium and severe depression. Much of this teaching involved individual staff members responsible for particular patients, but several didactic lectures were given to the entire staff. By helping staff members learn new skills and develop greater competence, these interventions were expected to increase staff independence, decrease work pressure and time urgency, and promote more innovative approaches to patient care.

As with most intervention programs, the group process did not always proceed smoothly. Meetings were sometimes canceled, and attendance varied from one meeting to another. Some meetings were marked by silence or superficial discussion rather than by meaningful exploration of issues. In the overall course of the intervention, however, nursing staff members achieved a greater sense of being a team (increased involvement and cohesion), better individual techniques for coping with work stressors, greater acceptance of the inevitability of mistakes, and reasonable solutions to many administrative problems (such as moving from an eight-hour to a ten-hour shift pattern, arranging regular times to meet with staff physicians, and changing the content of the nursing report). The staff successfully worked through feelings of anger toward an antisocial patient, and feelings of grief when a favorite patient died unexpectedly on the unit.

The Postintervention Work Environment

The results of the WES real and ideal forms after the 12th meeting gave some support to the liaison psychiatrist's impression that many of the initial problems had been resolved satisfactorily. The response rate was 72% for R.N.'s and 94% for all other staff.

Of the eight WES dimensions on which staff perceptions changed, seven (all but physical comfort) changed in the direction of the staff's preferred work setting (see Figure 2). The increase in autonomy was statistically significant ($t = 2.17$; $p < .05$), whereas the increases in involvement ($t = 1.65$; $p = .05$) and peer cohesion ($t = 1.68$; $p = .05$) were marginally significant.* Perceptions of the ideal work environment remained generally stable, although preferred peer cohesion exhibited some decrease ($t = 1.93$; $p < .05$), as did autonomy ($t = 1.62$; $p < .06$), and clarity ($t = 2.04$; $p < .05$). Real–ideal discrepancies were reduced on nine of the ten WES subscales (there was no change on physical comfort). The real/ideal discrepancies decreased significantly on involvement ($t = 2.17$; $p < .05$), peer cohesion $t = 2.79$; $p < .01$), and autonomy ($t = 3.85$; $p < .01$).

A more detailed analysis revealed some differential changes among the three shifts. The day shift staff, which had the highest attendance at the meetings, showed the largest number of statistically significant changes. For instance, in addition to the changes noted for the entire staff, the day staff perceived significantly more clarity and innovation and significantly less work pressure. We believe the greater changes perceived by the day shift reflect their greater participation in the group problem solving and, as a

*In these comparisons $df = 47$; p is one tailed.

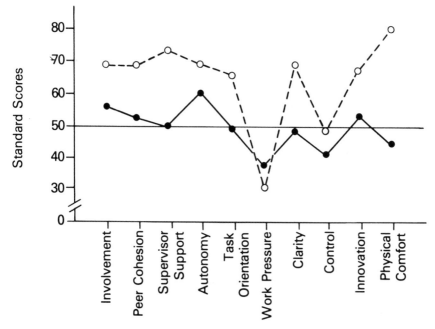

Figure 2. Postintervention WES profiles for burn unit staff (●—● = Real, o---o = Ideal).

result, greater actual changes in the work environment on their shift.

Although this liaison intervention produced measurable change in the work environment, Figure 2 testifies to the abundant room for additional improvement. The moderate size of the changes fits the limited magnitude of the intervention and gives evidence of the stability and slow rates of change of social systems.

Discussion

The present study suggests that a structured feedback procedure is a useful addition to the armamentarium of liaison psychiatrists and others who work with hospital staff. The feedback appeared relevant and helped staff focus on stressful aspects of the work setting and develop practical changes. The WES profile provided a comfortable and nonthreatening way to begin group discussions. It helped the staff focus on group norms and conflicts and realize they could control aspects of their work environment.

At the end of the intervention period, the liaison psychiatrist, the head nurse, and the medical director all felt that morale on the unit had improved substantially. The quality of patient care seemed better. The psychosocial aspects of patients' problems received more systematic attention, nursing and medical staff communicated more openly regrading these problems and the feelings they evoked, and staff showed more skill in dealing with pain and psychiatric disorders. The WES results indicate that the staff shared these impressions, and that they perceived substantial changes in the initial target areas (involvement, peer cohesion, autonomy, and innovation).

These changes are consonant with the problems discussed and resolved through the liaison group meetings, didactic seminars, and consultations with the unit's head nurse and medical director. We believe involvement and peer cohesion increased because of the staff's success in airing and resolving the disruptive interpersonal and administrative issues previously noted. Staff autonomy and innovation increased because the group meetings clarified role expectations and responsibilities. The increased clarity encouraged administrative staff to allow more autonomy and innovation, and permitted patient care staff to be comfortable with this additional freedom.

Finally, the changes in staff values about cohesion, autonomy, and clarity may have resulted from the lessened deprivation experienced in these aspects of the work environment as the liaison intervention progressed. Although these explanations are reasonable, we cannot be certain, in the absence of a controlled experiment, that the changes resulted from the liaison intervention.

The process of assessment, feedback, liaison consultation, and reassessment was also conducted with the hospital's surgical unit and its neonatal intensive care unit. After an intervention similar to the burn unit procedures, staff members in these two units perceived greater congruence between the actual and preferred work setting with regard to task orientation, work pressure, and two of the three relationship dimensions (involvement and cohesion in the neonatal ICU; involvement and supervisor support on the surgical unit).

Although these findings are promising, there is a need to

identify the relationship between changes in WES dimensions and measures of staff morale, absenteeism and turnover, patient satisfaction with care, and possibly even length of patient stay (an index of productivity). The development of a satisfactory medical work environment is itself an important goal, but how this environment influences the quality of patient care needs to be clarified. The WES dimensions are a tool to explore associations between changes in work atmosphere and changes in the quality and outcome of patient care.

Information about the work environment can help a liaison consultant better understand a medical unit. Just as therapists create mental models of their patients to guide therapy, consultants create a model of the social setting to assist them in their task. This model includes observations and speculations about the structure, function, and dynamics of the staff. The WES can contribute to this working image. A discrepancy between the WES and other information can generate new hypotheses. Moreover, obtaining a WES profile involves assessing factors relevant to the consultant's task, such as the degree of resistance to change, the resources for generating and maintaining innovations, and the staff's values and priorities.

Staff members' values are reflected in their portrayal of an ideal work environment, whereas their priorities are indicated by the size of the discrepancies between real and ideal scores on the WES dimensions. The staff's resources are reflected in WES dimensions, such as real peer cohesion, involvement, supervisor support, and clarity. High resistance to change may be foreshadowed by low WES real autonomy and innovation and by high real control.

The measurement-feedback-planning process has a number of benefits:

1. Staff members are encouraged to think about their work setting along the ten dimensions of the WES instead of in a one-dimensional space extending from "nonstressful" to "stressful."
2. Important but often overlooked work setting characteristics, such as the clarity of expectations and the emphasis on staff autonomy, become explicit.
3. Focusing staff members' change efforts on a few com-

monly defined areas reduces confusion and conflicting behavior and enhances the likelihood of orderly change.

4. Involvement is often increased simply because staff members are working together to change their work setting.

5. Finally, the intervention procedure provides an opportunity for staff members to expand their concern from caring for individual patients to considering the impact of the setting as a whole on all patients as well as on staff. Suddenly, for example, staff members are regarded as responsible for the policies and procedures of their unit and are considered competent to include program planning within their roles.

These procedures, however, are no panacea. The evaluation and change process can encounter serious resistance, especially when existing social relationships are ignored; when staff members feel that change may compromise patient care, increase work pressure, or decrease clarity in staff roles and responsibilities; or when staff members disagree on the type of program change desired.[25,26] Notwithstanding these problems, we believe that liaison programs that incorporate systematic assessment and feedback procedures can enhance staff morale and motivation and contribute to the quality of patient care.

References

1. Imparato, N. Job satisfaction patterns among nurses: An Overview. *Supervisor Nurse,* 1972, *3,* 53–57.
2. Nichols, G. A. Job satisfaction and nurses' intentions to remain with or to leave an organization. *Nursing Research,* 1971, *20,* 218–228.
3. Cartwright, L. Sources and effects of stress in health careers. In G. Stone, F. Cohen, & N. Adler (Eds.), *Health psychology: A handbook.* San Francisco: Jossey-Bass, 1979.
4. Cherniss, C. *Professional burnout in human service organizations.* New York: Praeger, 1980.
5. Pines, A., & Aronson, E. *Burnout: From tedium to personal growth.* New York: Free Press, 1981.
6. Artiss, K., & Levine, A. Doctor–patient relations in severe illness. A seminar for oncology fellows. *New England Journal of Medicine,* 1973, *288,* 1210–1214.
7. Weiner, M. F., & Caldwell, T. Stresses and coping in ICU Nursing. II. Nurse support groups on intensive care units. *General Hospital Psychiatry,* 1981, *3* 129–134.
8. Klagsbrun, S. Cancer, emotions and nurses. *American Journal of Psychiatry,* 1970, *126,* 1237–1244.

9. Cassem, N. H., & Hackett, T. P. Stress on the nurse and therapist in the intensive-care unit and the coronary-care unit. *Heart Lung*, 1975, *4*, 252–259.

10. Dubovsky, S. L., Getto, C. J., Gross, S. A., & Paley, J. A. Impact on nursing care and mortality: Psychiatrists on the coronary care unit. *Psychomatics*, 1977, *18*, 18–26.

11. Hay, D., & Oken, D. The psychological stresses of intensive care unit nursing. *Psychosomatic Medicine*, 1972, *34*, 109–118.

12. Mohl, P. C. Group process interpretations in liaison psychiatry nurse groups. *General Hospital Psychiatry*, 1980, *2*, 104–111.

13. Quinby, S., & Bernstein, N. R. Identity problems and the adaptation of nurses to severely burned children. *American Journal of Psychiatry*, 1971, *128*, 58–63.

14. Andreasen, N. J. C., Noyes, R., Hartford, C. E., Brodland, G., & Procter, S. Management of emotional reactions in seriously bruned adults. *New England Journal of Medicine*, 1972, *286*, 65–69.

15. Seligman, R. A psychiatric classification system for burned children. *American Journal of Psychiatry*, 1974, *131*, 41–46.

16. Steiner, H., & Clark, W. R. Psychiatric complications of burned adults: A classification. *Journal of Trauma*, 1977, *17*, 134–143.

17. Bailey, J. T., Steffen, S. M., & Grout, J. W. The stress audit: Identifying the stressors of ICU nursing. *Journal of Nursing Education*, 1980, *19*, 15–25.

18. Curtiss, S. The comparability of humanistic and behavioristic approaches in a mental hospital. In A. Wandersman, P. Poppen, & D. Ricks (Eds.), *Humanism and behaviorism: Dialog and growth*. New York: Pergamon, 1976.

19. Moos, R. H. Changing the social milieus of psychiatric treatment settings. *Journal of Applied Behavioral Science* 1973, *9*, 575–593.

20. Verinis, J., & Flaherty, J. Using the ward atmosphere scale to help change the treatment environment. *Hospital and Community Psychiatry*, 1978, *29*, 238–240.

21. Moos, R., Clayton, J., & Max, W. *The social climate scales: An annotated bibliography* (2nd ed.). Palo Alto, Calif.: Consulting Psychologists Press, 1979.

22. Moos, R. *Work environment scale manual*. Palo Alto, Calif.: Consulting Psychologists Press, 1981.

23. Moos, R., & Moos, B. Adaptation and the quality of life in work and family settings. *Journal of Community Psychology*, 1983, *11*, 158–170.

24. Billowitz, A., Friedson, W., & Schubert, D. S. P. Liaison psychiatry on a burn unit. *General Hospital Psychiatry*, 1980 *2*, 300–305.

25. Moos, R. *Evaluating treatment environments: A social ecological approach*. New York: Wiley, 1974.

26. Moos, R. Improving social settings by social climate measurement and feedback. In R. Munoz, L. Snowden, & J. Kelly (Eds.), *Social and psychological research in community settings*. San Francisco: Jossey-Bass, 1979.

XI

The Final Crisis
Death and the Fear of Dying

Death is life's final crisis. For some, death comes swiftly in an accident; others slip away silently in their sleep. Deaths like these are viewed as easy: They are quick and relatively painless. But many patients face the prospect of an extended period of time between the first abruptly imparted knowledge that they will die and actual death—the "living-dying interval." Though some of the coping tasks embedded in this crisis are similar to those we have seen earlier, the stark irrefutable reality of death makes the confrontation a unique challenge. Moreover, there are wide variations in the way individuals experience the dying process, in the ebb and flow of their emotions.[4]

The dying person must come to grips with many losses—future plans must be abandoned and significant relationships with family and friends must end. The psychiatrist Erich Lindemann spent his life trying to understand life crisis and the adaptation process. He has described ways of coping with impending death and of grieving for the most significant loss of all—the "losing of oneself." In facing his own painful death from a sacral chordoma, Lindemann noted the value of seeking information in response to the uncertainty of the situation, of learning from other people in a similar predicament, of structuring an acceptable future for those who are left behind, and of creating a lasting image of oneself that can survive one's own death and be remembered by family and friends. He recommends that staff promote these coping skills by forming a therapeutic alliance with

385

patients and by trying to understand their unique construction of reality.[1]

Dying patients face the difficult challenge of balancing anticipatory grief and disengagement while still creating a meaningful life during the unknown amount of time they have remaining.[6] Despite the dependent and helpless position in which they may find themselves, the terminally ill can maintain their dignity and individual identity by being responsible for decisions about their day-to-day lives and by setting realistic goals that can provide a sense of achievement when the usual work and family functions are relinquished. The mobilization of hope is one of the most significant coping mechanisms for the terminally ill. Even patients who have understood and accepted their prognosis can usually find some basis for hope, and staff should be careful not to be so absolute as to eliminate this possibility.

If patients can negotiate life's final crisis successfully, the process of coping with dying may enable them to achieve deeper self-awareness and closer relationships with their families. In the first article, Sylvia Poss identifies six overlapping, problem-solving tasks that dying patients confront as they prepare for death. The first task is to become emotionally aware of approaching death; such awareness may wax and wane from day to day. Patients sometimes dwell on the chance of recovery even though they "know" they only have a short time to live. The dying person also needs to strike a balance between hope and fear. More than death itself, patients may fear pain, abandonment, or uncertainty. Reassurance that they will not suffer or be isolated and belief in an afterlife in which they will be reunited with family members may enable patients to control their fears and counter their despair.

In Chapter 10, Alice Stewart Trillin spoke of the will to live as a valuable coping resource for cancer patients. But when death is near, a person must relinquish the will to live and make a conscious decision to accept death. The dying person's third task is to make an active decision to reverse the physical struggle to live. A related task is that of relinquishing responsibility and independence by letting go of life, giving up control, and allowing caregivers to make decisions. During this part of the dying process, patients may fight to survive for an important occasion, such as a last birthday or holiday. The final tasks entail disengagement from personal relationships and spiritual preparation for death. Faith offers the comfort and support that sustains many patients as they cope with the crisis of dying. Caregivers who understand these six tasks can help patients attain a sense of closure and die with dignity.

As concern about the process of dying has widened, health care professionals have communicated more directly with patients about their diagnosis, prognosis, and prospect of death. Even children may participate in making decisions about whether they would like further experimental treatment or supportive care.[3] Open communication not only promotes coping during the living-dying interval, but it can also lead to better family adjustment following the death of a family member, as was the case for parents who talked openly with their dying children.[7] Groups led by health care professionals or patients can provide a channel for addressing common issues and thus facilitate coping with dying. Such groups offer terminally ill patients a chance to share their experiences and learn how to make their remaining life meaningful and to come to terms with death.

In the second article, David Spiegel and Irvin D. Yalom describe a support group for women with metastatic breast cancer. The group enabled the women to put death in perspective and adapt to "living in the context of dying." As the women learned how other members coped, dying was "detoxified" and their fears of death diminished. The women became more assertive and set new priorities based on the knowledge that time was short and should be used wisely. For some women, marital relationships and communication improved as they became more assertive about meeting their needs. The women also established better working relationships with their doctors and taught them to be more responsive to their needs and the needs of cancer patients in general. By enabling them to make such contributions, the group helped the women achieve a sense of purpose as they slowly approached their death. The members found new meaning in life and taught their families and friends about living with cancer and dying with dignity.

In recent years, health care staff have become more aware of the special needs of dying persons and their families. Physicians' traditional emphasis on sustaining life and longevity has been augmented by programs such as Comfort Care Only[5] in which the aim is to alleviate pain and make patients as comfortable as possible as they approach death. The hospice movement has developed, and it is now more common for patients to be cared for and to die at home.[2]

In the final article, Courtney Rogers Malone writes movingly of her sister Bobby's death from cancer. Bobby's family helped her to fulfill her last wish—to die at home. When Bobby learned she had only a brief time to live, she decided she wanted to die at home without heroic life-support measures. She got together with her family in a house by the sea to spend her last Christmas. The family was aided by a physician friend who provided emotional support and helped to make Bobby comfortable by supplying oxygen equipment and pain medication.

By Christmas Eve, Bobby had become very weak. But there were brief periods when she made a special effort to participate in life, as on Christmas Day when she shared some final happy moments with her family. On New Year's Eve, Bobby had difficulty breathing and needed oxygen continuously. Family members bathed and fed her and played music and sang for her—expressions of their love, and in turn, ways to cope with their grief. Finally, Bobby took off her oxygen mask and said, "Let's get on with it." We see here the conscious decision to give up the physical fight and go about the business of dying of which Sylvia Poss spoke in Chapter 27. The family was led in prayer by their clergyman and each person said goodbye to Bobby. Bobby died peacefully the next afternoon. The family gathered together for a toast "to life" and rejoiced in the fact that Bobby had succeeded in dying as she wished. The family had succeeded too—they helped Bobby to negotiate her last crisis. In the process, they learned much about life, love, and caring.

References

1. Lindemann, E. Reactions to one's own fatal illness. In E. Lindemann & E. Lindemann (Eds.), *Beyond grief: Studies in crisis intervention*. New York: Jason Aronson, 1979.
2. Murphy, L. B. *The home hospital: How a family can cope with catastrophic illness*. New York: Basic Books, 1982.
3. Nitschke, R., Wunder, S., Sexauer, C. L., & Humphrey, G. B. The final-stage con-

ference: The patient's decision on research drugs in pediatric oncology. *Journal of Pediatric Psychology*, 1977, *2*, 58–64.
4. Pattison, E. M. The living–dying process. In C. A. Garfield (Ed.), *The dying patient.* New York: McGraw-Hill, 1978.
5. Schmale, A. H. The dying patient. *Advances in Psychosomatic Medicine*, 1980, *10*, 99–110.
6. Sourkes, B. *The deepening shade: Psychological aspects of life-threatening illness.* Pittsburg: University of Pittsburg Press, 1982.
7. Spinetta, J. J., Swarner, J. A., & Sheposh, J. P. Effective parental coping following the death of a child from cancer. *Journal of Pediatric Psychology*, 1981, *6*, 251–263.

27

How the Terminal Patient Accepts Dying

SYLVIA POSS

Introduction

Crisis theory has alerted us to the work that people have to do for themselves to master any life crisis.[1] Dying is life's terminal crisis. It demands of the dying patient a great deal of physical, social, intellectual, spiritual, and emotional effort to achieve death with dignity.

Although much has been written about isolated aspects of the terminal crisis, no one has brought these ideas together into a unified definition of the crisis. This article is based on earlier works and links them with my own observations[2] in an attempt to define the work required of the terminal patient in progressing toward an acceptance of death.

The dying patient's work comprises six problem-solving tasks. Although they are outlined here as though they are discrete and self-contained, in practice the distinctions are not clear, since the tasks overlap and shade into one another. Accepting one's

Reprinted with permission from *Patient Counseling and Health Education*, 1980, 2 (2), 72–77. Copyright *Excerpta Medica*, 1980.

SYLVIA POSS • Chief Social Worker, Johannesburg Hospital, Johannesburg, South Africa.

dying does not necessitate work on all six tasks; each individual will have to master different areas, depending on the issues that have been crucial in living.

The terminal crisis is complicated, and we do not fully comprehend it. Some uncertainty is present in every terminal situation: unexpected events—miracles do occur; pain, physical debility, and medical technology may interfere with the patient's dying work, and lay and professional caregivers may conspire to block the patient's work by confusing and contradicting the realization of imminent death.[3] It is important to keep these variables in mind while reading the description of the dying person's tasks.

The tasks are these:

1. To become aware of impending death
2. To balance hope and fear throughout the crisis
3. To make an active decision to reverse physical survival processes in order to die
4. To relinquish responsibility and independence
5. To separate the self from former experiences
6. To prepare the soul for death

Kübler-Ross's[4] description of the phases through which patients pass as they cope with death—denial, isolation, anger, bargaining, depression, and acceptance—defines the patient's emotional responses to the work of dying.

Becoming Aware of Impending Death

Although one's entire life may be viewed as an opportunity to equip oneself for death, one can begin to prepare for death only after becoming aware that it is approaching. This realization may become apparent at any stage of life, although for many it arises consciously only when the process of dying actually commences.

The internal cognitive and emotional internal processes of becoming aware that death is approaching may be complicated by external issues beyond the patient's control. At the same time that clues are offered to the discerning patient many environmental pressures thwart his acknowledgement of the fact that he is dying.[5] Glaser and Strauss[3] have identified open and closed awareness contexts and have highlighted the element of uncertainty in any terminal situation. In addition, a "conspiracy of silence" surrounds the dying patient's struggle for a definition of himself as a dying person.

In contrast, Kübler-Ross[4] observed that the act of becoming aware of impending death is more than a mere exercise of intellectual calculation: If the patient is to tolerate the new knowledge, emotional readiness has to accompany the mental discovery.

Awareness may take several forms. It might, for example, consist of acknowledging that death *may* be at hand, which possibility then becomes certain knowledge once acceptance is achieved. Or awareness may take the form of a suspicion or realization that death is approaching, accompanied either by an inability to verbalize this knowledge openly or by limited or sometimes open discussion of it.

Awareness of dying is, however, seldom consistently maintained over an extended period.[4] As with other emotional awareness, the patient is capable of tolerating different degrees of revelation at different times. A patient may know that he is dying yet behave at times as though he believes that he will recover.

The following example shows the struggle involved in becoming aware of and remaining in touch with realization of approaching death and illustrates one of the many forms that awareness may take.

Case 1. Mrs. F., a 58-year-old divorcee with carcinoma of the lung, was told by the consultant surgeon, in response to her persistent questioning, that she had a malignant growth in her lung and that a "gland" had been removed. The next day when the social worker visited, Mrs. F. insisted on knowing what was wrong with her and what the outcome would be. She told the social worker that the surgeon had said there was a growth. She had asked whether it was malignant, and he had said, "They always are." "So now," said Mrs. F. challengingly, "I still want to know whether mine is malignant."

Difficulty in becoming aware of dying is likely to be experienced by persons who are afraid of death and by those whose life pattern has been one of denial, withdrawal, or avoidance. Although it is not known whether unresolved awareness issues inhibit parallel work on other tasks, I believe that they do.

Balancing Hope and Fear

Both hope and fear prevail throughout the terminal crisis. The patient's task is to keep the two balanced.

The dying person has much to fear in approaching death: pain and suffering, disfigurement, abandonment, uncertainty, helplessness, loss, deprivation, impending judgment, and death itself.[6–8] Fear may, however, be balanced by hope.[9] These two emotions may be diminished or modified according to the state of dying work in which the patient is engaged. For example, once acceptance has been reached, the patient may be more anxious about his family's well-being than about his own. Such fearless dying is relatively rare and is possible only if hope is allowed to balance each emerging fear.

Hope provides the terminal situation with some meaning from which the patient may gain strength to persevere in the face of fear. For example, the patient may appropriately hope that he will be spared undue suffering, that he will not be isolated, that he will be adequately cared for, that his efforts will be rewarded, that life after death is a reality, that he will be reunited with his loved ones, and that his family will manage without him. Although hope of being cured is often inappropriate when the prognosis is uncertain, hope of recovery may not only be appropriate but also, paradoxically, keep despair at bay sufficiently to enable the patient to work on some other aspects of dying.

The patient should never be left without hope, for when hope is absent fear may reign. If the suffering is perceived as meaningless, feelings of hopelessness or despair may set in. Despair may result from the recognition that no human being can alter the terminal situation, while hope may lie in acknowledging that God can equip one to cope with it.

Case 2. Fluctuating hope is demonstrated by Mrs. I., a 41-year-old wife and mother with disseminated carcinoma. At first she hoped to get better: "I still have much work to do"; then to go home just once more to complete her tasks as mother: "There are many things I want to tell my [adolescent] daughter, things that she should hear from her mother"; then to be allowed to retain her position in the ward: "As least I can face the wall when I am sad so that no one else can see"; and then that her family would be looked after: "But don't upset them when you speak to them." (See also Case 6.)

The task of balancing hope and fear is likely to present difficulties to patients whose fears pervade the situation and those who are unbelieving, despairing, and hopeless.

Making an Active Decision to Reverse Physical Survival Processes

The ability to die appears to require some volition on the part of the patient. Unless the patient is heavily sedated this decision may be made consciously. Acceptance of dying has been described as a positive act, not mere capitulation,[10,11] yet, paradoxically, it involves an active cessation of former patterns of control.[11]

Similarly, the act of dying requires more than mere resignation: It is the very opposite of doing nothing.[12] According to Rayner[13]: "Perhaps a day or so before the end, the patient seems to give up interest and lets death take him. Many people lapse into unconsciousness; others may remain awake but simply withdraw; a subtle change takes place so that those around usually recognize that death is very close."

The will to live has been described in terms of the individual's hopefulness of what life has to offer.[14] Once a person loses hope, he may wish to stop living. The dying patient, on the other hand, relinquishes his will to live not because he has lost all hope but because he has consciously decided to move with the natural maturation processes, which at this stage lead to death. In so doing, the will to live is challenged, a struggle ensues, and a reversal process is set in motion. The resolution of the conflict marks the commencement of the patient's transition from an acceptance of dying to death itself.

At this point physical growth is reversed, and the patient diverts his energy from the fight for physical survival to accelerated emotional and spiritual development. It is not known whether this physical reversal process causes the patient to lose his will to live or whether giving up the fight causes the reversal.

Kübler-Ross[4] has described the reversal process and the struggle preceding it: "There are a few patients who fight [right] to the end . . . The day they stop fighting, the fight is over. The harder they struggle to avoid inevitable death . . . the more difficult it will be for them to reach this final stage of acceptance with peace and dignity."

The following case is a striking example of the decision to give up the struggle to live:

Case 3. Mr. G., a 64-year-old retired bank manager, married and father of three adult children, had had carcinoma of the rectum for 11 years. From the time of the onset of his illness, Mr. G. was aware of his terminal condition and made realistic preparation for his death. For months preceding his death, he was in the hospital, sleeping a great deal, in pain, and immobile but conscious and lucid. For two months his condition remained static. This period of waiting confused and distressed him, as he had been prepared to die and could not understand the delay. A week before he died, without provocation, Mr. G. said to his wife, "I have got to decide: Do I give up or carry on, or what do I do?" Thereafter he was calmer, appeared to be giving over, spoke very little, went into a coma, and died three days later.

The decision-making element is seldom as clearly demonstrated as in Mr. G.'s case, where reversal lay in his active acknowledgement that he would not recover. Thereafter he permitted physical deterioration to take its course while he concentrated on bringing other aspects of his being to fulfillment. The freeing of the self from the fight for physical survival thus allows the terminal patient to use his limited time creatively and to live his remaining life with meaning and fulfillment.[15]

The reversal process is likely to be resisted by patients who fear death and by those who do not yet view death as appropriate.

Relinquishing Responsibility and Independence

Occurring almost simultaneously with the reversal of the physical survival process is the task of relinquishing responsibility and independence. As the patient reverses his will to live, he appears to relinquish the characteristics that enabled him to function as a separate entity: autonomy, control of responsibility, and independence. He thus appears to be engaged in recapturing a childlike dependence and fearlessness,[4] which is not to be confused with excessive dependence in adulthood.

Weisman[11] views this relinquishing process as a transition from autonomous control to "counter-control," in which the patient yields to the decision making of selected caregivers. In this sense, dying may be regarded as a letting go in order to merge with something more extensive than the former limits of the ego have permitted. There is a quality of ecstasy, expansion, and growth to this experience so that dying need not be viewed as a restricting process. Many patients welcome the expansion and release of death and regret resuscitative measures that bring them back.[16]

In giving over, the dying patient submits to a force beyond himself. In this sense, yielding control is not giving in or giving up, both of which denote weakness, but is a positive act. Rather than feeling defeated, the patient has come to perceive his impending death as appropriate.[11]

Case 4. A 43-year-old wife and mother was desperately ill with disseminated carcinoma. She experienced extreme difficulty in breathing but fought with determination for several weeks to stay alive until her last ambition, that of spending Christmas with her family, had been realized. Content at having achieved her wish, she gave over her struggle for life and died the following day.

This example shows the patient's struggle for physical survival followed by her active decision to "stop the fight." By contrast, the next example illustrates the difficulty that may be experienced in relinquishing the will to live.

Case 5. Mr. H., 51, with carcinoma of the lung, had throughout his life fought for control of himself and his situation. While terminally ill, he struggled to maintain conscious control over his breathing and thus of his life. For five months he lay medically ready to die but determined not to give over. The medical staff were baffled by Mr. H.'s continuing struggle until they understood that he was emotionally unready to die because of fear of losing control. Eventually, although weak and emaciated, Mr. H. remained sitting upright and awake for 48 hours to continue his breathing. Then he keeled over. Even at the end there was no acceptance. He had not relinquished life; it had been taken from him.

This example reminds us that human beings are taught from

childhood to exert control over their affairs. The difficult task of relinquishing control is further complicated when society misinterprets it as an act of resignation or failure.[11] It is likely to prove difficult for those to whom control and independence have been essential elements of life.

Separating Oneself from Former Experience

In moving from one life phase to the next, the individual has a sense of progression, of leaving something behind. The same propulsion appears in approaching death. Death can be accepted only when the patient is prepared to leave life behind him and to detach himself from the former, familiar experiences. Kübler-Ross[4] expressed that death may be contemplated "with expectation."

Disengagement may be viewed as a process of decreased social involvement. Kübler-Ross[4] conceives of this gradual separation process as "detachment." Her work stresses this aspect of acceptance, which is devoid of emotion: The pain is gone. The struggle is over. The patient awaits the long-anticipated event and prepares for it by withdrawing from former relationships and emotions. Decathexis, therefore, leads to an emotion-free readiness to die.

Weisman[11] points out that once the patient is engaged in the process of separation, he can no longer be expected to bear responsibility or to maintain intense relationships, since he feels a reduced capacity for life and is responding to it appropriately by disengaging himself from it. It is not his intention to rebuff relatives, although this action may be misinterpreted and have a hurtful effect.

For some patients, however, disengagement can be a liberating experience, one of freeing the self from worldly ties and responsibilities.

In the following case, notice the active part Mrs. I. played in giving over responsibility and separating herself from life:

Case 6. (See also Case 2.) The 41-year-old mother with disseminated carcinoma had formerly expressed concern over "deserting" her two sickly

*children. After some weeks of lingering, Mrs. I. began to disengage her
concern for her children as she had come to realize that God could take far
better care of them than she could have done. She said that she was happy to
entrust them to Him. Having thus been relieved of responsibility, Mrs. I.
seemed to detach herself and died two days later.*

The following is another example of a patient who detaches
herself from earthly ties. Notice again, the active part Mrs. J.
played in withdrawing from life in order to die:

*Case 7. Mrs. J., a 62-year-old mother of adult children, had an advanced
malignant disease. She wanted "to go" and felt that those who tended her
(loved ones in her family) were holding her back. She asked them not to do
anything more for her, saying, "Leave me" and "Let me go." Since Mrs. J.
had detached herself from most human relationships, she refused to be
restrained in her departure, and therefore greeted visitors with, "Thank you
for coming. Goodbye." On her last day, Mrs. J. responded to her husband's
enquiry with, "Fine, thank you. Leave me." Mrs. J.'s disengagement was
facilitated by her keen anticipation of going to heaven. Her last words were,
"There is my dear Lord; there He comes already . . . and my dad . . . "*

Disengagement is likely to be more easily accomplished by the
patient who believes that he is going to heaven. In contrast, detachment may be difficult if the patient fears that he is going to
hell.

Spiritual Preparation

Once the patient becomes aware of impending death, he is
likely to ponder on what lies beyond life. Hinton[17] reports that
many patients have been observed to turn, return, or draw closer
to God in preparation for death. Consequently, concern and discussions about religious issues are appropriate during this stage of
adjustment.[6] In some cases, acceptance of death is synonymous
with calm faith or peace.[4] Religious faith does not obviate the
conflicts of the crisis, but it helps give the patient strength to
resolve them.

Are patients with religious faith or without it more likely to
reach an acceptance of death? According to Abrams,[18] "Religious

faith comforts and supports many patients and should be considered in any program for optimum management, especially in the terminal stage." While many terminal-care workers support this point of view, both Hinton[17] and Kübler-Ross[4] have observed that religious patients differ little from those without religion. The religious belief of most patients is not enough to relieve them of conflict and fear. These patients need help to make the best possible use of the faith they have.[19]

In my own experience of rendering social work service to 50 patients with terminal malignant disease and their families, 76% of the sample thought that their religious faith had aided them in their dying work. Using the patients' own assessments and the observations of staff, it was found that 60% of those with some faith or knowledge of life after death reached some acceptance of their dying, while only 6% of those without faith accomplished some resolution of the terminal crisis. I have concluded that the patient's religious faith does play a potentially dynamic role in facilitating his mastery of the crisis and that difficulty in this task is likely to affect work in every other aspect of the crisis.[2]

Spiritual preparation is likely to prove difficult for unbelieving patients, those who do not believe in life after death, those who have insufficient faith to aid them through this crisis, those who have rejected God, those who experience guilt in relation to their lives, and those who fear impending judgment, punishment, or hell.[6] This does not mean that those who do not believe in an existence after death do not also have need of some integration of their life experiences. Their reflective and contemplative work may, however, take the form of a search for meaning in life or of work on some other related terminal crisis task.

A Sense of Achievement and Completion

Dying can be a positive experience. There is no defeat in dignified dying. On the contrary, great fortitude is needed to lay down what has become familiar and to move calmly into the future.

Though dying is sad and often difficult, for the patient who has completed his dying work and reached acceptance there is a justifiable sense of achievement. Saunders[12] writes, "A whole life has been gathered together . . . (Here) is the moment of fullest individuality." She also highlights "the achievements that people continually make in their dying." Weisman[11] refers to a sense of completeness, and Kübler-Ross[4] uses the phrase "the monumental task" of reaching the acceptance of death. All three writers seem to support my view in communicating a sense of dignity and self-respect in which there is victory over death.

The following case exemplifies achievement in dying:

Case 8. Mr. K., a 65-year-old widower with carcinoma of the lung had lived a hard, deprived life. He had struggled to cope with life's demands and had suffered physical disability, a troubled marriage, and then, after a reconciliation, the death of his wife.

Once ill and himself in need of care, Mr. K. undertook to care for his stepson and grandchildren who had come to live with him. Mr. K. refused the offer of his sister to have him in her home where she could tend him, as he did not want to be a burden to her and because he was concerned that his pet would be neglected once he left home.

During the 17 months of his illness, Mr. K. changed from a helpless, depressed man into a person who, with relatively little social work help, was able to cope with his financial, domestic, and medical affairs. He obtained an old-age pension, paid off his house, and kept house for his stepson and family.

Mr. K. decided on his own terminal care, thinking in terms of the needs of others rather than himself. Throughout the terminal period he remained calm and accepting, experiencing only short periods of depression. Mr. K. died in his sleep without fuss, attention, or inconvenience to others. In mastering his own terminal situation, Mr. K.'s sense of deprivation appeared to have been dispelled. Herein lay achievement.

Integrating the Elements Involved in the Terminal Crisis

In some cases these six tasks appear to require attention in sequence. For example, any of the subsequent work will appear unnecessary to the patient who has no awareness of his dying. The separation and relinquishing work cannot be undertaken before the physical struggle is over, and for many, the act of commending the soul to God is the final one. On the other hand, these tasks may appear to demand simultaneous attention and seem to exist parallel to each other.

Complete resolution of the terminal crisis may require problem-solving work on all six tasks, thus indicating that the act of dying work may require effort in physical, psychological, intellectual, spiritual, and social spheres of functioning. Few patients appear to do equal battle in all six areas. While work in some areas appears vital to the mastery of the terminal crisis, other tasks may require little or no work. The tasks do appear to be linked and to influence the outcome of each other. For example, spiritual difficulties may provoke denial, fear, and resistance to the relinquishing and separation work required to reach acceptance.

It is not yet clear whether the psychosocial tasks required of the terminal patient arise during the appropriate stage of emotional adjustment to death, as outlined by Kübler-Ross,[4] or whether the problem-solving work provokes the relevant emotional response. I believe the latter is true.

The particular issues that require an individual's attention will be determined by his physical condition and by his patterns of functioning during former life phases. Thus, the way the patient has lived will influence the way he dies.

Timing may be a complicating factor: The patient who gives over too early may continue in as much distress as the patient who holds on for too long.[20] The actual timing of a person's death is beyond his control, but he is given some control by his own preparation for it. Thus, while any one of these tasks remains unresolved, the patient will either linger at the point of death, unready to die, or he will not be able to retain his dignity in dying.

Many issues in understanding the nature of the terminal crisis remain unresolved. Glaser and Strauss's words reflect my own experience: "Persons who are present when a death actually occurs are often struck by the remarkably thin line that stretches between life and death."[3]

Clearly, the caregiver's full understanding of the terminal crisis will equip her to help the patient in his resolution of the crisis.

References

1. Rapoport, L. Crisis intervention as a mode of brief treatment. In R. W. Romerts & R. H. Nee (Eds.), *Theories of social casework*. Chicago: University of Chicago Press, 1970.

2. Poss, S. *Towards death with dignity: Caring for dying people.* London: George Allen & Unwin, 1981.
3. Glaser, B. G., & Strauss, A. L. *Awareness of dying.* London: Weidenfeld & Nicolson, 1966.
4. Kübler-Ross, E. *On death and dying.* London: Tavistock, 1970.
5. Kalish, R. A. The onset of the dying process. *Omega 1,* 1970, 1, 57–59.
6. Carlozzi, C. G. *Death and contemporary man, the crisis of terminal illness.* Grand Rapids, Mich.: William B. Eerdmans, 1968.
7. Wahl, C. W. The fear of death. In R. Fulton (Ed.), *Death and identity.* New York: Wiley, 1966.
8. Rosenthal, H. R. Psychotherapy for the dying. In H. M. Ruitenbeek (Ed.), *Death: Interpretations.* New York: Delta, 1966.
9. Kübler-Ross, E. Hope and the dying patient. In B. Schoenberg *et al.* (Eds.), *Psychosocial aspects of terminal care.* New York: Columbia University Press, 1972.
10. Weisman, A. D., & Kastenbaum, R. A. The psychological autopsy—A study of the terminal phase of life. *Community Mental Health Journal Monograph,* no. 4. New York: Behavioral Publications, 1968.
11. Weisman, A. D. *On dying and denying: A psychiatric study of terminality.* New York: Behavioral Publications, 1972.
12. Saunders, C. Death and responsibility: A medical director's view. *Psychiatric Opinion,* 1966, *3,* 28–34.
13. Rayner, E. *Human development.* London: George Allen & Unwin.
14. Salzberger-Wittenberg, I. *Psycho-analytic insight and relationships: A Kleinian approach.* London: Routledge & Kegan Paul, 1970.
15. Hineman, J. H. *Counselling with the terminally ill: A clinical study.* Unpublished doctoral dissertation. University of Utah, Salt Lake City, 1971.
16. Osis, R. *Deathbed observations by physicians.* New York: Parapsychology Foundation, 1961.
17. Hinton, J. *Dying.* London: Penguin Books, 1968.
18. Abrams, R. D. *Not alone with cancer.* Springfield, Ill.: Charles C Thomas, 1974.
19. Leslie, B. *Helping the dying patient and his family* (Reprint). National Association of Social Workers, 1960 (pp. 11–15).
20. Oppenheimer, J. R. Use of crisis intervention in casework with the cancer patient and his family. *Social Work,* 1967, *12* (2), 44–52.

28

A Support Group for Dying Patients

DAVID SPIEGEL and IRVIN D. YALOM

Confrontation with the inevitability of one's death has long been considered a necessary part of authentic living. Philosophers from Plato to the twentieth-century existential thinkers have held that in order to learn to live well, one must first learn to die. But only comparatively recently have clinicians sought to help dying patients and their families integrate the knowledge of impending death with they way they live their lives. The time of facing death is one of sadness and mourning, but it is also a time of reorientation and a time of reconsidering one's values, one's priorities, and one's sense of meaning in life. In this article, we shall describe a group approach to the care of the dying patient, an approach which ministers both to the anguish of dying and to the vitality which a confrontation with death may stimulate in the life which remains to the patient.

Treatment Perspective

Our approach draws from three distinct clinical fields: group psychotherapy, self-help and community support systems, and

Reprinted from the *International Journal of Group Psychotherapy*, 1978, *28*, 233–245.

DAVID SPIEGEL and IRVIN D. YALOM • Department of Psychiatry and Behavioral Sciences, Stanford University School of Medicine, Stanford, California 94305.

the individual treatment of the dying patient. The research on group therapy suggests that there are features inherent in the group approach which are potent and not available in individual therapy.[1] In particular, certain curative factors in the group situation would seem particularly relevant to the group treatment of individuals with matastatic carcinoma. Among these factors are universality; the sense that group members develop a being "all in the same boat" can diminish the feeling of being singled out and alienated from the rest of humanity. A second factor is altruism, the experience which emerges in groups of helping oneself by helping others. A third is instillation of hope. Group members can see other people who have had the same problems, for example, anxiety, anger, or isolation and who have moved past these problems. Identification is important. Group members may learn to overcome specific problems in their lives by modeling their behavior in accordance with the successful example of another group member. Finally, group cohesiveness, the sense of unconditional acceptance and belonging, is important to offset the dreadful isolation so many terminal patients experience.

Many of the helping factors in self-help and mutual support groups such as Alcoholics Anonymous, Parents without Partners, and Reach for Recovery, among hundreds of others, overlap with features of group therapy, particularly in the area of what has been defined as "the helper-therapy principle."[2,3] It has been observed that many members of self-help groups find an enhanced sense of interpersonal confidence and self-worth through being of help to other people. But there are important differences between self-help and therapy groups as well. As Caplan[4] has noted, support systems provide a kind of concrete guidance and support to an individual which is not common to psychotherapy situations, and they do so for an indefinite period of time. Secondly, the members are recruited because they share a specific and often stigmatized attribute, such as alcoholism, compulsive gambling, or a medical illness. Thirdly, public confession of the stigma is often an important criterion of membership. The reasons for entering psychotherapy groups are more varied and, as a result, confession is not as specific or ritualized. Some behavior therapy groups are composed of patients with a specific common problem, but they are structured by a nonmember therapist.

Fourthly, mutual support groups are more often in a position to make real changes in the outside life of the patient. Many of them move in the direction of public and political involvement and thereby enhance the members' sense of self-esteem and assertiveness.[5] As will be discussed later, the fact that metastatic cancer was the ticket of admission to this group and that some group members were willing to involve themselves in such broad public issues as the education of professionals were of great importance to the overall group experience.

Finally, in recent years there has been a growing literature on individual treatment of the dying patient. Changes in our religious, political, and social institutions have been proposed as reasons for the growing public and professional interest in thanatology.[6] Writers such as Kübler-Ross[7] have helped focus attention on the importance of direct and honest communication with patients about the course of their disease in helping to minimize their sense of isolation. In our group, direct talk about death and dying is a necessary part of the experience for each member. However, it is only one of many factors in the treatment: Group support, family involvement, and the self-help aspects of the program vastly enrich the treatment experience. What follows is a description of the program and then a series of clinical themes which have emerged during the course of the group.

Treatment Structure

The group was organized over four years ago in an effort to provide support for cancer patients. Metastatic carcinoma was the criterion of admission to the group and was the major common bond among the members. The majority of group members had carcinoma of the breast. The therapists and the group members collaboratively determined the direction of the group. It has met weekly for 90 minutes, with at times special one-hour sessions preceding the regular group meetings during which training in self-hypnosis or meditation has been offered. The patients have all been fully aware of the nature and prognosis of their illness. Those patients who massively deny their illness and its implications and those patients considered by their doctors free of metastatic disease have not been included. The group has been an open one, and members come as often as their physical condition permits and as long as they continue to benefit from the experience. Almost all are outpatients, although several have attended while hospitalized. The number attending the meetings has varied from three to twelve, averaging between six and seven members. We have found that the maximum effective size is approximately seven, and when more than eight members have attended, we have often divided the group into two small groups for an hour and reconvened as a large group for the final thirty minutes.

Patients have usually entered the group by referral from another member of the group or from cancer organizations, such as the American Cancer Society. At first, physicians were reluctant to refer patients since they feared that a group which discussed death and dying would severely unsettle them. However, after observing the group and finding that it was life oriented and that patients found it enormously supportive, many physicians have referred their patients.

During the course of some four years, more than forty patients have attended at least one meeting. The group maintains an active roster of approximately ten members, some of whom attend regularly and some of whom attend only periodically when in despair. Fifteen members have died. There have been several therapists during the course of the group: two faculty members of the Department of Psychiatry, three psychiatric residents, a psychiatric social worker, and two counselors. One of the therapists is herself a victim of breast cancer, now in remission. Generally, there have been as many as three to four therapists present at every meeting, primarily because of student interest in the group.

The group is regularly observed through a one-way mirror by mental health workers and occasionally by family members of the women in the group. All observation is made with the consent and knowledge of the group members. The therapy program has also included family members. On occasion, we have had individual or conjoint meetings with families, but our most effective mode of working with families has been large family group sessions. The group consists of four to six weekly evening sessions led by the group therapists. In general, the index patients have not been involved in these family meetings, although usually, once in the course of a series of family meetings, they are invited to participate. The group has, on several occasions, also met with the families of members who have recently died.

Putting Dying in Perspective

Having a terminal disease has many implications for an individual's life. It affects her family, her work, her friends, her priorities in life as well as her relationship with her body. Fears grow—of loss of function, pain, and death. The group has focused not on dying per se but rather on living in the context of dying. The task has been not merely to face the fact of one's own death but to live in the face of it, to maintain meaningful family and social relationships and, in some instances, careers, and to live resolutely with neither denial nor depressive preoccupation—in short, to maintain a sense of purpose in life.

A major task of the group involved a search for the answer to the question: "What remains of myself when I give up highly valued functions and attributes?" These women had been quite active physically and were faced with loss of ability and energy in these areas. It had been easy for them to identify themselves as a parent, a counselor, or a lover of the outdoors. When their illness forced them to relinquish these attributes, much of the mourning of their loss was done in the group. They were forced to reflect on what was left, to give up thinking of themselves in terms of these categories and view themselves more in the Kierkegaardian sense as that person who gives up attributes.[8] At one meeting, an exercise was done in which members composed a list of their ten central attributes, ranked in order of importance. The members then meditated on the giving up of these attributes one by one and feeling that part of themselves which remained. The women were, almost without exception, deeply moved. A few simply stopped and said they could not do the exercise, that there were certain things they could not give up. Most members saw a self which remained beyond objective attributes, but the depth of the sadness in the room made it clear that they were mourning parts of their lives which were slipping away.

Detoxifying Dying

One of the major tasks of the group has been mourning and coping with the death of group members. This process has had important implications for the cohesiveness of the group as a whole and for each group member's capacity to face her own death. At the time of this writing, four members of the group have died within the last eight months. The first was a relatively new member with metastatic lesions in the brain. Her general proclivity within the group was to deny; she courageously "kept her chin up" and dressed with elaborate clothing and makeup to conceal her physical debilitation. She died while on a vacation with her husband. At first, the group briefly noted her death with sadness and then quickly moved on to other issues. Immediately afterwards, however, considerable anger and bickering emerged. Over the course of a month, it became clear that considerable fear lay under the anger. When the death of this member was discussed openly and in depth, the fighting in the group diminished, and a strong sense of mutual support emerged.

Shortly after that, a woman who had been very important to the group died rather suddenly. She was a dramatic, vital woman whose sense of engagement with life was striking. She had had some indication that her death was near and demonstrated great courage and serenity toward the end of her life. The dead woman's daughters came to the meeting after her death, and with simplicity and directness discussed their last contact with their mother and the arrangements they were making for a memorial service. These two daughters confronted the group both with the finality of their mother's loss and with those aspects of her forceful personality which survived in her children. The emotional tone of this meeting was intense, and one might have expected it to frighten or overwhelm the members of the group. Instead, this woman's manner of dying and the dignity of her children seemed to convey to the other members a sense that the way one died was significant and that even the last moments of life carry with them important choices.

Shortly after this, another central member of the group became sicker and suffered cerebral metasteses. She emphasized to all that she had acquired great strength from the dignified way in which the woman just described had faced her death. Forced to relinquish her hope that she would have a spontaneous remission, she felt that her contact with the group had enhanced her ability to face her imminent death. She took pride in the manner in which her own children were prepared to carry on their lives; she was able to face her death with her caring husband; and she mustered the courage to discuss with him her wish that, after he recovered from her death, he should find another woman to love. In a brief period of time she passed from panic and despair to a state of openness and acceptance. At the end of her life, she ministered to others, comforted her family, and died with lucidity and tranquility. She had come to desire a quick and peaceful death and had felt that she would not live until Thanksgiving. She died at 5:00 P.M. the day before. At a powerful group meeting after her death, her husband and daughter spoke tearfully of how much the group support had meant to her and how much the family support had meant to them. They then had the group read a note she had written to herself a year previously. It concluded with these words: "You're going to die and now you know it. Admit it. You feel it. You feel afraid of the uncertainties about debilitating things that might happen in the course of the disease—*and* you feel cheated of the future for which you've always had a hog's appetite. Admit it and find some way to express it or your happy face will be only a facade and you really will have cheated yourself out of this year." In fact, she did not cheat herself of this last year and found the courage to live fully until the end of her life. This patient's family reminded the other group members that in many ways the task for the living is harder than that for the dying. In this sense, dying was put in perspective. Many group members discovered that they feared dying more than death, and death less than the painful task of living without a loved one.

It is often noted in psychotherapy that fantasies are worse than reality, and this even holds true in the face of dying. The process of dying was detoxified and demystified for the group through their experience with it. Another group member died in a most graphic way. While increasing cerebral involvement, she first became cachectic, and then gradually lost the use of her extremities. After a time, she had to be carried to the meetings and at her final regular meeting, she required assistance to hold her head upright. Shortly before her death, she was bedridden, and the meeting was held in her bedroom. This woman was the target of more anger than her participation in the group would seem to warrant. Gradually, the members realized that she graphically represented what they feared most of all: absolute loss of control over their own bodies. With this realization, much of the anger dissolved, and the group emerged the stronger for having faced and survived this confrontation with some of their worst fears.

Impact on Families

The group has had a significant effect on the families of members, both through direct contact with the families, as described earlier, and through the members sharing experiences and ideas about how to deal with their families. One mother of two latency-aged children was encouraged to discuss her illness more directly with them in language they could understand, which she did and which led to a decrease in her personal and family tension. An older member who felt that too many demands were being placed on her by her husband was urged to seek help from other members of her extended family.

In general, the families have felt very close to the group members, and there has been much informal contact between meetings. One widower spoke warmly about the group, many of whose members attended his wife's funeral service. He noted that in her last year the group had become a focal point in his wife's life because many friends had drifted away after she was forced to leave work and had become more invalided by her physical problems. In this sense, the group shared his burden of providing emotional support and understanding.

Just as the women felt a sense of setting an example in the way they died for other members of the group, this sense also developed in regard to their families. In the group, they discussed the way their parents had died and the impact this had had on their subsequent life. These shared memories helped them realize that the manner in which they lived the remainder of their lives would have a profound impact on their husbands and children.

Developing a Sense of Meaning in Life

During the course of the group, the members came to feel less like passive victims of a disease process and more like experts on living. They discovered, often to their surprise, that they had something to teach others, both those who had more recently discovered that they had cancer and also people who had not yet confronted death. For many group members, the increased awareness of the passage of time brought about by the diagnosis of cancer seemed to accelerate the process of personal growth. Many of them said that they had learned to say "no" and mean it for the first time in their lives, and they often expressed the wish that they had had this kind of confrontation with themselves when they were younger and healthier. This was part of their sense that they had something to teach their husbands and children about living. A member with young children had serious difficulties with her marriage but developed a deep sense of purpose in life by deciding her major remaining task was to impart significant life values to her children.

The group was eager to have observers; they especially wanted to influence the medical profession, to change physicians' attitudes toward the metastatic cancer patient. One woman made a major project out of altering her oncologist, a distant, authoritarian man who, thanks to her efforts, became much more empathic with his terminal patients. They wanted other women to know that the diagnosis of breast cancer was not the end of one's life but, rather, the beginning of a different kind of life. The notion that through their experience they had something to teach as well as something to learn seemed to have a significant effect on their self-esteem and their sense of meaning in what remained of their lives.

The Pressure to Do Psychotherapy

At times during the course of the group, there was pressure from the patients on the therapists to turn the group into a more traditional psychotherapy group focusing on characterological issues and family problems. Some of this pressure reflected an effort to maximize the pleasure derived from dealing with close friends and relatives. Sometimes personality conflict was a diversion from coping with an impending or recent death.

Some members felt that psychotherapeutic personality change could influence the course of their cancer. They were impressed with the mass media promulgation of the psychosomatic hypothesis concerning cancer, i.e., that cancer develops as a result of stress and from maladaptive methods of coping with stress. This hypothesis holds that if one brings on cancer through poorly handled emotions, one can stop cancer through psychological means. One woman, for example, was convinced that her metastases developed because of her sense of frustration at her husband's having changed jobs, thereby giving up a good pension shortly before retirement. Some members employed the approach to the treatment of cancer advocated by Carl Simonton which emphasizes meditation and visual imagery of the patient's body defenses destroying cancer cells. Some women found that the psychosomatic hypothesis gave them strength, while others found themselves additionally burdened with the guilt of having brought cancer upon themselves.

Some members worked on their ways of coping with stress, learning to be more assertive. Some got more in touch with their sense of anger at being viewed as "damaged merchandise" by their husbands. This was a special problem for women who had been recently married. In general, these characterological issues, while important, took second place to the life choices forced upon the members by terminal illness.

The Cohesiveness of the Group

The group members developed a strong sense of cohesiveness as attested to by regular attendance at the group meetings and their frequent contact with one another between meetings. Certainly their common experience of having cancer provided an immediate rapport among the members, but it was not the sole explanation of the ongoing emotional impact of the group. The shared experience of the members helped them put in perspective their own emotional responses to this crisis in their lives. Each member had her own fears and guilt and other reactions to discovering that her disease had spread and there was the need for additional surgery, but these were modified by the responses of the other women in a similar situation. The individual often acquired a sense of being less strange and isolated from the rest of humanity. Often, also, a member gathered information from those who had been through an experience and could gain the kind of reassurance only available from such a person. One anxious new member tearfully spoke about how, when she learned of her cancer, she had thought sadly: "I will not live to see my grandchildren." Another member looked at her and said, "That's what I thought three years ago when I was told. I now have a lovely grandson."

But even this kind of realistic counseling and reassurance is not enough to explain the intense solidarity in the group. The women often visit with one another between group meetings or when one member is in despair. Loving gifts—plants, books, a poem—are exchanged. The very message of joining a group at this time in a patient's life conveys the idea that the person has not been put out to pasture, that she is not without importance because she is dying, that what she does still matters. Finally, these women have gone through the experience of genuinely mourning the loss of members. Coping with the harsh realities of life is an experience which happens only occasionally in a traditional psychotherapy group, but it is part of the life of this group of women with cancer. Going through such deep experiences together creates a powerful bond among the members.

Changes in the Group Members

While there has been considerable variation in the response of members of the group to their experience with it, we have noted the following types of changes in members who have been with the group for at least six months. There is, in general, a decrease in denial about having cancer, and talk about dying is detoxified. Time is seen as precious, too precious to be wasted on unwanted social commitments or "pleasing others." Very often the women have felt that they were treated as objects by their physicians and were not given the information they were entitled to have. The group provided support to its members in developing ways to work more effectively with their doctors and, in particular, to insist that they become part of the decision-making process about the course of treatment. Many of the patients reported improved communication with their doctors and a heightened sense of assertiveness with many other people in their lives. Several of the women who had been engaged in constant struggles with their spouses reported that they made major improvements in their marriages by simply learning to say no and to value their own time and energy as being equally important to that of others. Some members reported improved communication with their families, an improvement corroborated by family members. Others who had a less rewarding family situation used the group as an alternative focus of intimacy and support. For many, the group countered a sense of loneliness and isolation. In general, group members became less depressed, although more overtly sad at times, as the task of facing personal illness and the illness of others engaged them. Finally, many members acquired a sense of importance and found new meaning in their lives in the sense that how they lived the remainder of their lives and how they died came to seem significant. They realized that they had something to teach others and that other group members, their families, and their friends were looking to them as an example. This helped to lessen the inevitable sense of meaninglessness in dying.

Conclusion

The structure and outcome of a group organized for women with metastatic breast carcinoma have been described. The group met regularly on a weekly basis, and the group members often had informal contacts with one another and among their families. The therapists' role involved clarifying major themes in the group, which included putting dying in perspective, detoxifying dying, coping with the death of group members, the impact of cancer on family, friends, and doctors, and the expertise in living acquired by these cancer patients. The work of the group involved both mourning loss of abilities and involvement in life and focusing on what remained and the importance of the time left and how it was spent. The group seemed able to help its members face their death realistically without denial but also without morbid rumination. In the process of doing this grief work, the group members were able to plan and live through the remainder of their lives with an enhanced sense of meaning and dignity.

ACKNOWLEDGEMENTS

The authors gratefully acknowledge the assistance of Regina Kriss in reviewing the manuscript.

References

1. Yalom, I. D. *The theory and practice of group psychotherapy* (2nd ed.). New York: Basic Books, 1975.
2. Killilea, M. Mutual help organizations: Interpretations in the literature. In G. Kaplan & M. Killilea (Eds.), *Support systems and mutual help: Multidisciplinary explorations.* New York: Grune & Stratton.
3. Riessman, F. The "helper" therapy principle. *Social Work.* 1965, *10*, 27–32.
4. Caplan, G. *Support systems and community mental health: Lectures on concept development.* New York: Behavioral Publications, 1974.
5. Spiegel, D. Going public and self-help. In G. Caplan & M. Killilea (Eds.), *Support systems and mutual help: Multidisciplinary explorations.* New York: Grune & Stratton, 1976.
6. Cohen, R. J. Is dying being worked to death? *American Journal of Psychiatry,* 1976, *133*, 575–577.
7. Kübler-Ross, E. *On death and dying.* New York: Macmillan, 1969.

29

A Special Christmas
An Account of the Last Christmas of Barbara Mackenzie Rogers Hepner

COURTNEY ROGERS MALONE

It was getting-ready time—the week before Christmas when our three families were preparing to gather at our home near the sea in order to celebrate Christmas together in our usual fashion. As the house was decorated, presents wrapped, and food cooked, mixed feelings occupied our hearts and minds. We knew there would be a great deal of love. We hoped there would be some laughter and joy. We prayed there would be strength and courage, for this was to be my sister Bobby's last Christmas. She had been told by her doctor on December 17 that the cancer she had suffered had spread to her lungs. She would probably have two to three more months to live.

Bobby's Final Wish: Death with Dignity

Bobby was not particularly surprised by her doctor's prognosis for her, although she had felt well most of the fall. She had

Reprinted from *Topics in Clinical Nursing*, 1981, *3*, 39–43, with permission by Aspen Systems Corporation.

COURTNEY ROGERS MALONE • Learning Disabilities Specialist, Public School System, Falmouth, Massachusetts 02540.

419

spent two years battling the physical demon as well as the mental ones. From time to time, she had experienced severe grief, anger, and depression as well as long periods of serenity. But she also had been getting ready. By December 17, serenity had won over, and she asked us to help her to die as she had lived—with dignity and graciousness.

She told us that if it were possible, she would like to die at home. She signed a paper saying that she did not want life support systems to be used. She did not want to linger on, and she wanted to remain conscious if the pain could be kept within bearable bounds. Bobby prefaced each request with the statement that she did not want to burden anyone and would understand if some of her wishes could not be carried out.

There were two other wishes that I was asked to help fulfill. Dick, her husband, wanted to give her a warm bathrobe that would be lightweight and smooth next to her skin. Through my daughter in Boston, we found a perfect one which was filled with down. Bobby wanted to give Dick a fine gold watch, as he had never had one. She pulled her waning strength together for what had to be a very short outing. I fervently hoped there would be one she could afford in the village. We walked into the store, and there was just one. The perfect one. Bobby had it engraved to show their marriage dates: BRH-RHH, 1952–1980.

Christmas Day

And so we gathered together. Bobby and Dick and their four grown children drove down from New Hampshire. Ray, her brother, and his wife Lois and their four children came from New Jersey. Al and I, with my children, welcomed them, and Christmas began.

Although we usually go to the midnight service together on Christmas Eve, Bobby was not strong enough to do so. Instead, on Christmas Day, we gathered in a circle in the living room to celebrate the Christmas Eucharist. Al, an Episcopal clergyman, led us in prayer, and Ray led us in song. In spite of the sorrow, we felt deeply thankful for the love our close-knit family had always shared. A great feeling of peace prevaded the house.

By Christmas night it was apparent that Bobby was weakening much more quickly than had been expected. We made her as comfortable as possible and propped her up on a myriad of pillows on a reclining chair to aid her breathing. She announced that she would stay there for the night, and Dick kept vigil on the couch.

It was as if Bobby had decided that now was the time, for she was with the people she loved most, and she was by the sea, which she loved. So she set about orchestrating her last days. Each day and through the nights we could see the life draining from her. Yet there were certain times when she willed herself to rally. On Christmas Day, we mustered up some of our usual jollity, and Bobby joined in the fun, albeit from her chair of pillows. One could almost imagine that she might indeed have a few more months.

New Year's Eve

By New Year's Eve, however, Bobby needed constant oxygen for two days and was exhausted by her efforts to breathe. Yet she wished to remain among us. Her sense of humor was still with her, as she smiled in appreciation of some of the jokes being told in the movie we were watching on television. However, she was determined to move on.

We asked for the help of a physician friend. Along with the oxygen machine, he supplied us with a painkilling medicine and the encouraging words that no one could do more for her than we were doing. He also offered us options that we could take if the nursing became too difficult for us: We could get the help of a homemaker or visiting nurse; he would arrange for a room at the local hospital, where we could be with Bobby as much as we wished; or we could have a hospital bed installed at home. He offered these options, but he did not insist on them. They were available if needed. We chose to order a bed and to nurse her ourselves. He also let us know where he would be at all times so that we could contact him personally if we needed him. We were very grateful for his support and understanding.

New Year's Day

By New Year's Day, Bobby's suffering was acute. We scheduled watches so that some could rest while others cared for her. But the watches went by the board, as no one would go to bed. Various members of the family, from a 16-year-old nephew on up, stayed by Bobby's side hour by hour. We felt that everything we did for her was a present so full of love that it was beyond measure. And yet they were all little things in themselves. We tenderly bathed her and fed her small spoonfuls of gelatin, which tasted refreshing to her. We held her hands and caressed her forehead. We played Chopin and Beethoven for her, and we cooled her lips with chunks of ice. We bought her the loveliest nightgown that could be found. We picked a green tiger lily leaf from our beloved summer home, "Lazy Lawn," and brought it to her. We sang carols around the piano and played duets on our recorders. Each in his or her own way told her and showed her what she meant to him or her and she in turn responded to each of us. It was a holy time.

That night Bobby's suffering became more acute. At the same time, her resolution grew firmer. As her lungs filled with fluid, she said, "Pray for courage."

We replied, "You have it."

Her response was, "I know it."

At 10:30, she tore off her oxygen mask and said, "Let's get on with it." She would not put it back on again.

Feeling the power of her spirit fighting to free itself from her body, we all gathered around her in the quiet light of the Christmas window candles. Al led us in prayers of thanks for her presence in our lives. He ended with, "Into thy hands, O merciful Savior, we commend thy servant." A daughter led us in singing "Amazing Grace." Each of us said goodbye. Then Bobby looked at Dick, and as was her wont, whispered, "See you in the morning."

However, the battle was not yet won, and we continued to keep vigil throughout that long, still night. We were thankful for the beauty of the sky, with its brilliant stars and full moon, which augmented the candles. From time to time, we would step out onto the deck to catch a breath of fresh air and gather our thoughts. We found that we were still able to laugh a little when we discussed the evening meal, which Lois had named "God knows casserole." As the night waned, Bobby chose to take no more medicine. She was determined to remain lucid. And so she did. She was able to whisper an occasional word to us between her efforts to breathe.

Bobby's Death

The next afternoon, Bobby suddenly started breathing normally. She turned over on her side and arranged herself in her usual sleeping position. She opened her eyes wide and looked as if she was seeing something beyond us. Then she shut them and died. Although it was a very sad moment, we also felt triumphant. She was victorious, through sheer will and prayer, in living her last days as she had wished and in dying among us as she had hoped.

One of us proposed that we have a toast. I got out the best crystal goblets, and we filled them with sherry or ginger ale. We gathered around this dear person who had been our beloved wife, mother, sister, and aunt. Then we raised our glasses as a son declared, "To life!"

Bobby's Funeral

The funeral was a celebration. Bobby had planned it. Al and a family friend officiated. The simple pine casket was draped with our ancestral tartan with the family crest pinned to it. On top of this was a small bouquet of heather and mums from Dick. We sang the hymns lustily, and Ray played "Amazing Grace" on the bagpipes, because Bobby had asked him to. Al gave the sermon. Because it was the day before Epiphany, he talked about gifts and reminded us that the Magi had had to go home another way after visiting the Christ child. It was fitting, because we realized that not only had Bobby's presence among us over the years been a gift beyond measure, but the intangible gifts we had all been giving and receiving during that Christmas season were mighty treasures. Because we would no longer have Bobby among us and because of our experiences, we all knew that life would be different, and we indeed would be going home another way.

Bobby's Victory: Allowing the Terminally Ill to Die at Home

I have written this account in hopes that the experience of our family may be of some help to others. As death after long illness has become so common in our modern age, we all wonder before the fact how best to deal with it. Medicine can do much, but the time comes when life and death, and the quality of them, transcend science. This can be a fearful realization, but it can also be a glorious one. Not every family can manage death, or might want to, as we did. We were given several options by our physician friend. There is also the hospice movement, which is devoted to enabling the terminally ill to live more fully their last days. We discovered inner strength we were not sure we had by committing ourselves to Bobby's wish to die at home. We are all very glad we did. We thank her for teaching us so much about life as she let go of hers.

Author Index

425

Subject Index

431